# SLEEPING AND WAKING DISORDERS: INDICATIONS AND TECHNIQUES

# SLEEPING AND WAKING DISORDERS: INDICATIONS AND TECHNIQUES

*Edited by*
## Christian Guilleminault, M.D. (D. Med.)

Association of Sleep Disorders Centers
Chairman, Committee on Somnology and Clinical Polysomnography

Associate Professor
Department of Psychiatry and Behavioral Sciences
Stanford University School of Medicine

Maître de Recherche
Institut National de la Santé et Recherche Médicale

ADDISON-WESLEY PUBLISHING COMPANY
Medical/Nursing Division • Menlo Park, California
Reading, Massachusetts • London • Amsterdam
Don Mills, Ontario • Sydney

*Sponsoring Editor:* Richard W. Mixter

Copyright © 1982 by Addison-Wesley Publishing Company, Inc.
Philippines copyright 1982 by Addison-Wesley Publishing Company, Inc.

All rights reserved. No part of this publication may be reproduced, stored in a retrieval system, or transmitted, in any form or by any means, electronic, mechanical, photocopying, recording, or otherwise, without the prior written permission of the publisher. Printed in the United States of America. Published simultaneously in Canada.

**Library of Congress Cataloging in Publication Data**
Main entry under title:

Sleeping and waking disorders.

Includes index.
1. Sleep disorders.   2. Sleep—Physiological aspects.
I. Guilleminault, Christian.
RC547.S57        616.8'49         81-14888
ISBN 0-201-10500-4              AACR2

ABCDEFGHIJ-MA-8987654321

The authors and publishers have exerted every effort to ensure that drug selection and dosage set forth in this text are in accord with current recommendations and practice at the time of publication. However, in view of ongoing research, changes in government regulations, and the constant flow of information relating to drug therapy and drug reactions, the reader is urged to check the package insert for each drug for any change in indications of dosage and for added warnings and precautions. This is particularly important where the recommended agent is a new and/or infrequently employed drug.

---

The paper in this book meets the guidelines for permanence and durability of the Committee on Production Guidelines for Book Longevity of the Council on Library Resources.

---

Addison-Wesley Publishing Company
Medical/Nursing Division
2725 Sand Hill Road
Menlo Park, California 94025

# LIST OF CONTRIBUTORS

**Bollinger, Cynthia,** Sleep Disorders Center, Presbyterian Hospital, Oklahoma City, Oklahoma 73104.

**Bornstein, Sharon Keenan, B.S., R.EEGT.,** Sleep Disorders Clinic and Research Center, Stanford University School of Medicine, Stanford, California 94305.

**Carskadon, Mary A., Ph.D.,** Sleep Disorders Clinic and Research Center, Stanford University School of Medicine, Stanford, California 94305.

**Coble, Patricia A., R.N.,** Department of Psychiatry, Western Psychiatry Institute and Clinic, University of Pittsburgh School of Medicine, Pittsburgh, Pennsylvania 15261.

**Cohn, Martin, M.D.,** Sleep Disorders Center, Mount Sinai Medical Center, Miami Beach, Florida 33140.

**Coleman, Richard M., Ph.D.,** Sleep Disorders Clinic and Research Center, Stanford University School of Medicine, Stanford, California 94305.

**Czeisler, Charles A., Ph.D.,** Sleep-Wake Disorders Center, Laboratory of Human Chronophysiology, Department of Neurology, Montefiore Hospital and Medical Center and The Albert Einstein College of Medicine, Bronx, New York 10467.

**Dement, William C., M.D., Ph.D.,** Sleep Disorders Clinic and Research Center, Stanford University School of Medicine, Stanford, California 94305. (President, Association of Sleep Disorders Centers.)

**Fortin, Linda D., R.EEGT.,** Sleep Disorders Evaluation Center, College of Medicine, Ohio State University, Columbus, Ohio 43210.

**Geidel, Sue, R.N., M.S.,** SIDS Research, LAC/USC Medical Center, Los Angeles, California 90033.

**Guilleminault, Christian, M.D.,** Sleep Disorders Clinic and Research Center, Stanford University School of Medicine, Stanford, California 94305.

**Hauri, Peter J., Ph.D.,** Dartmouth-Hitchcock Sleep Disorders Center, Dartmouth Medical School, Hanover, New Hampshire 03755.

**Hoppenbrouwers, Toke, Ph.D.,** SIDS Research, LAC/USC Medical Center, Los Angeles, California 90033.

**Judson, Lorie, R.N., M.N.,** SIDS Research, LAC/USC Medical Center, Los Angeles, California 90033.

**Karacan, Ismet, M.D.,** Department of Psychiatry, Baylor College of Medicine and Research Service, Veterans Administration Medical Center, Houston, Texas 77211.

*List of Contributors*

**Knauer, Richard S., B.S.,** Sleep-Wake Disorders Center, Laboratory of Human Chronophysiology, Department of Neurology, Montefiore Hospital and Medical Center and The Albert Einstein College of Medicine, Bronx, New York 10467.

**Miles, Laughton, M.D., Ph.D.,** Sleep Disorders Clinic and Research Center, Stanford University School of Medicine, Stanford, California 94305.

**Mitler, Merrill M., Ph.D.,** Sleep Disorders Program, State University of New York at Stony Brook, Stony Brook, New York 11794.

**Orr, William C., Ph.D.,** Sleep Disorders Center, Presbyterian Hospital, Oklahoma City, Oklahoma 73104.

**Reynolds, Charles F. III, M.D.,** Department of Psychiatry, Western Psychiatric Institute and Clinic, University of Pittsburgh School of Medicine, Pittsburgh, Pennsylvania 15261.

**Ronda, Joseph M., B.A.,** Sleep-Wake Disorders Center, Laboratory of Human Chronophysiology, Department of Neurology, Montefiore Hospital and Medical Center and The Albert Einstein College of Medicine, Bronx, New York 10467.

**Ruiz, Maria Elena, R.N.,** SIDS Research, LAC/USC Medical Center, Los Angeles, California 90033.

**Schmidt, Helmut S., M.D.,** Sleep Disorders Evaluation Center, College of Medicine, Ohio State University, Columbus, Ohio 43210.

**Shaw, David H., M.S.,** Department of Psychiatry, Western Psychiatric Institute and Clinic, University of Pittsburgh School of Medicine, Pittsburgh, Pennsylvania 15261.

**Stahl, Monte,** Sleep Disorders Center, Presbyterian Hospital, Oklahoma City, Oklahoma 73104.

**Tharp, Barry R., M.D.,** Department of Neurology, Stanford University Medical Center, Stanford, California 94305.

**Weitzman, Elliot D., M.D.,** Sleep-Wake Disorders Center, Laboratory of Human Chronophysiology, Department of Neurology, Montefiore Hospital and Medical Center and The Albert Einstein College of Medicine, Bronx, New York 10467.

**Zimmerman, Janet C., Ph.D.,** Sleep-Wake Disorders Center, Laboratory of Human Chronophysiology, Department of Neurology, Montefiore Hospital and Medical Center and The Albert Einstein College of Medicine, Bronx, New York 10467.

# PREFACE

Sleep disorders medicine is a new and rapidly expanding field. With the development of many sleep disorders centers, new diagnostic techniques and protocols have been developed and refined; unfortunately, much valuable information has either remained unpublished or has been published in different journals. There has been no single volume containing the latest clinical and technical information in the sleep disorders field available to the scientific community.

The need for this book was pointed out by many researchers and clinicians to the Association of Sleep Disorders Centers. The Executive Committee asked that the Committee on Somnology and Clinical Polysomnography undertake the project; as chairman of that committee, I am solely responsible for the contents, as arbitrary as my selections may appear. I recognize that this book is not complete, but I believe it will prove valuable to sleep researchers and clinicians and will aid in training those new to our field. I am deeply indebted to the many talented and skilled professionals who have contributed to this endeavor.

I also wish to thank Eileen Gunther, whose careful editing has resulted in a cohesive and coherent collection of papers. I am grateful to Deena Dickenson for help in preparing the manuscript. Finally, the publication of this book was supported in part by the Josiah Macy, Jr. Foundation.

**Christian Guilleminault, M.D.**

# CONTENTS

|  | Foreword<br>*William C. Dement* | xi |
|---|---|---|
| **Chapter 1** | Basics for polygraphic monitoring of sleep<br>*Mary A. Carskadon* | 1 |
| **Chapter 2** | Electronic monitoring in the newborn and young infant: theoretical considerations<br>*Toke Hoppenbrouwers* | 17 |
| **Chapter 3** | Electronic monitoring in the newborn and young infant: technical guidelines<br>*Toke Hoppenbrouwers, Sue Geidel, Maria Elena Ruiz, Lorie Judson* | 61 |
| **Chapter 4** | The second decade<br>*Mary A. Carskadon* | 99 |
| **Chapter 5** | Electronic pupillography in disorders of arousal<br>*Helmut S. Schmidt, Linda D. Fortin* | 127 |
| **Chapter 6** | The multiple sleep latency test as an evaluation for excessive somnolence<br>*Merrill M. Mitler* | 145 |
| **Chapter 7** | Sleep and breathing<br>*Christian Guilleminault* | 155 |
| **Chapter 8** | Respiratory monitoring during sleep: polysomnography<br>*Sharon Keenan Bornstein* | 183 |
| **Chapter 9** | Respiratory monitoring during sleep: respiratory inductive plethysmography<br>*Martin Cohn* | 213 |
| **Chapter 10** | Evaluating disorders of initiating and maintaining sleep (DIMS)<br>*Peter J. Hauri* | 225 |

| | | |
|---|---|---|
| **Chapter 11** | Depressive patients and the sleep laboratory<br>*Charles F. Reynolds III, Patricia A. Coble,*<br>*David J. Kupfer, David H. Shaw* | **245** |
| **Chapter 12** | Periodic movements in sleep (nocturnal myoclonus) and restless legs syndrome<br>*Richard M. Coleman* | **265** |
| **Chapter 13** | Chronobiological disorders: analytic and therapeutic techniques<br>*Elliot D. Weitzman, Charles A. Czeisler,*<br>*Janet C. Zimmerman, Joseph M. Ronda,*<br>*Richard S. Knauer* | **297** |
| **Chapter 14** | Measurement of gastroesophageal reflux during sleep by esophageal pH monitoring<br>*William C. Orr, Cynthia Bollinger, Monte Stahl* | **331** |
| **Chapter 15** | Evaluation of nocturnal penile tumescence and impotence<br>*Ismet Karacan* | **343** |
| **Chapter 16** | Epilepsy and sleep<br>*Barry R. Tharp* | **373** |
| **General Appendix I** | A sleep questionnaire<br>*Laughton Miles* | **383** |
| **General Appendix II** | A sleep/wake scoring system for infants during the first year of life<br>*Christian Guilleminault, Marianne Souquet* | **415** |
| **Index** | | **427** |

# FOREWORD

In its origin, a clinical discipline generally passes through several stages. Practitioners begin to gather in little groups to discuss their patients; they then found a society and have formal meetings; they begin to solve problems of clinical training and quality assurance; they foster standardization of procedures and terminology; finally, someone must write a comprehensive textbook. These steps have all been taken by sleep disorders specialists, except for the last and most difficult. This volume is not a comprehensive textbook. Nonetheless, as the first attempt to assemble some of the material we collectively feel practitioners must know, it is a major accomplishment for the development of our discipline.

What is this "new discipline"? Is it simply the diagnosis and treatment of sleep disorders patients? Is it chronobiology in a very broad sense? Is it clinical and basic sleep research? The precise definition of our field and the clear delineation of its boundaries are not possible here. There is, however, an urgent practical question to which the best possible answer must be formulated and reformulated on a continuing basis: what does the clinical practitioner of sleep disorders medicine need to know in order to obtain the best possible results for his patients? Where does he find what he needs to know? At the present time, although books on sleep, dreams, and other aspects of the discipline proliferate, there is no single, truly authoritative cumulation of what the clinical practitioner must know. There is no book that could be read and studied, and if everything in it were known, that could equip the practitioner to practice his craft. Such a book ought to contain the core body of knowledge, special technology, and diagnosis and treatment information that pertains to the discipline. I am now speaking of something like Cecil's or Harrison's Textbooks of Medicine. *Sleeping and Waking Disorders: Indications and Techniques* is not nearly so comprehensive and authoritative in every area, detail, and minutia of the discipline as those time-honored tomes. Yet it is a beginning, and it is badly needed.

The initial concept of the Association of Sleep Disorders Centers in sponsoring this book was to assemble a standard manual of techniques utilized in polysomnographic testing. This goal was deemed important because of its potential usefulness in the development of sleep disorders centers. Heretofore, the model of clinical practice in sleep disorders centers and the specific techniques of the polysomnography laboratory have been inculcated essentially by apprenticeship. This is highly inefficient and is an obstacle to rapid dissemination of the clinical practice of sleep disorders medicine.

*Foreword*

The concept of a technical manual has remained, although under the leadership of the ASDC Committee on Somnology and Clinical Polysomnography it has become much broader and more clearly discipline-oriented. The authors of the various chapters are among the most experienced and expert, if not *the* most experienced and expert, in their topic areas. They have each contributed selflessly to this effort. The result is our best effort to date to provide a resource that will guide neophytes, trainees, and new enthusiasts; will help them to diagnose and treat their patients; will prepare them for our examinations; and will enable them to participate in the further development of their special professional identity. Furthermore, having taken the presumptuous step of declaring what everyone ought to know, we expect to see healthy reaction, revision, improvement, and refinement, out of which we will see further progress, consensus, and coalescence in our discipline.

## Some Historical Highlights in the Development of the Discipline of Basic and Clinical Sleep Research and Sleep Disorders Clinical Practice

Perhaps the first person to devote essentially his entire scientific career to sleep research is University of Chicago physiologist Nathaniel Kleitman.* Professor Kleitman's professional life spanned the 1920s, 30s, 40s, and 50s, and his work truly established sleep research as a legitimate field of study. His contributions include detailed attention to the ontogeny of sleep, systematic studies of sleep deprivation, careful observations of the sleep characteristics of populations, and key contributions to electroencephalographic studies of sleep, culminating in his historic discovery of rapid eye movements during sleep with Eugene Aserinsky in 1953 *(2)*. Finally, he published the first comprehensive scientific monograph on sleep and wakefulness in 1939 and a second completely revised and updated edition in 1963 *(3)*.

The development of the electroencephalogram and other polygraphic techniques as the primary descriptors of sleep and wakefulness was also extraordinarily important in establishing the field. These techniques were not fully exploited until the decade following the post-war years when we saw, in rapid succession, the discovery of rapid eye movements, description of the basic sleep cycle *(4)*, discovery of REM sleep in animals and newborns *(5,6)*, and application of the Horsely-Clark stereotaxic apparatus to work on the brainstem reticular formation with an emphasis on sleep and arousal *(7,8)*. The 1960s saw the first real clinical approaches, including the discovery of sleep-onset REM periods in narcolepsy *(9,10)*, the first sleep laboratory studies of the effects

---

*Outside of the United States, Henri Pieron should be mentioned, though he had several other very important career interests. Nonetheless, his book on sleep *(1)* was an important landmark.

of sleeping pills *(11)*, and, perhaps of paramount importance, the description of sleep apnea independently by Gastaut and his colleagues *(12)*, and by Jung and Kuhlo (13).

From an organizational point of view, March 1961 was important because the first general meeting of sleep researchers took place then at the University of Chicago. This group, which met to seek agreement on some of the sleep stage and EEG stage terminology, was later to become the Association for the Psychophysiological Study of Sleep (APSS).

Although Kleitman's monograph was the most scholarly and comprehensive work in the field of sleep research, the first major effort that was intended solely as a service to the field was the 1962–1968 Sleep and Dream Research Bibliography compiled by Allan Rechtschaffen and Dottie Eakin, published in 1968 by the UCLA Brain Information Service. Indeed, it is worth pointing out that in its formative years, the Brain Information Service utilized the small and identifiable group of sleep laboratory proprietors in preparing one of its first models of information dissemination, the *Sleep Bulletin*.

Three conferences should be singled out as having landmark significance in the development of sleep disorders medicine. All three took place in Europe. The first was held in France in 1963 and published as *Sommeil de Nuit, Normal et Pathologique: Etudes Electroencéphalographiques (14)*. The second, convened at the University of Bologna in 1967, utilized the occasion of the Fifteenth European Meeting on Electroencephalography for a truly international conference dealing with abnormalities of sleep in man, and the proceedings contained a number of important and original reports on sleep-related pathophysiology, particularly respiratory disturbances and abnormal leg movements *(15)*. Finally, although seven years had elapsed since the initial description, an explosion in the development of knowledge about sleep apnea syndromes and their clinical relevance was touched off by the Rimini Symposium on *Les Hypersomnies avec Respiration Périodique* in 1972 *(16)*.

The first truly disciplinary consensus exercise in the field of sleep research took place during 1967 and 1968, when a broadly representative committee of leading sleep researchers produced a standard manual of scoring sleep stages. This manual was published by the Brain Information Service in 1968 and is still the authoritative rule book *(17)*. It is to be hoped that the participants in the meetings that produced the manual will someday publish an account of those disputations and hard-working sessions full of high purpose, low blows, compromise, and finally consensus—all totally in the service of the discipline of sleep research. A similar attempt to standardize scoring rules and procedures in infants was published in 1971 *(18)*, but has been less successful, probably because the impetus to obtain consensus was lower.

The First International Symposium on Narcolepsy took place in the French Languedoc in the summer of 1975 immediately after the Second International Congress of the APSS in Edinburgh. This meeting, in addition to being scientifically productive, had landmark significance because it produced the first consensus definition of a specific sleep pathology *(19)*. The definition was drafted, revised, and unanimously endorsed by 65 narcoleptologists of international reputation. Thus, the diagnostic ambiguity of

*Foreword*

narcolepsy was finally eliminated. (The American Narcolepsy Association, a patient volunteer organization, also was formed in 1975.)

In the fall of 1975, a group of clinical sleep researchers interested in the diagnosis and treatment of sleep pathology met at Chicago's O'Hare Airport. An informal meeting had taken place in Edinburgh that summer. The group agreed that clinical sleep disorders had advanced to the point where a more formal approach was desirable, and the Association of Sleep Disorders Centers (ASDC) came into being at the 1976 APSS meeting in Cincinnati. The goals of the organization were the enhancement of patient care, introduction of standards and standardization in clinical practice, and formulation and development of a standard diagnostic classification system. The certification standards and guidelines for sleep disorders centers were published by the ASDC early in 1978 *(20)*, and later in the same year, a brief guideline for the use of polysomnography in sleep disorders centers was published *(21)*. The first examination of candidates to qualify for certification as "clinical polysomnographers" was held in December, 1977, in Cincinnati. In the autumn of 1978, the first edition of the scientific journal *Sleep* was published, sponsored jointly by the APSS, the European Society for Sleep Research, and the ASDC. At the same time, the United States Institute of Medicine of the National Academy of Science, at the specific request of the White House and the National Institute of Drug Abuse, initiated a study of sleeping pills, insomnia, and medical practice.

Nineteen seventy-nine was a banner year for our field. The United States Institute of Medicine report was published and had a great impact *(22)*. Among its recommendations were calls for additional sleep research and a national education program. The ASDC/APSS *Diagnostic Classification of Sleep and Arousal Disorders* was published in the fall of 1979 *(23)* after three years of extraordinary effort by the small group of dedicated individuals who comprised the "nosology" committee. To cap this banner year, on December 17 the Surgeon General of the United States, Dr. Julius Richmond, announced the inauguration of "Project Sleep: The National Program on Insomnia and Sleep Disorders" at a press conference in Washington, D.C. To quote the Surgeon General, this project will be "a major educational and research effort aimed at increasing the level of knowledge of physicians, their patients, and the public about the nature of insomnia and sleep disorders and their treatment. Our primary aim will be to influence physicians' diagnostic and treatment practices, including their prescribing habits. The second aim is to improve the knowledge, attitude, and pill-taking practices of all persons who use sleeping pills. The third is to identify the gaps in our medical knowledge of sleep disorders and medications with the research necessary to expand our treatment." Also at the press conference was Dr. Gerald L. Klerman, head of the Alcohol, Drug Abuse, and Mental Health Administration (ADAMHA) who said, "Project Sleep is a major attempt by ADAMHA to upgrade medical practices and to educate patients about sleep disorders and their treatment. This is a unique nonregulatory and cooperative endeavor of the federal government and the private sector joined together to address a mutually perceived serious health problem."

# The Challenge of the Future

What can we expect for our discipline in the years ahead? We can reasonably expect that the practice of sleep disorders medicine will grow rapidly. Project Sleep is under way and should have a national impact. The Association of Sleep Disorders Centers will increase its membership, and member centers will continue to implement and upgrade the clinical practice of sleep disorders medicine. By the end of the decade of the 1980s, the benefits of this clinical discipline could be readily available to everyone.

What must be done to realize these possibilities? It is absolutely crucial that researchers and practitioners of sleep disorders medicine accept and proclaim their discipline's identity, practice their craft with excellence, and promote their discipline conceptually and politically in every way possible. At the present writing, in spite of self-congratulatory scientific meetings and scientific successes, sleep disorders medicine is not well established. There is no widespread public mandate for teaching and research; public and professional awareness remain virtually nonexistent; and, in spite of a clinically relevant body of knowledge, there is no systematic, independent teaching of sleep-related matters in American or other medical schools. The precarious state of sleep disorders medicine is all the more surprising when one considers the ubiquity of serious problems relating to sleep and biological rhythms. If one carefully peruses all the surveys (24), it appears that more than half of all adults claim to have difficulty sleeping, and only specialists in our field have a clear idea of the many specific causes of these complaints. I contend that the major problem was a failure about 20 years ago of individuals engaged in basic and clinical sleep research to coalesce into a formal discipline. Without such a discipline identity, lobbying for and securing such things as curriculum time in medical schools, questions on National Board Examinations, third-party payment, and so forth, is extremely difficult.

There is an urgent need to recruit, train, and examine additional sleep disorders clinical researchers and clinical practitioners with a career commitment. We may expect this book to be helpful in this enterprise. Unfortunately, there is no ready academic home for a person who identifies himself as a somnologist, a sleep researcher, or a sleep disorders expert. Perhaps the first truly fertile soil for career growth is in sleep disorders centers, which must have *somnologist–clinical polysomnographers* in order to function and be fully certified by the ASDC.

In addition, we must continue to confront the conceptual problems of defining our discipline. Though sleep research—and particularly clinical sleep research—interfaces with many other disciplines, is there a sufficient core body of knowledge, and are the core problems of sleep research sufficiently compelling? I think the answers to both questions are resounding affirmatives. In addition to everything involved in the diagnosis and treatment of sleep disorders patients, the core body of knowledge includes all the descriptive information on normal sleep and wakefulness, survey studies of sleep habits, clinical sleep laboratory studies, sleep laboratory descriptions of sleep in various populations and/or species, and so forth. A true scholar might also include the minutiae of sleep and wakefulness, such as knowledge about sleep positions, sleep surfaces, sleep clothing, sleep companions, etc. The massive literature on experimental sleep loss also belongs to our discipline. Why does sleep exist? What, if anything, does it accomplish? The hygiene of sleep is our special problem. We must know how much and what kind of sleep is best for each individual; this aspect of knowledge about sleep and wakefulness would affect every man, woman, and child on the face of the earth. The investigation of sleep mechanisms is central to our discipline. How does the brain organize and maintain the states of sleep and wakefulness? How do these mechanisms interact with circadian oscillators? The treatment of sleep with hypnotics is particularly ours, though we nearly lost it by default. We have many problems facing us in regard to how sleep produces or is essential to the occurrence or development or manifestation of respiratory pathology, cardiac pathology, etc. We must include our hard-won knowledge of the psychophysiology of dreaming and, to some extent, of dream content. Finally, a true discipline is concerned about its history. *All information pertaining to the above issues should be disseminated in the training process of somnologist–clinical polysomnographers, and graduates should demonstrate their broad scholarship.*

Particularly in the area of regulatory (homeostatic) processes during sleep, and the many techniques adapted from other fields to study these processes, there is overlap with many other fields. I cannot emphasize enough that the main issue is not to worry about these interfaces, but to define our own unique core as precisely and possessively as possible and then work outward. However, we must also retain as much as possible of the areas that overlap with other disciplines. We can even foresee, at some time in the future, a pulmonary medicine of sleep, a cardiology of sleep, a neurology of sleep, a gastroenterology of sleep, and so forth. Sheer efficiency and cost containment demand that these areas of sleep-related function be investigated in central polysomnography laboratories rather than in many small laboratories that exist as ancillary components of the various waking biomedical disciplines. In this sense, sleep disorders medicine must necessarily include both a unique core of knowledge and skills and a broad interdisciplinary expertise. Precedents for this type of scientific and clinical organization already have been set by geriatric medicine and pediatrics.

## What Will Be the Benefits of the Widespread Existence and Active Practice of Somnology–Clinical Polysomnography?

We assume that increasing knowledge about sleep hygiene will lead to improved daytime function for all human beings. Many human beings will also profit by an increased life expectancy when serious and potentially lethal sleep problems are solved. We believe that there are important relationships between aging and sleep processes. We expect to see enormous benefits from an effective integration of chronobiology, chronopathology, and chronotherapy into the diagnosis and treatment of sleep disorders patients. We expect that as the mechanisms are better understood, people may have some freedom from the inexorable internal clock and may be better and more flexibly able to organize their time and travel. Finally, we are now beginning to enter the enormous arena of unsuspected asymptomatic sleep disorders. Sleep apnea and its potentially dangerous interaction with casual sleeping pill use, sleep-related asymptomatic cardiac arrhythmias, and all the chronopathology generated by modern society and culture are a few examples.

Once there is a true discipline, with professionals who practice the discipline as a career and earn their living from it, many necessary activities will be greatly facilitated: effective lobbying with the federal government, widespread public education, cooperative group efforts, tackling of problems that affect practitioners, and so forth. It is not necessary that sleep research and sleep disorders medicine expand continually, but we must reach an equilibrium at which we can respond effectively to the needs of millions of citizens with serious sleep disorders.

Thus, the future rests with the men and women in the trenches—the clinicians who, as in all of medicine, are motivated chiefly by the desire to alleviate the suffering of their individual patients, who want to do the best possible job, and who want their art to be continually better and more effective. This means better training, better skills, and prompt solutions to urgent problems. As said earlier, this book is only a small part of the process, but it is a beginning.

**William C. Dement, M.D. Ph.D.**
President, Association of Sleep Disorders Centers
Stanford, California

## References

1. Pieron H. Le problème physiologique du sommeil. Paris: Masson and Cie, 1913.
2. Aserinsky E, Kleitman N. Regularly occurring periods of eye motility, and concomitant phenomena, during sleep. Science 1953; 118:273–4.
3. Kleitman N. Sleep and wakefulness. Chicago: University of Chicago Press, 1963.
4. Dement W, Kleitman N. Cyclic variations in EEG during sleep and their relation to eye movements, body motility, and dreaming. Electroencephalogr Clin Neurophysiol 1957; 9:673–90.
5. Dement W. The occurrence of low voltage, fast electroencephalogram patterns during behavioral sleep in the cat. Electroencephalogr Clin Neurophysiol 1958; 10:291–6.
6. Roffwarg H, Dement W, Fisher C. Preliminary observations of the sleep-dream pattern in neonates, infants, children, and adults. Monogr Child Psychol 1964; 2:60–72.
7. Moruzzi G, Magoun H. Brain stem reticular formation and activation of the EEG. Electroencephalogr Clin Neurophysiol 1949; 1:455–73.

8. Lindsley D, Schreiner L, Knowles W, Magoun H. Behavioral and EEG changes following chronic brain stem lesions in the cat. Electroencephalogr Clin Neurophysiol 1950; 2:483–98.
9. Rechtschaffen A, Wolpert E, Dement W, Mitchell S, Fisher C. Nocturnal sleep of narcoleptics. Electroencephalogr Clin Neurophysiol 1963; 15:599–609.
10. Takahashi Y, Jimbo M. Polygraphic study of narcoleptic syndrome, with special reference to hypnagogic hallucinations and cataplexy. Folia Psychiatr Neurol Jpn [Suppl] 1963; 7:343.
11. Oswald I, Priest R. Five weeks to escape the sleeping pill habit. Br Med J 1965; 2:1093–5.
12. Gastaut H, Tassinari C, Duron B. Etude polygraphique des manifestations épisodiques (hypniques et respiratoires) du syndrome de Pickwick. Rev Neurol 1965; 112:568–79.
13. Jung R, Kuhlo W. Neurophysiological studies of abnormal night sleep and the Pickwickian syndrome. Prog Brain Res 1965; 18:140–59.
14. La Société d'Eletroencéphalographie et de Neurophysiologie Clinique de la Langue Française. Le sommeil de nuit normal et pathologique: études électroencéphalographiques. Paris: Masson and Cie, 1965.
15. Gastaut H, Lugaresi E, Berti-Ceroni G, Coccagna G, eds. The abnormalities of sleep in man. Bologna: Aulo Gaggi Editore, 1968.
16. Sadoul P, Lugaresi E, eds. Hypersomnia with periodic breathing (les hypersomnies avec respiration périodique). Bull Physio-path Resp 1972; 8:967–1292.
17. Rechtschaffen A, Kales A, eds. A manual of standardized terminology, techniques and scoring system for sleep stages of human subjects. Los Angeles: UCLA Brain Information Service/Brain Research Institute, 1968.
18. Anders T, Emde R, Parmalee A, eds. A manual of standardized terminology, techniques, and criteria for scoring of states of sleep and wakefulness in newborn infants. Los Angeles: UCLA Brain Information Service/Brain Research Institute, 1971.
19. Guilleminault C, Dement W, Passouant P, eds. Narcolepsy. New York: Spectrum, 1976.
20. Association of Sleep Disorders Centers. Certification standards and guidelines for sleep disorders centers. Prepared by the Certification Committee, 1978.
21. Association of Sleep Disorders Centers. Guidelines in the use of polysomnography. Prepared by the Committee on Techniques of Clinical Polysomnography, 1978.
22. Institute of Medicine. Report of a study: sleeping pills, insomnia, and medical practice. Washington, D.C.: National Academy of Sciences, 1979.

23. Association of Sleep Disorders Centers. Diagnostic classification of sleep and arousal disorders. 1st ed. Prepared by the Sleep Disorders Classification Committee, HP Roffwarg, chairman. Sleep 1979; 2:1–137.
24. Miles L, Dement W. Sleep and aging. Sleep 1981; 3:1–150.

# ONE
# BASICS FOR POLYGRAPHIC MONITORING OF SLEEP

MARY A. CARSKADON

## Introduction

Sleep recordings are performed in many laboratories, for many purposes. The material presented below is intended only as an introduction to certain basic techniques that may be helpful in establishing standard sleep laboratory practice. This presentation in no way represents an attempt to give an exhaustive review of the procedures, nor should it be considered the final word on sleep recording technology. To an extent the procedures reflect idiosyncratic approaches of the Stanford group, and we can only point out the rich historical roots of our laboratory. The procedures outlined in this chapter had their beginnings in the Dement and Kleitman *(1)* work and incorporate the suggestions of the Rechtschaffen and Kales *(2)* standard manual.

## Historical Notes

Richard Caton made the first recordings of EEG using a crude recording system in cats, rabbits, and monkeys. Caton presented his original findings to the British Medical Society in 1875 *(3)* and in 1887 was performing recordings in unanesthetized, restrained animals. Neurophysiology became a rapidly expanding field, and many other workers continued the investigation of mammalian electroencephalography.

Not until 1929 *(4)*, however, were EEGs first recorded in humans by Hans Berger, an Austrian psychiatrist. Berger was fortunate to have an excellent arrangement with neurologists who permitted him to work with patients in whom a piece of skull had been removed. Thus he could place his recording electrodes on the epidural surface. Nonetheless, Berger worked with many handicaps, not the least of which was the lack of suitable electrical amplification. The optically amplified tracings he obtained are quite foreign to the powerfully amplified and filtered signals we use today. Berger's patient work identified many EEG patterns, including the alpha rhythm of about 10 cycles per second.

Berger's work continued largely unappreciated for several years until his findings were confirmed by Adrian and Matthews *(5)*. One of the major reasons Berger's findings were not readily accepted was that the brain activity seemed to be unrelated to the expected physiologic activity. Based on existing knowledge of the electrical activity of the heart, most investigators expected brain waves to be largest and most active when subjects were thinking vigorously. Berger's data, however, showed that brain activity was greatest or most noticeable when the subjects were most relaxed. Individuals interested in further historical background on electroencephalography are referred to the English translation of Berger's original papers by Gloor *(6)* and to Brazier's *(7)* account of the early studies of brain electrical activity.

Among the earliest workers to utilize electroencephalography for studying the sleep of humans were Davis, Harvey, and Loomis, who in the late 1930s devised a classification system for the EEG during sleep *(8)*. They divided the brain waves into five patterns, which were described in the following manner:

- *Stage A:* an interrupted alpha pattern, with frequencies of 9–11 cycles per second and amplitude of approximately 60 $\mu$V. This pattern was found typically in relaxed wakefulness or drowsiness.
- *Stage B:* a low-voltage pattern in which the alpha rhythm is no longer present. This stage represented the onset of sleep.
- *Stage C:* characterized by spindle activity—waves of 14–15 cycles per second and 20–40 $\mu$V. The spindles were superimposed on slower background activity.
- *Stage D:* a pattern combining spindles with occasional, much slower waves of very high amplitude (as high as 300 $\mu$V).
- *Stage E:* mainly slow, high-amplitude waves, with virtually no spindles.

These investigators also identified a large biphasic wave pattern that occurred in stages B and C and could be seen following auditory stimuli. This wave form was assigned the letter K.

In the early 1950s, the University of Chicago group (Kleitman, Aserinsky, and Dement) began to study the eye movement patterns of sleeping subjects. Initially, these investigations were carried out using direct visual observation of the eyes moving beneath the lids. Subsequently, these investigators used electrical recording of eye movements in conjunction with the brain wave recordings and identified a pattern of low-voltage, fast EEG activity accompanied by bursts of rapid eye movements. A number of their early studies attempted to localize dreaming to these periods and found a high correlation of dreaming mentation associated with arousals from this state of sleep. In 1957, Dement and Kleitman *(1)* published their classic description of the EEG and eye movement patterns of overnight sleep in humans, coining the term REM sleep and describing the cyclic nature of REM and NREM sleep.

Another discovery of interest to basic polysomnography was reported by Jouvet's group in 1959 *(9)*. They noted that the periods of low-voltage, fast EEG activity and rapid eye movements that Dement *(10)* had described in cats were accompanied by postural relaxation. That is, the animals maintained their initial sleeping posture until the occurrence of the activated EEG pattern, whereupon there was a total postural relaxation, usually seen as the dropping of the head. Again, the observational finding was supported by direct electrical recording. Electrical activity of the neck muscles, recorded in combination with brain wave and eye movement activity, enabled Jouvet and his colleagues to show that electrical silence of the muscles accompanied REM sleep.

The developments outlined above combined to give us the three measures that are now used to characterize sleep: electroencephalography, electro-oculography, and electromyography. These three measures, recorded in a standard manner, form the basis of polysomnography. In 1968, a group of sleep researchers undertook the first consensus exercise in the field, which resulted in the Rechtschaffen and Kales *(2)* manual for recording and scoring sleep stages in human subjects.

# Electrode Placements for Recording Sleep

## Electroencephalogram (EEG)

Most sleep researchers have adopted the nomenclature of the 10–20 electrode placement system recommended for use in electroencephalography by the International Federation of Societies for EEG and Clinical Neurophysiology. The international 10–20 electrode placement system was developed by Jasper *(11)* in Montreal. Although other placement systems have been proposed, the 10–20 system enjoys the most widespread use. The 10–20 electrode placement system permits replicable placement of electrodes with great accuracy. Placements in different patients do not necessarily overlie identical cortical regions, although they are usually quite similar. Not all 10–20 placements are used routinely for recording sleep, but their locations and names should be known in case they are needed (for recording sleep in patients with epilepsy, for example).

The system of EEG electrode placement used for sleep recording is based on the 10–20 system but is a greatly simplified montage. To identify the stages of sleep it is not necessary to obtain measures of focal activity or to make regional comparisons. Sleep stage scoring relies on more widespread electrical activity that can usually be identified from placements in the central region of the scalp. This activity includes vertex sharp waves, sleep spindles, alpha rhythm, K complexes, and the high-amplitude slow waves of stages 3 and 4 sleep. Thus, in general, only $C_3$ and $C_4$ are used to record the stages of sleep, one or the other being recorded at a given time. (Both $C_3$ and $C_4$ are applied at the beginning of the night to ensure an adequate recording all through the night.) In many cases, especially when precise determination of sleep onset is required or when subjects have poorly visualized central alpha activity, an occipital ($O_1$ or $O_2$) electrode is also applied because of its usefulness in determining sleep onset. Certain laboratories also routinely record from frontal placements.

*Sleeping and waking disorders: indications and techniques*

The 10–20 system is based upon measurements from four standard points on the head: the *nasion,* the *inion,* and the left and right *preauricular points.* These points are also the referents used for measuring placements in sleep recordings. Before applying electrodes, each position is marked with a skin pencil. For minimal standards of practice in sleep laboratories, we suggest that these measurements be performed as a standard practice. Standard textbooks of electroencephalography *(12)* provide descriptions of measuring techniques. The following material describes measuring techniques for the placement of $C_3$, $C_4$, $O_1$, and $O_2$.

- Measure the distance from nasion to inion along the midline through the vertex and make a preliminary mark at the midpoint, $C_z$. No electrode will be placed on this spot, but it will be used as a landmark.
- Check that this point is midway between the preauricular points.
- Reapply the tape at the midline and mark the point at 10% from the inion ($O_z$). No electrode will be placed on this spot, but it will be used as a landmark.
- Reapply the tape transversely through $C_z$ and mark $T_3$ (10% up from the left preauricular point), $C_3$ (30% up from the left preauricular point), $T_4$ (10% up from the right preauricular point), and $C_4$ (30% up from the right preauricular point). (Only $C_3$ and $C_4$ will be used as placements; $T_3$ and $T_4$ are landmarks.)
- Measure the distance between $T_3$ and $O_z$ and mark a point at 20% from $O_z$. This is the position of $O_1$. $O_2$ is placed in the same way on the right side of the head, between $T_4$ and $O_z$.

Application of EEG electrodes so that they maintain excellent contact throughout the night or longer—as in the case of a night recording followed by multiple sleep latency tests—requires a certain amount of care. Many laboratories use collodion-soaked gauze patches dried with compressed air to form an airtight seal around the jelly-filled electrode cup. When applied correctly, excellent contact with the scalp can be maintained for 24 to 36 hours using this technique. An alternate method involves using scalp electrodes with a hole in the center. The electrode is similarly sealed to the scalp with a collodion-soaked gauze patch, but the electrode jelly is applied using a blunt-tip needle after the electrode is affixed. The advantage of the latter technique is that it allows the technologist to "prime" the electrode at any time without having to remove and replace it entirely.

## Electro-oculogram (EOG)

There are two general reasons for recording eye movements during sleep. First, the onset of sleep in most subjects is heralded or accompanied by slow, rolling eye movements. Second, a cardinal sign of REM sleep is the phasic bursts of rapid eye movements, which are an essential criterion for scoring REM sleep. The slow eye movements of sleep onset are not essential for scoring; however, they are very helpful in many subjects.

In the eyeball, there is a small electropotential difference from the front to the back. Thus the eyeball exists in the head as a potential field within a volume conductor.

The front (cornea) of the eyeball is positive with respect to the back (retina) of the eye. Because of this constant potential difference, movement of the eyes can be measured from electrodes placed on the skin surrounding the eye. An electrode nearest the cornea will register a positive potential; an electrode nearest the retina will register a negative potential. As the eye moves left, right, up, or down, the position of the cornea and retina will change with respect to the fixed position of the electrode. Thus a potential change will register as a pen deflection on the polygraph, corresponding in direction to the changing position of the eyeball.

Each corner of the eye is referred to as the canthus. The lateral corners of the eyes (nearest the temporal bone) are called outer canthi. Inner canthi are the corners nearest the nose. Standard EOG placements are the right outer canthus (ROC) and the left outer canthus (LOC). According to the standard manual *(2)*, the EOG electrodes should be offset from horizontal, with one slightly (about 1 cm) above and the other slightly below horizontal. In this manner, the electrodes can sense both horizontal and vertical eye movements. Electrodes placed precisely on the horizontal plane would record only horizontal and oblique eye movements. At Stanford, EOG electrodes are referred to the opposite earlobe or mastoid reference electrodes. (This referencing system is *not* as shown in the standard manual.) This technique has proved helpful for evaluating electrode artifact in the EOG or reference electrode. In addition, a standard orientation of EOG channels is used, with $ROC/A_1$ always on the channel above $LOC/A_2$. With this setup, conjugate eye movements will always register as out-of-phase pen deflections on these two channels. Given the standard "negative up" rule, when the subject looks to the right or up, the $ROC/A_1$ pen will deflect downward (positive) and the $LOC/A_2$ pen will move upward (negative). When the subject looks left or down, the $ROC/A_1$ pen will move up and the $LOC/A_2$ pen will move down.

Standard recording procedure calls for two eye-movement channels. Single-channel recordings are sometimes used, however, when recording channels are limited. One technique for single-channel eye-movement recording, the differential EOG, uses two split electrodes. Each is applied to the outer canthus of one eye and the inner canthus of the other. A single-channel EOG can also be obtained by referencing the ROC and LOC to one another.

When a major goal of an experiment is to determine the precise direction of eye movements, the EOG may be simultaneously recorded from both horizontal and vertical placements. In addition to placements on the outer canthi, electrodes would be placed above (supraorbital) and below (infraorbital) the eyes. This technique has been used most frequently in studies relating eye movements to dream content.

## Electromyogram (EMG)

In a standard polysomnographic recording, the EMG from the chin is used as a criterion for scoring REM sleep *(2)*. EMG recordings from other muscles may also be used to evaluate certain sleep disorders. For example, EMG from the anterior tibialis muscles is important in evaluating patients who have nocturnal myoclonus. The intercostal EMG is used in certain laboratories to monitor respiratory effort. Clinical EMG recordings used to evaluate muscle disorders are far more complex than the recordings used in sleep. Frequently such recordings involve inserting small wires directly into a muscle fiber. Most EMG recordings during sleep require simply placing electrodes over the skin above the muscle group of interest.

Three electrodes are taped on the chin for recording EMG. The primary reason for using three electrodes (even though only two are recorded at any given time) is to ensure that there is always a backup electrode in case of failure of one placement. This is even more important for chin EMG than most other placements because the likelihood of failure is greater, especially if electrodes remain on in the daytime when subjects are eating and talking. EMG electrodes are referenced to one another; any combination of the three placements can be used. In general, the combination that is selected depends on the quality of the recording.

Patients with beards may pose a problem when EMG is recorded from skin electrodes taped to the chin. Depending upon the extent of the beard, the EMG electrodes may be placed in a manner that is not too inconsistent with the standard procedure. If the beard is extensive and a precise EMG recording is essential, the subject will sometimes agree to shave the portion of the beard beneath the chin. If all else fails, it is possible to use cup electrodes applied with collodion patches (in the manner of the EEG) to record chin EMG from a bearded subject.

## Summary of Electrode Placements

Twelve electrodes are attached to record sufficient parameters for scoring sleep stages. Not all of the placements will be recorded at all times, since a number of the electrodes are applied as backups in case of failure. The hookup presented above will include four EEG placements at $C_3$, $C_4$, $O_1$, and $C_2$; two placements for EOG, offset at ROC and LOC; three EMG electrodes on the chin; two reference electrodes—one each on the right ($A_2$) and left ($A_1$) earlobe or mastoid; and one electrode (GND) placed on the forehead as a common ground. Most laboratories find that a standard electrode-numbering system is useful for keeping procedures uniform within a group and avoiding problems that can arise when each individual has his own system. The numbering system used at Stanford is listed in Table 1–1. Note that the numbering system maintains the left-odd/right-even logic of the 10–20 system.

Minimal four-channel montages for recording sleep with these electrode placements are shown in Table 1–2. A number of laboratories use $A_1$ and $A_2$ together as a common reference for EEG and EOG channels. At Stanford, this common reference is used only as a technique to reduce ECG artifact in subjects where the artifact is especially severe. In addition to the four channels needed for scoring sleep stages, we suggest that a continuous recording of heart rate should be added to these parameters, even if no other additional variables are to be recorded. (Heart rates can easily be obtained by taping electrodes on both shoulders or right shoulder and left lower rib cage.)

Additional techniques can be used to ensure high-quality, accurate recordings. When the hookup is complete, electrode impedances should be checked. Impedances

*Basics for polygraphic monitoring of sleep*

**Table 1–1** Suggested Numbering System for Electrodes

| Lead | Electrode Number |
|---|---|
| $C_3$ | 1 |
| $C_4$ | 2 |
| LOC | 3 |
| ROC | 4 |
| $O_1$ | 5 |
| $O_2$ | 6 |
| $A_1$ | 7 |
| $A_2$ | 8 |
| EMG (chin) | 9, 10, 11 |
| GND | unnumbered |
| (Heart rate) | (12,13) |

below 10,000 ohms will result in an adequate recording, although many laboratories require impedances of 5,000 ohms or less. (Devices for easily and reliably testing impedances are available commercially. They include the Grass Instruments Company impedance meter series.) For laboratories performing multiple sleep latency testing, impedances should be tested before each nap.

Several techniques may be helpful in achieving low impedances. Thorough cleansing of the scalp and skin with acetone or alcohol is necessary to remove oils and dead

**Table 1–2** Montages for Four-Channel Sleep Recordings

| Channel | Derivation |
|---|---|
| *Recording Montage at Sleep Onset* | |
| 1 | $C_3/A_2$ (with $C_4/A_1$ as backup) |
| 2 | $O_2/A_1$ (with $O_1/A_2$ as backup) |
| 3 | ROC/LOC |
| 4 | EMG/EMG (with third EMG as backup) |
| (5) | (Heart rate) |
| *Recording Montage After Sleep Onset* | |
| 1 | $C_3/A_2$ (with $C_4/A_1$ as backup) |
| 2 | ROC/$A_1$ |
| 3 | LOC/$A_2$ |
| 4 | EMG/EMG (with third EMG as backup) |
| (5) | (Heart rate) |

skin. (Water is usually sufficient on the faces of prepubertal subjects.) We also vigorously rub a small dab of electrode conductive jelly onto the electrode placement site. If using a blunt-tip needle to apply electrode jelly through a center-hole electrode, a gentle abrading of the scalp with the needle will improve the conductive surface.

If the subject is expected to be very active during sleep (e.g., suspected sleep apnea syndrome) or if multiple sleep latency testing is performed, the integrity of the electrode placements can be assisted by affixing the electrode wire bundle to the scalp. All wires are brought to the nape of the neck and taped together with a comfortable amount of slack for head movements. The wires are then affixed to the scalp atop the head with a collodion-soaked gauze patch. This patch serves as an anchor for the wires and prevents movement from affecting the electrode placements.

# Polygraph Settings

The primary function of the polygraph is to permit monitoring of the bioelectric activity of the body. The polygraph amplifies and records the tiny fluctuating potential differences between the two inputs and simultaneously compares them to a common ground. In addition to amplifying the bioelectric signal, the polygraph also enables one to focus the signal by filtering out data that are not relevant to the signal of interest. Thus the frequency range selected by filtering is determined by the frequencies of the potentials that will be recorded and the frequencies of extraneous potentials that one wishes to eliminate.

Most sleep laboratories use a standard paper speed of 10 or 15 mm/sec. Slower speeds are discouraged because clear visualization of alpha rhythm and sleep spindles becomes extremely difficult. Faster paper speeds are unusual because of the generally prohibitive length of the recording period. A calibration that gives a pen deflection of 7.5 to 10.0 mm for a 50-$\mu$V signal is recommended for the EEG and EOG channels. The chin EMG is often adjusted after the recording has begun so that an acceptable EMG signal is obtained. We generally use a 1-cm pen deflection for a 50-$\mu$V signal. Greater amplification of the EEG may result in pen blocking during slow-wave sleep (stages 3 and 4), especially in younger subjects. Less amplification may result in difficulty observing small-amplitude spindles.

Table 1–3 lists settings for the various sleep parameters. These settings are available on the Grass model 7 series driver amplifiers and wide-band AC preamplifiers. If these settings are not available, the most similar settings should be chosen. Occasional modification of these settings is required by a particular circumstance, as listed in Table 1–3. In certain subjects (especially older individuals), the amplitude of the EEG using the standard gain may be so small that the record is extremely difficult to evaluate. The gain may be increased so that a 50-$\mu$V pulse gives a pen deflection of 15 mm. By contrast, the amplitude of the EEG in some young children is so great that the pen sweep is not large enough to register the signal. If severe, the gain on the EEG channels (and on EOG channels) may be reduced so that a 50-$\mu$V pulse causes a pen deflection of 5 mm. In every case, it is important to mark the changes on the recording chart paper and to recalibrate the channel when necessary.

**Table 1-3** Polygraph Settings Using Grass Series 7 Amplifiers

| Parameter | Deflection at 50 μV Signal | ½ Amp High Freq | ½ Amp Low Freq | Time Constant |
|---|---|---|---|---|
| *Standard* | | | | |
| EEG | 10 mm | 35 Hz | 0.3 Hz | 0.24 sec |
| EOG | 10 mm | 35 Hz | 0.3 Hz | 0.24 sec |
| EMG | * | 75 Hz | 10.0 Hz | 0.015 sec |
| Heart rate | † | 15 Hz | 1.0 Hz | 0.1 sec |
| *Patient with Low-Amplitude EEG* | | | | |
| EEG | 15 mm | 35 Hz | 0.3 Hz | 0.24 sec |
| *Child with High-Amplitude EEG* | | | | |
| EEG | 5 mm | 35 Hz | 0.3 Hz | 0.24 sec |
| *Child with "Sweat" Artifact* | | | | |
| EEG | 5 or 10 mm | 35 Hz | 1.0 Hz | 0.1 sec |
| EOG | 5 or 10 mm | 35 Hz | 1.0 Hz | 0.1 sec |

*Sensitivity of the chin EMG is 20 μV/cm.
†Sensitivity of heart rate will vary with electrode placements. Adjust as necessary to obtain a suitable tracing.

EEG and EOG channels may pick up a very low frequency artifact caused by sweat. If extreme, "sweat artifact" can make the record virtually unscorable. When a correction cannot be made by re-referencing or lowering the room temperature, the low-frequency cutoff may be set at 1.0 Hz. Take this step only in extreme cases and be sure to mark the chart paper. Frequent checks of the problem should be made by returning the low frequency to 0.3 Hz (time constant to 0.24 sec). Especially in adults, the 0.3 Hz low-frequency filter setting (time constant 0.24 sec) should be used whenever possible. In children, sweat artifact does not need to be extreme to justify changing the low-frequency filter because they have such pervasive slow waves in stages 3 and 4 sleep.

# The All-Night Recording

## Procedure Before Hookup

Before the subject arrives in the laboratory, all equipment will be assembled for the hookup, the polygraph will be calibrated, and the chart paper labeled. All pertinent information should be placed at the start of the recording chart and should include the

*Sleeping and waking disorders: indications and techniques*

subject's name, room number, date of recording, purpose of the recording or name of the experiment, type of polygraph, calibration signal, paper speed, and technician's name. Each channel should be labeled with the derivation to be recorded and the high- and low-frequency filter settings.

## Putting the Subject to Bed and Subject Calibrations

The following points are intended as general reminders. Each laboratory has its own procedures, and a good technologist will have a checklist similar to the list below.

1. Have the subject complete the bedtime questionnaire. Check to make sure he has not neglected to complete any items. (Make this check before lights-out.)
2. Make sure the subject has completed his presleep rituals and is ready to go to bed. Has he brushed his teeth, gone to the bathroom, etc.?
3. Ask the subject to remove his watch; place it out of sight and out of reach. (In a hospital setting, one might request that the individual put his watch in a safe place with his other valuables.)
4. When the subject is in bed and comfortable, plug the electrode leads into the appropriate jacks on the electrode box. Count them. Are there as many electrodes plugged in as were applied? Make sure the subject is not lying on the wires. Let the subject know that he has considerable freedom of movement and should not feel constrained to lie in one position for the entire night.
5. Assure the subject that he will be monitored throughout the recording. Show him the intercom (or other system) and make sure he knows how to operate it. Assure the subject that he should call at any time if he wishes to get up or has any problem. Ask him not to unplug the electrodes himself.
6. Explain that he will be asked to perform several tasks to see if the hookup is working properly. Ask him to lie quietly on his back and listen for instructions.
7. *Subject calibrations*. The subject calibrations serve two general purposes. First, they enable the technician to determine if any problems are immediately apparent in the recording. These problems will be resolved before the recording begins. Second, the calibration tracings are invaluable to the person who will score the record. They allow the scorer to compare, for example, a questionable epoch of wakefulness during the night to the unquestioned waking record at the beginning of the night. They also allow the scorer to assess any peculiarities that may be present in the basic recording, such as a misalignment of pens.
    a. "With your eyes open, please look straight ahead." This condition should be maintained for at least 30 seconds of movement-free record.
    b. "Please close your eyes." Once again, the condition should be maintained for at least 30 movement-free seconds. If no alpha rhythm can

be seen, even in the occipital trace, look in on the subject to make sure his eyes are closed.
   c. "Open your eyes . . . without moving your head, look to the right . . . look to the left . . . look to the right . . . look to the left . . . look straight ahead . . . look up . . . look down . . . look up . . . look down . . . relax." Watch the polygraph carefully to make sure the pens are deflecting appropriately (out-of-phase) with each eye movement.
   d. "Holding your head still, please blink your eyes slowly five times." Blink artifact will be seen in the EEG and EOG traces.
   e. "Please grit your teeth (or clench your jaw) . . . relax." This procedure will cause an increase in the EMG amplitude and muscle artifact in the EEG and EOG channels.
   f. If respiration is being recorded, ask the subject to "inhale and hold your breath . . . exhale and breathe normally."
   g. The anterior tibialis EMG channels are calibrated by asking the subject to "flex your left (right) leg . . . relax."
   h. While the subject is relaxed, put the 60-Hz notch filters on "out" to determine if there are any loose electrodes or other problems.
8. Correct any problems indicated by the subject calibrations and 60-Hz check.
9. Make a final check on the subject's well-being, wish him good night, turn out the lights, and close the door. If there is a preset bedtime, lights-out should be as close to this time as possible.
10. Throughout all the hookup procedures and subject calibration procedures, be sure the subject does not fall asleep before lights-out.

## Overnight Procedures

The recording will require constant vigilance during the night. Thus a key concern is to stay awake and alert. As soon as the recording is going well, complete the experimenter's evening questionnaire and/or make a log entry detailing the conditions at lights-out. Note the subject's relative level of vigilance. Was he alert or sleepy? Did he fall asleep before lights-out? Also note the subject's mood. Did he seem depressed, anxious, calm, etc.? Note also whether the windows were open, fan on, how many blankets were used, the subject's sleeping attire, and so forth.

At the Stanford laboratories, the following procedures are performed at set intervals. Every 30 minutes, the exact time is written on the recording chart paper. (This procedure allows adjustments to be made for inexact paper-drive speed.) Every 60 minutes, a 60-Hz check is performed on each channel. Adjustments are made to the recording as necessary.

Other procedures are to be used as required. The recording must be observed very frequently to check for paper jams, ink clogs, recording artifacts, changes in pen alignment, etc. Whenever the recording is altered in any fashion, the changes (filter settings, sensitivity, electrode derivations, etc.) should be noted very clearly on the chart paper.

### End of Night

At the appropriate time, open the subject's bedroom door and awaken him. Give the subject a little warning before turning on a bright overhead light. Note the difficulty of arousing the subject. Subject calibrations may be repeated at this time. Depending on the protocol requirements, a number of other procedures should be performed before the subject gets out of bed. These may include various questionnaires, temperature, pulse, blood pressure, etc.

The night recording is not complete until notations regarding the recording are made by the overnight technologist. Notations will include an account of any unusual occurrences during the night, the subject's mood on awakening, recording difficulties, and electrodes that will need to be reapplied before daytime recordings are performed.

# GLOSSARY OF COMMON EEG AND PSG TERMS

(From: EEG Journal 1966; 20:293 & Rechtschaffen/Kales manual, 1968.)

**Activated sleep:** sometimes used as a synonym for REM sleep.
**Activity:** any sequence of waves.
**Alpha rhythm:** EEG rhythm, usually with frequency of 8–13 cps in adults; most prominent in the posterior areas; present most markedly when the eyes are closed; attenuated during attention, especially visual. (Characteristic of relaxed wakefulness with the eyes closed.)
**Alpha wave:** individual component of an alpha rhythm.
**Artifact:** a nonbiological signal that appears in an EEG or sleep recording or a signal that interferes with the derivations being recorded.
**Attenuation:** decrease in amplitude of activity.
**Background activity:** more or less general and continuous activity in contrast with paroxysmal or focal activities.
**Beta:** used to indicate a frequency band, i.e., EEG frequencies higher than 13 cps.
**Beta rhythm:** EEG rhythm with a frequency higher than 13 cps.
**Body movement:** scored during any sleep stage when a phasic increase in the amplitude of the EMG lead of 1 sec or longer is accompanied by muscle artifact in an EEG or EOG trace.
**Burst:** see paroxysm.
**Canthus:** corner of the eye (plural: canthi).
**Common average reference lead:** a common lead that is the average of potential differences at a number of electrodes.

*Basics for polygraphic monitoring of sleep*

**Common reference lead:** lead that is the same in all derivations of a montage.
**Complex:** group of two or more waves, clearly distinguished from background activity and occurring with a well-recognized form or recurring with consistent form.
**Cycle:** the complete series of potential changes undergone by a wave before the same series is repeated.
**Delta:** used to indicate a frequency band or a period, i.e., EEG frequency of less than 4 cps and period of more than ¼ second.
**Delta activity:** series of regular or irregular EEG waves with durations of more than ¼ second.
**Delta rhythm:** EEG rhythm with frequency of less than 4 cps.
**Delta sleep:** sometimes used as a synonym for stages 3 and 4 sleep. (Note that the frequency criterion for scoring slow EEG waves in stages 3 and 4 sleep is 2 cps or slower.)
**Delta wave:** EEG wave with duration of more than ¼ second.
**Depth EEG:** EEG derived from electrodes in direct contact with subcortical structures.
**Derivation:** recording from a pair of leads.
**Desynchronized sleep:** sometimes used as a synonym for REM sleep.
**Diffuse:** occurring over large areas without constant location. Used to describe activity occurring more or less simultaneously (without necessarily being synchronous) in large areas.
**Driving:** occurrence of waves phase-locked with rhythmic stimuli.
**Drowsy sleep:** sometimes used as a synonym for stage 1 sleep.
**Duration of a wave:** time interval from beginning to end of a wave.
**Electrical silence:** absence of electrical activity.
**Electrocorticogram (ECoG):** record of electrical activity derived from electrodes in direct contact with the cortex.
**Electroencephalogram (EEG):** record of the electrical activity of the brain.
**Electromyogram (EMG):** record of the electrical activity of muscles.
**Electro-oculogram (EOG):** record of the electrical activity of eye movements.
**Fast sleep:** sometimes used as a synonym for REM sleep.
**Frequency:** the number of complete cycles of a rhythm in 1 second.
**Index:** the percentage of time occupied by the wave specified (e.g., alpha index) with larger than specified amplitude (usually 10 µV) in a given sample (usually of 1 minute's duration).
**K complex:** EEG wave forms having a well-delineated negative sharp wave immediately followed by a positive component; duration exceeds 0.5 seconds; waves of 12–14 cps (sleep spindles) may or may not constitute a part of the complex; generally maximal over vertex regions; occurring during sleep either spontaneously or in response to sudden (usually auditory) stimuli. (Characteristic of stage 2 sleep.)
**Lambda wave:** sharp wave in the occipital areas, mainly positive in relation to other areas and usually evoked by visual exploration.
**Lead:** term used to denote a single electrode placement.
**Light sleep:** sometimes used as a synonym for stage 2 sleep.

**Location:** refers to a brain area.

**Low-voltage EEG:** EEG in which no activity larger than 20 μV can be recorded between any two points on the scalp.

**Montage:** combination of a number of derivations.

**Morphology:** the shape (form) of a wave or activity.

**Movement time:** sleep-scoring epoch during which the polygraph record is obscured by movements of the subject.

**Mu rhythm:** EEG rhythm at 7–11 cps in central region, often with arcade or comb form; associated with beta rhythm; attenuated by real, imagined, or intended movement or tactile stimulation, particularly of the hands.

**NREM sleep:** sleep stages 1, 2, 3, and 4.

**Paradoxical sleep:** sometimes used as a synonym for REM sleep.

**Paroxysm:** group of waves that appears and disappears abruptly and that is clearly distinguished from background activity by different frequency, morphology, or amplitude.

**Period:** duration of a cycle. The period is the reciprocal of the frequency of a rhythm.

**Phase:** strictly, amplitude time relations of sinusoidal waves; loosely, time relations of different parts of a wave (or waves) in a single trace, or of a wave (or waves) as recorded simultaneously in different traces.

**Quantity:** amount of activity, in terms of amplitude and number of waves, with respect to time.

**Quiet sleep:** sometimes used as a synonym for stages 3 and 4 sleep.

**Random:** occurring at unconstant time intervals.

**Reactivity:** changeability of the EEG following change in the environment.

**REM sleep:** a relatively low-voltage, mixed-frequency EEG in conjunction with episodic rapid eye movements and a low-amplitude EMG.

**Rhythm:** activity of approximately constant period and morphology, but not necessarily of amplitude.

**Saw-tooth waves:** notched wave forms in vertex and frontal regions that sometimes occur in conjunction with bursts of rapid eye movements in REM sleep.

**Sleep spindle:** a waxing and waning wave form with a frequency of 12–14 cps, most prominent in stage 2 sleep.

**Slow-wave sleep:** sometimes used as a synonym for stages 3 and 4 sleep.

**Spike:** wave distinguished from background activity and having a duration of 1/12 second or less.

**Spike and wave complex:** complex of two waves, one with a duration of 1/12 second or less (spike) and the other with a duration of 1/5 to 1/2 second (wave).

**Spindle sleep:** sometimes used as a synonym for stage 2 sleep.

**Stage B:** sometimes used as a synonym for stage 1 sleep.

**Stage C:** sometimes used as a synonym for stage 2 sleep.

**Stage D:** sometimes used as a synonym for stage 3 sleep.

**Stage E:** sometimes used as a synonym for stage 4 sleep.

**Stage W (wakefulness):** EEG contains alpha activity and/or low-voltage, mixed-frequency activity. (The subject is responsive to the environment.)

**Stage 1 sleep:** relatively low-voltage, mixed-frequency EEG without rapid eye movements; slow eye movements are often present; vertex sharp waves may be seen; EMG activity is not suppressed.

**Stage 2 sleep:** 12–14 cps sleep spindles and K complexes on a background of relatively low-voltage, mixed-frequency EEG activity.

**Stage 3 sleep:** moderate amounts (20%–50%) of high-amplitude (75 $\mu$V or greater), slow-wave (2 cps or slower) EEG activity.

**Stage 4 sleep:** predominance (greater than 50%) of high-amplitude (75 $\mu$V or greater), slow-wave (2 cps or slower) EEG activity.

**Theta:** used to indicate a frequency band or a period, i.e., an EEG frequency of 4 cps to less than 8 cps or a period of ¼ second to more than ⅛ second.

**Theta activity:** series of regular or irregular EEG waves with durations of ¼ to more than ⅛ seconds. (May be seen in stage 1 or REM sleep.)

**Theta rhythm:** EEG rhythm with a frequency of 4 cps to less than 8 cps.

**Theta wave:** EEG wave with a duration of ¼ second to more than ⅛ second.

**Topography:** distribution of activity with respect to anatomic landmarks. (Synonym: spatial distribution.)

**Unilateral:** occurring on one side of the head.

**Vertex sharp wave:** sharp wave, maximal at the vertex and negative in relation to other areas (often occurring during later portions of stage 1 sleep).

**Wave:** any transient change of potential difference in the EEG.

# REFERENCES

1. Dement WC, Kleitman N. Cyclic variations of EEG during sleep and their relation to eye movements, body motility and dreaming. Electroencephalogr Clin Neurophysiol 1957; 9:673–90.
2. Rechtschaffen A, Kales A, eds. A manual of standardized terminology, techniques and scoring system for sleep stages of human subjects. Los Angeles: UCLA Brain Information Service/Brain Research Institute, 1968.
3. Caton R. The electric currents of the brain. Br. Med J 1875; 2:278.
4. Berger H. Uber das elektroenkephalogramm des menschen. Arch Psychiatr Nervenkr 1929; 87:527–70.
5. Adrian ED, Matthews BHC. Berger rhythms: potential changes from occipital lobes in man. Brain 1934; 57:355.
6. Gloor P. Hans Berger on the electroencephalogram of man. The fourteen original reports on the human electroencephalogram. Translated and edited by P. Gloor. Electroencephalogr Clin Neurophysiol (Suppl) 1969, Volume 28.

7. Brazier MAB. A history of electrical activity of the brain. London and New York: Macmillan, 1961.
8. Kleitman N. Sleep and wakefulness. Chicago: University of Chicago Press, 1963:25–6.
9. Jouvet M, Michel M, Courjon J. Sur un stade d'activité électrique cérébrale rapide au cours du sommeil physiologique. CR Soc Biol (Paris) 1959; 153:1024–8.
10. Dement WC. The occurrence of low voltage, fast electroencephalogram patterns during behavioral sleep in the cat. Electroencephalogr Clin Neurophysiol 1958; 10:291–6.
11. Jasper HH (Committee chairman). The ten twenty electrode system of the International Federation. Electroencephalogr Clin Neurophysiol 1958; 10:371–5.
12. Cooper R, Osselton JW, Shaw JC. EEG technology. London: Butterworths, 1974.

# TWO
# ELECTRONIC MONITORING IN THE NEWBORN AND YOUNG INFANT: THEORETICAL CONSIDERATIONS

TOKE HOPPENBROUWERS

## Introduction

Clinical electronic monitoring of various physiologic parameters is indicated when hypoventilation or prolonged apnea is observed or anticipated in infants. Such surveillance usually includes polygraphic recording of ECG, instantaneous heart rate (HR), HR variability, impedance respiration, temperature (1), and use of a transcutaneous oxygen sensor (tcPo$_2$) (2). For example, the premature infant with immature lungs and vacillating shunts exhibits unreliable oxygen transportation, which can produce severe hypoxia, causing insult to the developing central nervous system (CNS). Infants with unexplained prolonged apnea beyond the newborn period, sometimes referred to as near-miss for sudden infant death syndrome (SIDS) or aborted crib deaths, can suffer CNS damage as well. Electronic monitoring constitutes a noninvasive methodology to prevent life-threatening events and serious CNS insults.

Similarly, electronic monitoring can be utilized as an investigative tool to provide clues to the etiology of life-threatening physiologic behavior and to suggest methods of prophylaxis. Finally, clinical electronic monitoring can be used to determine the efficacy of a chosen treatment plan or modality. This has proven particularly valuable in documenting the effectiveness of xanthine-like drugs such as aminophylline, caffeine, and theophylline for preventing apnea (3) and tolazoline for reducing pulmonary hyperoxia (4). Monitoring of tcPo$_2$ has been particularly useful in determining the level and duration of supplemental oxygen for the ill, premature infant to prevent hyperoxemia and subsequent retrolental fibroplasia (3). The optimal level of assisted ventilation can also be more accurately defined (5).

A decade of experience with electronic monitoring has yielded information about adverse side effects and unexpected benefits. At present, the majority of signals that can be recorded require skin electrodes and transducers, which tend to restrict the infant's motility and the mother's inclination to cuddle or hold the infant. Such direct contact is important in premature-infant development, bonding between mother and child, and recovery from illness *(6-9)*. This hands-on policy has also been the traditional and time-proven way for physicians and caretakers to obtain vital information about the infant. Moreover, equipment output can give a false sense of security and can induce inordinate attention to instrumentation at the expense of the infant. One unexpected benefit has been the discovery that some of the diagnostic, therapeutic, or care procedures in the intensive care unit, such as endotracheal suctioning, intubation, and punctures, actually produced hypoxemia *(10,11)*. Preoxygenation can now prevent hypoxemia due to other intervention *(1,12)*. Bedside availability of continuous data has provided valuable feedback, allowing medical personnel to optimize movement patterns and to select the best position for the infant *(13)*.

With the increasing availability of sophisticated equipment and the incorporation of microprocessors, electronic monitoring technology is being utilized with greater frequency in the clinical setting. It is the purpose of this chapter to assist practitioners and investigators in weighing the benefits of electronic monitoring against the drawbacks and to suggest indications for clinical use.

# Objectives and Options in Electronic Monitoring

The ability to intervene promptly when an infant is in a life-threatening situation is the prime objective in the selection of surveillance equipment. Recently, for example, Peabody et al. *(14)* reported the inadequacy of conventional intensive care unit apnea monitors. Available evidence suggests that for accurate detection of hypoxemia, a $tcPo_2$ monitor is essential. Once hypoxemia—with or without apnea, periodic breathing, or bradycardia—has been detected, a number of options are available to determine etiology. If a central nervous system abnormality is suspected, continuously monitored EEG with examination for tracé alternant, immature patterns, or spindle development *(15-18)* can indicate maturity. A lack of spindles beyond three months of age has been associated with hypothyroidism *(19)*. With more sophisticated equipment, EEG power spectra and interhemispheric coherence can be determined *(20-23)*.

Auditory-evoked potentials are used to assess brainstem integrity *(24-29)*. Hypotonia can be electronically documented *(30)*. Finally sleep-waking patterns should reflect CNS maturation, whereas the correlation or *concordance* of individual sleep parameters, such as chin muscle tone, eye movements, EEG, and respiration, provide clues to CNS integrity *(31,32)*. Continuous ECG recordings can reveal cardiac anomalies, arrhythmias, tachycardia, or cardiac lability (Figure 2–1), and measurement of the

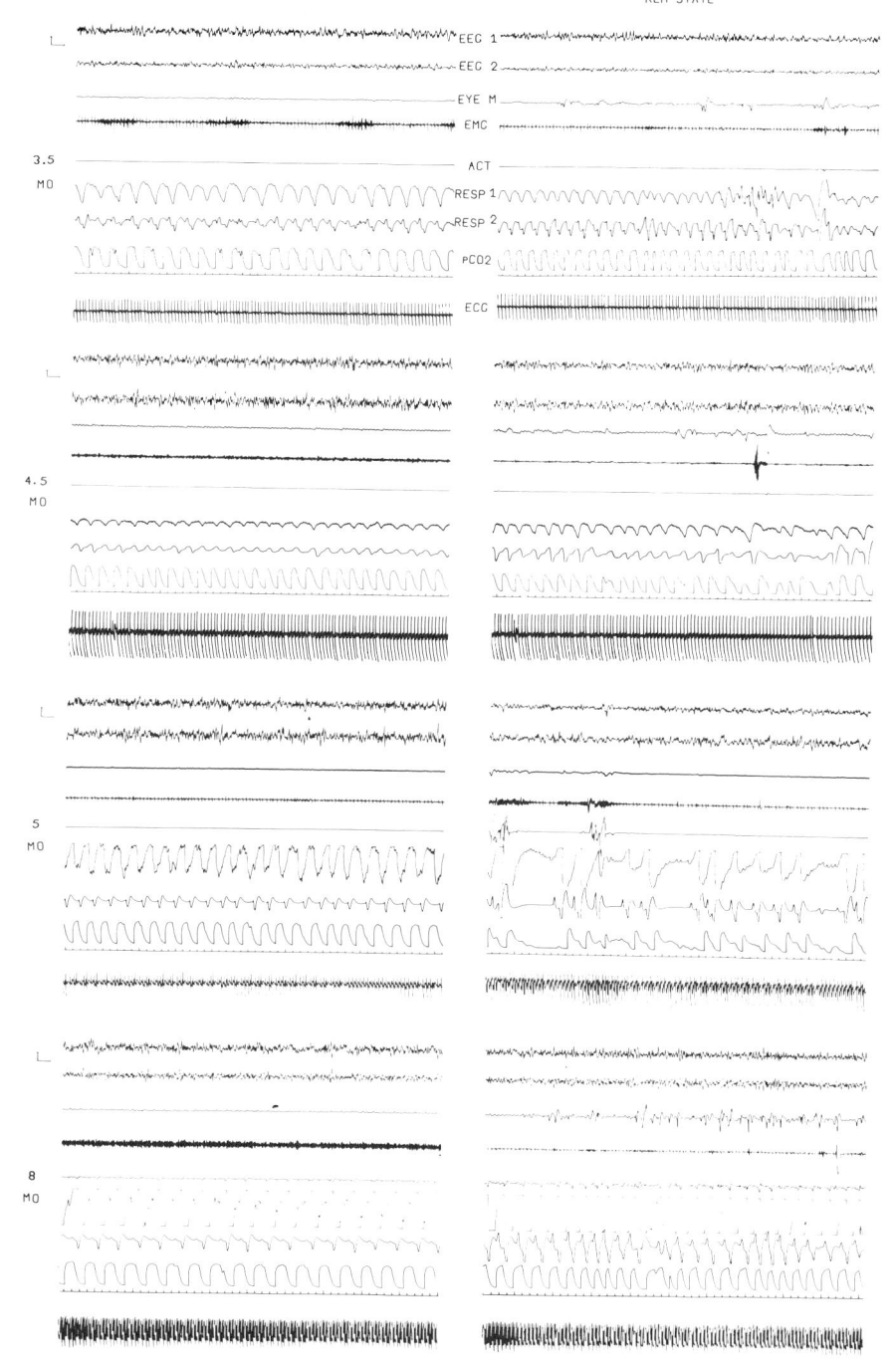

**Figure 2–1.** Spontaneous benign cardiac arrhythmia in AS and QS from the same infant between three and eight months of age. This pattern was first observed during perinatal FECG recordings.

electromechanical interval (EMI) has recently been introduced as a means of assessing the mechanical performance of the heart muscle *(33)*. Respiratory tracings can distinguish between breathing pauses due to cessation of respiratory muscle movements (central apnea) and breathing pauses due to partial or complete airway obstructions (obstructive apnea). Gastroesophageal reflux can sometimes explain the presence of apnea *(34)*. Further information on ventilatory performance can be derived from measurements of end-tidal $CO_2$ *(35,36)*, tachypnea *(37)*, paradoxical and disorganized breathing *(38–40)*, and the recently introduced transcutaneous measurement of arterial $CO_2$ *(41)*. Once the obstacles to spontaneous sleep that tend to accompany the measurement of end-tidal $CO_2$ have been removed, other ventilatory measures, such as oxygen consumption and compliance, can be obtained *(42,43)*. Two simultaneous estimates of $PO_2$ with transcutaneous electrodes can yield information about cardiac and pulmonary shunts *(44,45)*. Peabody reported an exploitable correlation between the skin $tcPO_2$ heating value and mean aortic blood pressure *(14)*.

# Reliability and Validity of Physiologic Measures

Although these noninvasive options are currently at our disposal, their usefulness in a given situation depends upon the validity and reliability of the measures and the availability of normative data. In Peabody et al.'s study of premature infants *(14)*, correlation of apnea duration and degree of hypoxemia was low ($r = 0.27$). Since apnea monitors are frequently set for an arbitrary time limit, the prevention of hypoxemia is accordingly not assured. Alarm failures are not uncommon. Only 38% of apneic periods ⩾ 15 seconds resulting in a $PO_2 < 40$ torr were detected. Sixty-one percent of apneas resulting in a $PO_2 < 40$ torr were accompanied by bradycardia. Therefore, adding bradycardia as a variable slightly improved the identification of apnea-induced hypoxemia. Hypoxemia was often observed during episodes of disorganized breathing that failed to trigger the alarm *(14)*. The additional monitoring of $tcPO_2$ provided a more reliable estimate of the significance of an apnea. We have stressed the presence of bradycardia without apnea in normal infants *(8)*. Bradycardia without apnea can sometimes induce a drop in $tcPO_2$. Pörksen et al. *(11)* studied 26 premature and newborn infants ranging in gestational age between 28 and 40 weeks. They divided episodes of bradycardia into groups lasting 1–30 seconds, 31–60 seconds, and > 60 seconds. The average drop in $tcPO_2$ in each category was significantly different. An episode lasting less than 30 seconds almost never led to a drop below 40 torr, whereas one in excess of a minute virtually always did. Hypoxemia can also occur unaccompanied by either apnea or bradycardia as a result of crying caused by pain and discomfort *(46,47)*.

These data indicate that apnea monitors cannot be relied upon to detect hypoxemia in the premature infant. Apnea detectors exhibit other shortcomings as well. Most episodes of central apnea during sleep can be detected adequately, but approximately one-third of the breathing pauses are accompanied by motility, and in these cases movement artifacts conceal the nature of the apnea or prevent alarm triggering (Figure 2–2). Reliable identification of obstructive apnea is more difficult and requires at least two simultaneous tracings. Recently we have obtained promising results with the combination of strain gauge and microphone (Figure 2–3).

The tcPO$_2$ measure is an estimate of PaO$_2$, and the majority of published reports have dealt with their correlation *(3,48,49)*. Correlation coefficients between tcPO$_2$ and PaO$_2$ for premature and fullterm newborns have been generally high, ranging between 0.89 and 0.98 *(50,51)*. An electrode temperature of 42.5–44 C has yielded optimal results in that adequate skin perfusion was obtained without producing skin lesions. Correlation coefficients decreased considerably with hypovolemia, arterial hypotension, anemic hypoxemia, and/or acidemia *(49)*. Systematic studies of tcPO$_2$ in older infants are sparse. Bompard et al. *(52)* reported data from 14 patients ranging in age between three months and 13 years. When a patient in shock was excluded, the correlation coefficient was found to be $r=0.907$. An increase in electrode temperature can counteract the reduction in diffusion that accompanies a thicker skin, but skin lesions almost inevitably ensue *(53)*. Although the majority of investigators consider tcPO$_2$ measurement a valuable adjunct to neonatal monitoring, technical problems such as drift still abound and require regular supplemental blood gas measurements by conventional methods *(54)*. This places limitations on the use of tcPO$_2$ measurements when invasive techniques cannot be tolerated, such as in research projects. Assessment of usefulness in the older infant awaits further studies.

Determination of end-expired CO$_2$ and CO$_2$ response curves during spontaneous sleep and wakefulness cannot be easily performed. Placing a hood over the infant invariably disturbs normal sleep, especially in the older infant, and closed systems involving rather bulky catheters are also not conducive to spontaneous sleep and waking behavior. Whole-body plethysmography in normal older infants has provided some limited data *(55)*. A canopy system, recently introduced for adults *(56)*, could possibly be adjusted for the older infant. Introduction of very soft rubber nasal prongs with minimal dead space, coupled to a miniaturized T system, may further improve ventilatory studies during normal sleep and wakefulness *(57)*. Epstein et al. *(58)* recently reported determinants of distortions in CO$_2$-catheter sampling systems. They demonstrated the significance of two variables in particular for the valid and reliable measurement of end-tidal CO$_2$. These were sample flow rate and sample cell volume.

Reports on evoked potentials in infants and children appeared in the literature in the 1950s and 1960s *(59,24)*. Recently, the brainstem auditory evoked potential (BAEP) in particular has been used clinically for early detection of hearing deficiencies and assessment of brainstem integrity *(28,29)*. Latency and amplitude of the multiple positive and negative deflections provide information about the integrity of the successive relay stations of the auditory system. Some investigators *(25)* recognize as many as seven peaks, reflecting in succession eighth nerve, cochlear nucleus, olivary complex, nucleus of the lateral lemniscus, inferior colliculus, medial geniculate, and cortical radiations. Others, less ambitious, categorize the multiple potentials into three, representing activity in the cochlear nerve, brainstem, and midbrain *(29)*. Stimulus char-

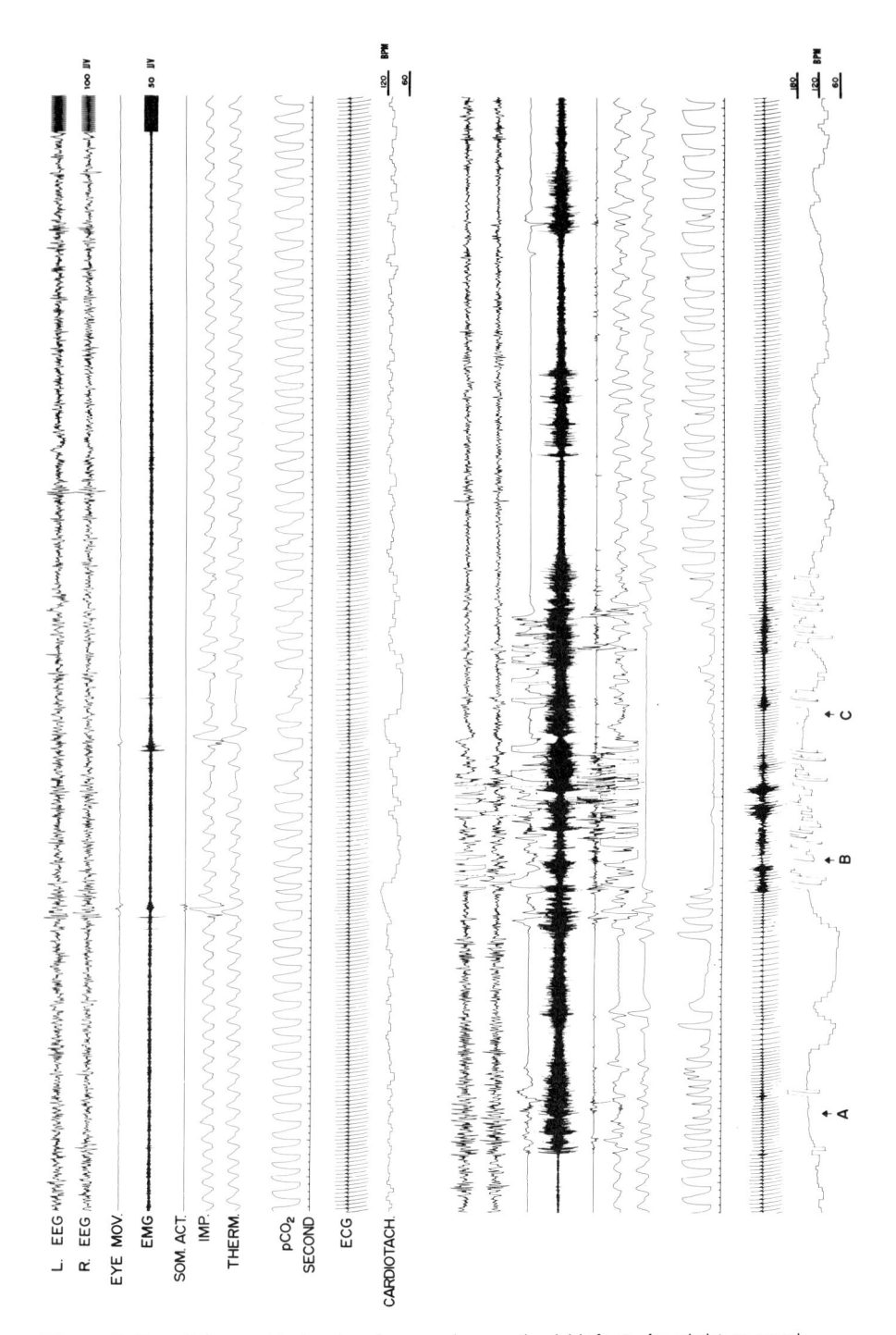

**Figure 2–2.** Polygraphic tracing from a six-month-old infant. An eight-second central apnea is followed by a cessation of airflow manifested in the P$co_2$ and thermistor tracings. The impedance tracing is affected by movement artifact, which precludes identification of the origin of the apnea. Nurse's notes: A, sucking; B, writhing; C, moving.

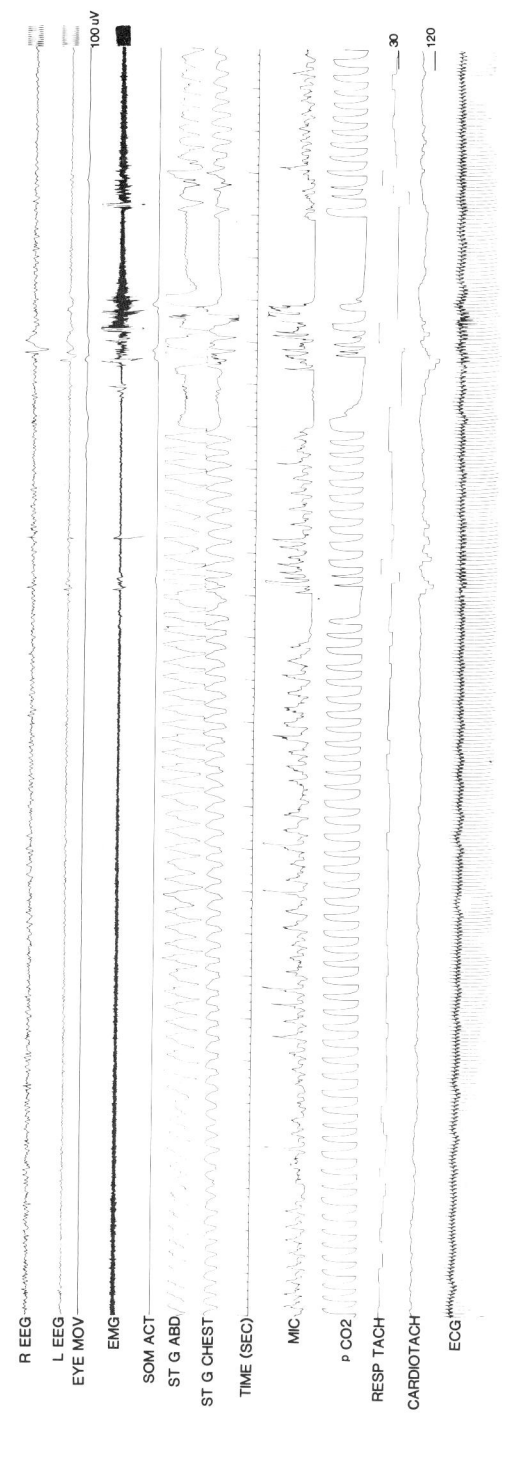

*Electronic monitoring in the newborn and young infant*

**Figure 2–3.** Polygraphic tracings from a three-month-old infant during AS. The microphone allows identification of a short obstructive pause (four seconds), followed by two central pauses of six and nine seconds respectively.

23

acteristics such as rate and intensity can partially explain the differences in results *(60)*. Despland and Galambos *(29)* reported their findings from 120 premature and fullterm infants between 26 and 42 weeks of gestational age. These authors discriminated between sensorineural- or ochlear-type responses indicating hearing deficits and purely neurologic deficits due, for instance, to intracranial pressure. Auditory threshold testing was an important feature of their diagnostic workup. Both Ellingson et al. *(61)* and Ohlrich et al. *(26)* have stressed the variability in BAEP amplitudes. Thus far, a systematic discriminative study indicating the validity and reliability of this technique, including false positive and negative diagnoses, has not been reported.

Although it is important to collect infant-state data to correctly interpret all other physiologic data, the outlook for identifying problem infants on the basis of polygraphically obtained sleep and waking parameters, such as percentages, is not promising. This statement may seem to belie the numerous findings of altered sleep and waking patterns under abnormal clinical and experimental conditions, but, on the contrary, it is based precisely on these findings. Table 2–1 delineates the conditions that have been demonstrated to affect aspects of sleep and wakefulness in infants. The only logical conclusion to be drawn from these findings is that alterations in sleep and wakefulness constitute a nonspecific response to a wide variety of stimuli and can therefore not add a great deal of specific diagnostic information. Monod and Guidasci *(62)* systematically studied the most abnormal set of infants in terms of CNS lesions. Even among their group, some infants exhibited normal sleep and waking patterns.

## Normative Data

Normative data, presently available for a number of variables, are summarized in Tables 2–2 *a, b, c, d*. Although these studies do not constitute an exhaustive list, they demonstrate a number of points. First, in some investigative areas data appear abundant, whereas in others they are sketchy or absent. A similar heterogeneity characterizes the ages studied. In general, more information is available for the premature or newborn infant than for older infants. Second, a number of studies are characterized by disagreement. Investigations on apnea, for instance, display frequent controversy concerning the definition and measurement of apnea and analysis strategies (Table 2–2 *b*). The effects of posture and temperature are seldom addressed *(93,94)*. Although gender distribution is noted, rarely has the influence of gender upon visceral functions been examined systematically. Thoman et al. *(95)* demonstrated a gender difference in breathing pauses, a finding we confirmed and extended to include respiratory rates as well *(96)*. Metabolic rate and skin stimulation can also affect respiratory behavior *(97,98)*. Third, the variability in physiologic data, both among different infants and within the same infant monitored at several consecutive times, is not always appreciated. Ellingson et al. *(61)* noticed this variability in their studies on visually evoked potential in human infants. Since then, other supportive evidence has been accumulated *(26,78)*.

**Table 2–1** Factors Affecting Sleep and Waking

| Laboratory Monitoring | Ambient Temperature and Humidity | Cold Symptoms | Sound and Noise |
|---|---|---|---|
| Unfamiliar Environment | Immunizations | Sleep Deprivation | Indigestion |
| Nature of Food | Feeding Schedule | Medication | Early or Late Cord Clamping |
| Blue Light | Teething, Wet Diaper, Pain | Fever and Illness | Light or Dark Environment |
| Time of Day | Activities During Wakefulness | Infant-Caretaker Interaction | Swaddling, Sleeping Position |

Another manifestation of this variability is found in the failure to confirm findings. An example is our intensive longitudinal overnight-monitoring sessions of 25 normal infants between the third trimester of pregnancy and the sixth month of life. The objective of a recent review of these data was to determine whether physiologic variables clustered in such a way that their interrelationship could provide insight into mechanisms operating during postnatal maturation. To that end, respiratory, cardiac, and somatic data during active sleep (AS), quiet sleep (QS), indeterminate (IN), and wakefulness (AW) of all infants were submitted to a computer sort program *(99)*. This set was supplemented with selected state data. Study groups consisted of infants one week, and one, three, and six months of age. Sorting consisted of identification of the 25% of infants who exhibited the highest score in each variable and the 25% who exhibited the lowest score. We will call these outliers. The results constitute rather dramatic proof of the variability indicated above. Pairs of variables consisting of respiratory rate (RR) and variability, RR and HR, HR and somatic activity, and RR and somatic activity, were examined first. Approximately two-thirds of the infants were outliers in one or more of these pairs at each age. Therefore, being an outlier proved to be rather common. But being an outlier once did not mean being one at every age. Only one infant exhibited an extreme value at every age. Ten percent of the infants were extreme in more than three variable pairs simultaneously; and an equal percent, though different infants, scored extremely low in one variable pair but extremely high in another. Sleep-state parameter pairs, such as percent of QS and number of episodes of QS, which theoretically are dependent, also showed a disappointing lack of patterning, an issue discussed in more detail elsewhere *(100)*. Two parameters constituted an exception to this variability. Infants who were outliers with respect to long breathing pauses ($\geq 6$ sec) in

**Table 2–2a** Normative Data*
Respiratory Rate, Variability; Heart Rate, Variability

| Ref | Subjects | Age at Monitoring | Gender | Transducer | Parameter | Method | Monitoring Time/ Duration | Comments |
|---|---|---|---|---|---|---|---|---|
| 63 | 22 fullterm | ≤ 3 days† | 10F; 12M | Strain gauge around lower chest | Mean RR/min | V | Morning sleep 3 hrs | Room temp 30 C |
| 64 | 14 fullterm | ≤ 5 days† | 6F; 8M | Trunk plethysmograph mask | Mean RR | C | Morning sleep NR | Primarily ventilatory study |
| 36 | 10 fullterm 11 SGA 10 preterm + RDS 8 preterm | 42, 52, 64 wks‡ | NR | NR | NR | V | Nighttime sleep 12 hrs | QS respiratory rate |
| 65 | 23 fullterm | 1, 2, 3, 4, 5 wks† | 9F; 14M | Pressure transducer under crib mattress | Mean RR based on 30-sec sample every 2 min R var = mean SD of RR | V | Daytime sleep 3.5 hrs | |

26

| Ref | Subjects | Ages | Sex | Method | Measurement | | Sleep | Temp |
|---|---|---|---|---|---|---|---|---|
| 66 | 8 fullterm | 1 wk, 1, 2, 3, 4, 6 mos† | 5F; 3M | Cannula for expired $CO_2$ | Median RR/min RR var: interquartile range of RR/min | C | Nighttime sleep 12 hrs | Room temp 23–25 C |
| 67 | 25 fullterm | 1 wk, 1, 2, 3, 4, 6 mos† | 9F; 16M | Cannula for expired $CO_2$ | same as ref 66 | | Nighttime sleep 12 hrs | Room temp 22–30 C |
| 68 | 9 preterm<br>14 preterm<br>9 fullterm | 27–33 wks‡<br>34–36 wks<br>37–40 wks | NR | Cannula for expired $CO_2$ | Mean RR/min<br>RR var = fastest to slowest RR | V | Daytime sleep 1 hr | Skin temp 36.5 C |
| 69 | 13 fullterm<br>8 preterm | 1, 10, 20, 30, 40, 50 wks | NR | Impedance pneumography | Mean RR based on 3 min | C | Daytime sleep 1–3 hrs | Room temp 24 C |
| 70 | 17 preterm | 25–34 wks<br>36–40 wks | NR | NR | Modal, minimal and maximal HR intervals | C | NR 3 hrs | |
| 71 | 8 fullterm | 1 wk, 1, 2, 3, 4, 6 mos | 2F; 6M | Bipolar chest leads | Median HR/min HR var: interquartile range | C | Nighttime sleep 12 hrs | Room temp 23–25 C |

27

Table 2-2a—Continued

| Ref | Subjects | Age at Monitoring | Gender | Transducer | Data Analysis Parameter | Method | Monitoring Time/ Duration | Comments |
|---|---|---|---|---|---|---|---|---|
| 67 | see above | see above | | Bipolar chest leads | Mean HR var: (a) SD of HR/min (b) SD of beat-to-beat HR differences | C | see above | |
| 69 | see above | see above | | Bipolar leads midaxillary lines in 3rd–5th intercostal space | Mean RR HR var: SD of HR | C | see above | |
| 72 | 38 preterm | 34 wks† | 20F; 18M | Standard skin electrodes | HR var: (a) difference maximum to minimum from two 2-min windows (b) see ref 74 | V | NR | Skin temp 36.5 C |
|  | 18 preterm mild RDS | 31 wks | 15F; 3M |  |  |  | 6 hrs and 1 hr |  |
|  | 20 preterm severe RDS | 31 wks | 6F; 14M |  |  |  |  |  |
|  | 16 preterm severe RDS expired | 30 wks | 9F; 7M |  |  |  |  |  |

| 73 | 8 fullterm | 2 wks, 1, 2, 3, 4 most† | NR | Surface electrodes | Mean HR var: beat-to-beat HR differences | C | Morning sleep 2 hrs | Study examined relation- ship between HR and HR var |

NOTES for Tables 2–2a through 2–2d:
* Only studies that incorporated states are included.
† Postnatal age.
‡ Conceptional age.
§ International 10–20 System.
C Computer analysis.
V Visual analysis.
F Female.
M Male.
HL Hearing level.
SL Sensation level.
HR Heart rate.
NR Not reported.
RR Respiratory rate.
SD Standard deviation.

RDS Respiratory distress syndrome.
SGA Small for gestational age.
SPR Stimulus presentation rate.
VAR Variability.

**Table 2–2b** Normative Data*
Breathing Pauses

| Ref | Subjects | Age at Monitoring | Gender | Transducer | Nature of Apnea | Analysis Method | Definition of Pause | Monitoring Time/Duration |
|---|---|---|---|---|---|---|---|---|
| 74 | 14 fullterm 15 preterm | 30 wks–3 mos‡ | | Conductive rubber strip | | | 2 apneic periods ≤ 3 sec within 20 sec Apnea ≥ 6 sec | Daytime 2–3 hrs |
| 75 | 8 preterm | 31–35 wks‡ | NR | Nasal thermistor; Cannula for expired $CO_2$ | NR | ∨ | > 10 sec | Daytime 2 hrs |
| 76 | 12 fullterm 15 fullterm | 1 wk 1.5–4.0 mos† | 6F; 6M 6F; 9M | Abdominal, thoracic strain gauges | Central | ∨ | ≥ 2 sec ≥ 5 sec ≥ 10 sec | Daytime 1.5 hrs |
| 65 | 23 fullterm | 1, 2, 3, 4, 5 wks† | 9F; 14M | Pressure transducer under crib | Central | ∨ | ≥ 2 sec | Daytime 3.5 hrs |
| 77 | 28 preterm 4 fullterm | 28–36 wks‡ 1 wk† | NR | Impedance pneumography | Central | ∨ | ≥ 10 sec | Daytime 1.5 hrs |
| 78 | 9 fullterm | 1 wk, 1, 2, 3, 4, 6 mos | 6F; 3M | Cannula for expired $CO_2$ Nasal thermistor Impedance pneumography | Central; periodic breathing | ∨ | ≥ 6 sec 2 central pauses (2–5 sec) within 20 sec | Nighttime 12 hrs |

| 79 | 18 twin sets | 40, 44, 52 wks‡ | 21F; 15M | Nasal thermistor | NR | V | 2–5 sec<br>20 sec<br>2.0–4.9 sec<br>5.0–9.9 sec<br>≥ 10 sec | Daytime 2–4 hrs |
| --- | --- | --- | --- | --- | --- | --- | --- | --- |
| 67 | 19 fullterm | 1 wk, 1, 2, 3, 4, 6 mos | NR | Cannula for $CO_2$<br>Nasal thermistor<br>Impedance pneumography | Central, obstructive, mixed | V | ≥ 6 sec | Nighttime 12 hrs |
| 80 | 32 fullterm | 2–45 wks | 16F; 16M | Impedance pneumography | Periodic breathing | V | Three or more pauses ≥ 3 sec | Nighttime 12 hrs |
| 81 | 30 fullterm | 3, 6 wks<br>3, 4, 5, 6 mos | NR | Abdominal, thoracic strain gauges<br>Nasal, oral thermistors<br>Cannula for expired $CO_2$ | Central, mixed, obstructive; periodic breathing | | 3–6 sec<br>7–10 sec<br>≥ 11 sec<br>two central pauses < 10 sec within 20 sec | 24 hrs |
| 82 | 25 fullterm | 1 wk, 1, 2, 3, 4, 6 mos | | Cannula for expired $CO_2$ | No differentiation | C | 2–5 sec<br>6–9 sec<br>≥ 10 sec | Nighttime 12 hrs |

NOTES: See bottom of Table 2–2a.

*Sleeping and waking disorders: indications and techniques*

**Table 2-2c** Normative Data*
EEG and Evoked Potentials

| Ref | Subjects | Age at Monitoring | Gender | Variables Analyzed | Analysis Method | Monitoring Time/Duration | Comments |
|---|---|---|---|---|---|---|---|
| 15 | 17 preterm 5 SGA 10 fullterm | 30–42 wks‡ 40–42 wks | NR | EEG patterns | V | Nighttime 2.5–3.0 hrs | $Fp_2/T_4$; $Fp_1/T_3$; $Fp_2/C_4$; $Fp_1/C_3$; $T_4/O_2$; $T_3/O_1$; $C_4/O_2$; $C_3/O_1$§ |
| 16 | 59 fullterm 51 preterm | 14 hrs–4 mos | NR | Sleep spindles | V | 1 hr | |
| 17 | 21 fullterm | 2 mos–2.25 yrs† | NR | Spindles 11–14 c/sec | V | Nighttime 1.5 hrs | $F_3/C_3$; $F_4/C_4$ |
| 19 | 19 normal infants | 34 wks–4 yrs† | NR | Spindles | C | NR 2–3 hrs | $Fp_2/C_4$; $Fp_1/C_3$; $C_4/O_2$; $C_3/O_1$; $O_2/T_4$; $O_1/T_3$ |
| 21 | 10 fullterm | 1 wk, 1, 2, 3, 4, 6 mos† | 6F; 4M | Coherence 0–3 c/sec 4–7 c/sec 8–11 c/sec 12–15 c/sec 16–19 c/sec | C | Nighttime 12 hrs | $C_3/T_3$ $C_4/T_4$ Circadian variation |
| 83 | 44 fullterm | 10 days–6 mos† | NR | Spindles 13–14 c/sec | V | Daytime 1.5 hrs | Derivations not reported; descriptive |

| | | | | | | |
|---|---|---|---|---|---|---|
| 84 | 26 normal infants | NR | NR | 8 frequency bands | C | Daytime 1.5–2.0 hrs | Study compares EEG from infants of alcoholic mothers $C_4/A_1$; $C_3/A_2$ |
| 22 | 19 fullterm | 21–70 hrs† | 17F; 2M | Interhemispheric coherence | C | Daytime 1.5–2.5 hrs | $Fp_1/Fp_2$; $C_3$, $C_4$, $T_3$, $T_4$, $O_1$, $O_2$ with reference to ipsilateral earlobe or mastoid |
| 85 | 26 preterm | 31–45 wks‡ | 17F; 9M | EEG patterns | V | 2–3 hrs | $F_4/C_4$; $F_3/C_3$; $C_4/T_4$; $C_3/T_3$; $P_4/O_2$; $P_3/O_1$ |
| 86 | 16 twin sets | 52 wks‡ | 19F; 13M | Spindles | V | 2–4 hrs | $Fp_1/T_3$ |
| 23 | 12 fullterm | 6–12 mos† | 1F; 11M | Auditory-evoked potentials | C | Nighttime 5 hrs | |
| 87 | 35 fullterm | 3 wks–3 yrs† | NR | Auditory-evoked potentials | C | NR | |
| 88 | 24 preterm | 34–42 wks‡ | NR | Auditory-evoked potentials | C | Daytime 1–2 hrs | |

## Table 2-2c—Continued

| Ref | Subjects | Age at Monitoring | Gender | Variables Analyzed | Analysis Method | Monitoring Time/Duration | Comments |
|---|---|---|---|---|---|---|---|
| 24 | 40<br>41<br>40<br>31<br>39<br>27 | 1–3 days†<br>2–4 wks<br>5–7 wks<br>2–4 mos<br>5–7 mos<br>9–15 mos | NR | Auditory-evoked potentials | C | Awake | 55 dB SL 20 μsec clicks; SPR 10/sec, binaurally |
| 25 | 16 | birth–3 yrs† | 5F; 11M | Auditory-evoked potentials | C | Daytime sleep | 100 65 dB SL clicks, binaurally; SPR 0.4/sec |
| 26 | 46 | 3–12 mos† | 21F; 25M | Auditory-evoked potentials | C | Daytime sleep | *see ref 32* |
| 27 | 6 | NR | NR | Auditory-evoked potentials | C | NR | 90 dB HL, monaurally; 100 μsec clicks; SPR 11.1/sec |
| 28 | 120 | 26–42 wks‡ | NR | Auditory-evoked potentials | C | NR | 60 dB; SPR 10/sec, monaurally; threshold testing |

NOTES: See bottom of Table 2–2a.

**Table 2–2d** Normative Data*
tcP$O_2$ and End-Tidal C$O_2$

| Ref | Subjects | Age at Monitoring | Gender | Variables Analyzed | Technique Employed | Monitoring Duration | Comments |
|---|---|---|---|---|---|---|---|
| 89 | 10 fullterm | 15–56 hrs† | NR | tcP$O_2$ Chest wall movement | Radiometer strain gauges | NR | |
| 90 | 10 fullterm 10 preterm | 6 days† 32.3 ± 2.3 wks‡ | 3F; 7M 4F; 6M | tcP$O_2$ | Drager tcP$O_2$ electrode | 3 hrs | |
| 91 | 12 infants | NR | NR | End-tidal C$O_2$ and C$O_2$ response | Nasal pneumotachygraph | NR | Ventilatory study |
| 35 | 10 preterm 10 fullterm | 31 ± 3 wks‡ 40 ± 1 wk | 8F; 2M 3F; 7M | End-tidal C$O_2$ and C$O_2$ response | Nasal pneumotachygraph | NR | Ventilatory study |
| 92 | 12 preterm | 32 ± 1 wk‡ | 8F; 4M | End-tidal C$O_2$ and C$O_2$ response | Nasal catheter Screen-flow meter | 2–3 hrs | Ventilatory study |
| 55 | 14 fullterm | 3–4 mos† | NR | C$O_2$ response | Whole-body plethysmograph | 2 hrs | Ventilatory study |
| 37 | 20 fullterm | 1–10 wks† | NR | Thoracic-abdominal phase relationships | Strain gauges | 3 hrs | |

NOTES: See bottom of Table 2–2a.

three or more states tended to be so in short pauses (2–5 sec). This relationship was previously demonstrated for all infants with the aid of correlation coefficients *(82)* and was also reported by Thoman et al. *(65)*. In conclusion, a search for an elusive maturational pattern or blueprint based on a select number of physiologic variables, although tempting, is thwarted by the extreme variability among and within infants. Although maturational trends can be clearly detected *(67,71,78)*, individuals follow a rather unpredictable course and frustrate our attempts to declare their behavior abnormal. In the case of multiple longitudinal recordings, we must of course compare the infant's physiologic tracings with those from previous and subsequent occasions. Large departures should always evoke careful scrutiny and analysis.

In summary, normative data for a number of variables have been reported in the literature. In general, less information is available for the older infant. Vast differences in objectives, methods, monitoring duration, and analysis techniques must be appreciated, and few variables lend themselves to such scaling as the standard growth curves. Identification of abnormal physiologic behaviors or patterns is further frustrated by the seemingly intrinsic feature of maturation: variability. Few normative studies on tcPO$_2$ have appeared so far. For clinical purposes, 40 torr is frequently used as the cutoff for hypoxemia. The range among normal infants is large, and whether or not infants exhibit levels in the lower range of the distribution may have clinical implications.

## Indications for Monitoring

Extensive longitudinal studies in normal infants as well as in infants at increased statistical risk for SIDS, including approximately 35 near-miss infants, have provided some basic information on respiratory behavior. Breathing pauses of less than 15 seconds in duration are an integral part of normal development. Very short breathing pauses (between 2 and 5 seconds) reflect normal breathing intervals, especially in infants beyond three months of age. Infants at risk exhibited fewer rather than more breathing pauses, accompanied by increased respiratory rates *(67)*. Thoman et al. *(65)* reported relative tachypnea in two infants, one of whom died of SIDS while the other had a near-miss event. We did not find an increased incidence of obstructive apnea or periodic breathing. Data from other investigators differ from our findings. Guilleminault et al. reported an increase in short obstructive apnea in near-miss infants *(81)*, and one infant who subsequently died of SIDS exhibited an increased incidence of obstructive apnea *(101)*. Monod et al. *(76)*, however, found no evidence of increased obstructive apnea in a number of infants who subsequently died. Kelly and Shannon *(80)* reported increased periodic breathing in near-miss infants, a finding not substantiated by our own data or those of Guilleminault et al. *(81)*. These findings are not surprising in light of the differences in techniques, data analyses, location, and length of recording. The true heterogeneity in physiologic findings in near-miss infants, an observation we have previously stressed *(102)*, has been confirmed by subsequent studies *(55)*. Despite these discrepancies, infants with prolonged apnea requiring resuscitation continue to present themselves and constitute a baffling problem for the physician. Polygraphic recording is indicated for these infants, as well as for prematures with prolonged apnea. In the remainder of this section, a workup involving only electronically monitored variables will be proposed. This is based on currently available information. A step-by-step process is diagrammatically presented in Tables 2–3 and 2–4. Additional information about pathogenesis and diagnosis of apnea can be found in Rigatto's report *(103)*. It should be emphasized that such a workup at present can only provide limited information. There is a probability of detecting or ruling out a truly treatable condition, such as a cardiac arrhythmia or seizure disorder. A second objective is to evaluate overall physiologic functioning. Benefits are bound to be more limited in this case, since detection of abnormalities does not necessarily dictate a remedy. Polygraphic recordings of sufficient duration can be analyzed for the presence of eight variables, as outlined in Table 2–3. The absence of each of these abnormal patterns provides the clinician with some assurance that the infant is functioning properly, at least at that point in time. Seizure activity is notoriously difficult to observe, but prolonged recordings increase the chance of detecting subclinical EEG abnormalities, including abnormal slow and spindle activity *(104)*. Evidence of immaturity, e.g., lack of spindle activity, presence of tracé alternant or other immature patterns at an inappropriate age, or a lack of concordance between parameters, in the absence of any other abnormalities,

**Table 2–3**  Physiologic Variables That May Provide Initial Clues to Etiology

| Presenting Sign | | Characteristics |
|---|---|---|
| I | Apnea | > 25 seconds in newborns and prematures |
| | | > 15 seconds in infants ⩾ 1 month |
| II | Bradycardia | Episodes of HR < 90 beats per minute lasting longer than 1 minute |
| III | Tachypnea | Respiratory rates > 2 standard deviations from the mean for the age group |
| IV | Obstruction or excessive disorganized breathing | Multiple episodes lasting in excess of 6 seconds, accompanied by stridor, with or without bradycardia |
| V | Hypoxemia | Episodes of $tcP_{O_2}$ ⩽ 40 torr lasting longer than 2 minutes and not explained by interventions |
| VI | Cardiac arrhythmias | |
| VII | Subclinical or clinical EEG seizure patterns | |
| VIII | Immature EEG and polygraphic patterns | |

suggest that increasing maturity with time will rectify the problems encountered. If, however, findings in one of the seven remaining variables are positive, a further search for etiology can be undertaken (Table 2–4).

Apnea, tachypnea, bradycardia, and hypoxemia can, but need not, occur simultaneously. If multiple prolonged central apnea is present, with or without bradycardia or hypoxemia, a number of tests can be performed. Gastroesophageal reflux and seizures must be ruled out as the etiology of apnea. Ventilatory studies and BAEP may further elucidate the problem. Immaturity in EEG and polygraphic tracings may well accompany the apnea. Bradycardia (with or without hypoxemia) calls for a partially different set of tests. Traces should be examined for the presence of obstructive apnea, disorganized or excessive paradoxical breathing, and cardiac abnormality. Hypotonia observed during a neurologic exam may explain functional obstructions, especially during AS. A BAEP may identify brainstem involvement in abnormal cardiac regulation. Premature infants, especially those who have had respiratory distress syndrome (RDS), continue to breath faster during infancy *(37)*. Tachypnea is also found with fever *(97)*. When these conditions are ruled out, ventilatory studies may elucidate the

**Table 2–4**  Electronic Monitoring in Search of Etiology

| Positive Findings | Further Examinations or Signs |
|---|---|
| Prolonged central apnea with or without bradycardia or hypoxemia | 1) Gastroesophageal reflux<br>2) Seizure<br>3) Immature EEG or polygraphic patterns<br>4) Ventilatory studies: $O_2$ and $CO_2$ response<br>5) BAEP |
| Bradycardia with or without hypoxemia | 1) Multiple short obstructions, disorganized or excessive paradoxical breathing<br>2) Cardiac abnormality<br>3) BAEP |
| Tachypnea | 1) Ventilatory studies<br>2) Immature EEG or polygraphic patterns |
| Prolonged obstructions with or without hypoxemia and bradycardia | 1) Ultrasound determination of pulmonary hypertension<br>2) Disorganized or excessive paradoxical breathing<br>3) Ventilatory studies: mechanical compliance |
| Hypoxemia | 1) Shunt<br>2) Disorganized breathing or excessive paradoxical breathing |

cause of the elevated respiratory rate. Excessive obstructive apnea, with or without hypoxemia, calls for an ultrasound determination of hypoxemic pulmonary hypertension *(105)*. Disorganized or paradoxical breathing may indicate the need to examine mechanical compliance. Again, hypotonia of chest or neck may accompany obstructions. Hypoxemia (< 40 torr) will not commonly occur without either bradycardia or apnea. It can occur as a result of shunts. Simultaneous monitoring of two $tcPO_2$ electrodes has been shown to be useful for detection of vacillating shunts *(44,45)*. Transient hypoxemia, not caused by therapeutic or care practices, and oxygen levels close to the lower normal range may indicate a reduced reserve. Little evidence is presently available, so the incidence and significance of these hypoxemic patterns are matters of conjecture. Finally, cardiac arrhythmias or seizure activities may reveal the need for some specific treatment. Our experience with near-miss infants has thus far not revealed patterns that lend themselves to etiologic diagnosis and unequivocal treatment plans. Only on one occasion have we found good grounds for home monitoring. Thus far we have not performed ventilatory studies. Shannon et al. *(91)* reported abnormal chemoreceptor responses in a number of near-miss infants, consisting of a lack of increase in minute ventilation in response to $CO_2$. Brady et al. *(106)* could not replicate these findings, but they did find altered responses to lowered oxygen in near-miss infants compared to control infants *(107)*. Haddad et al. *(55)* reported that near-miss infants tended to have a larger percentage increase in resting instantaneous minute ventilation ($VT/T_{tot}$) in response to 2% $CO_2$ when compared to normal infants. These authors advanced a number of explanations for the discrepancy between their results and those of Shannon et al. *(91)*: monitoring over a prolonged period of time; use of the barometric method, which avoids facial stimulation known to alter breathing *(98)*; and differences in $CO_2$ percentage. The last factor may be of more importance than thus far appreciated. In observations of infant monkeys during administration of $CO_2$ levels between 0% and 4%, Jacky *(108)* found that sleep-state differences in $CO_2$ response were present with low $FiCO_2$, but disappeared at 4%. This indicates that the evaluation of $CO_2$ responsiveness needs to be performed under conditions that approximate normal $CO_2$ levels during spontaneous sleep and wakefulness. Differential responses of sleep states to mild and severe hypoxia have also been reported *(109)*.

# Monitoring of Sleep and Waking States

Ample evidence indicates that it is desirable to obtain objective measures of both sleeping and waking states in the infant. Virtually every physiologic measure is modulated differently in AS, QS, and AW. These include respiration *(64,66)*, cardiac variables *(71)*, blood gases *(89,90)*, reflexes *(110,111)*, muscle tone *(30, 39)*, and evoked potentials *(24)*. Specification of states in the immature organism meets with various problems of definition. Whereas states in adults are characterized by recurrent constellations of physiologic and behavioral variables that show a relative degree of stability, in the immature organism individual variables demonstrate seemingly independent developmental changes and only gradually begin to give rise to the state concordance observed in the adult. This problem applies in particular to the premature infant *(32,112)* but is also evident in the full term infant between birth and three months of age. Solutions have varied depending on the purpose of each study and the variables available for state determination. Moreover, the duration of monitoring sessions, whether only one age or several ages were examined, and the availability of analytic tools have influenced the selection of state coding criteria.

Prechtl and Beintema *(113)* dealt with this problem by developing a behavioral scale for the newborn infant, which classified state exclusively on the basis of observable behaviors. Each minute of observation was classified into one of five states on the basis of the status of the eyes, respiration, general bodily movements, and vocalization (Table 2–5). Continuous observation is obviously not always possible. Parmelee and Stern *(112)* attempted to compare the state development of premature infants with that of full term infants across an age span of at least eight months. Such a developmental focus required that the same criteria were adhered to at each stage of evaluation. They chose a combination of observable and electronically recorded variables that consisted of eye status, motility, and respiration and eye movement signals. The results of our own studies were based on approximately 400 overnight recordings. The enormous volume of information thus generated dictated our strategy for sleep-state definition. Because reliable, continuous visual observation in long-term overnight recordings was not feasible, polygraphic signals were chosen as the primary state criteria, with observed behaviors used in a supplementary fashion (Table 2–6). Even this strategy will not always be practical in a clinical setting. The optimal choice of variables will be presented below.

Thus far we have examined objectives and indications for monitoring reliability and validity issues, and the availability of normative data. For ongoing surveillance of the neonate, three parameters are of paramount importance: apnea and bradycardia measures must be supplemented with $tcPo_2$ monitoring in order to detect hypoxemia. Diagnostic procedures are better done during a set and limited time period. This raises the next two questions: What is the best time to monitor? How long should the monitoring session last? Some recent information provides tentative answers to these questions.

**Table 2–5** Behavioral States According to Prechtl

| | |
|---|---|
| State 1: | Eyes closed, regular respiration, no gross movements |
| State 2: | Eyes closed, irregular respiration |
| State 3: | Eyes open, no gross movements |
| State 4: | Eyes open, gross movements |
| State 5: | Eyes open or closed, vocalization |

*Electronic monitoring in the newborn and young infant*

**Table 2-6** State Scoring Criteria and Decision-Making Rules for One-Minute Epochs

| Code | Criteria |
| --- | --- |
| AS | Absence of sustained EMG tonus together with three of the following criteria:<br>1. At least one eye movement, independent of chin and gross body movements<br>2. Within a given minute, breathing rate variation is greater than 25 breaths per minute as measured by the respiratory tachometer<br>3. Presence of twitches and brief head movements<br>4. Absence of EEG spindles or tracé alternant |
| QS | All the following criteria must be fulfilled:<br>1. Within a given minute, breathing variation is no greater than 25 breaths per minute as measured by the respiratory tachometer. However, if the variation is due to gross movement, startle, suck, or apnea, the change is disregarded. Also, allow one isolated irregular breath<br>2. No more than one isolated eye movement; eyes closed<br>3. Sustained EMG tonus and/or EEG spindles or tracé alternant |
| AW | Three of the following criteria must be fulfilled:<br>1. Sustained EMG tonus with activity bursts<br>2. Eyes open<br>3. Within a given minute, breathing-rate variation is greater than 45 breaths per minute as measured by the respiratory tachometer<br>4. Vocalization<br>5. Sustained gross movements |
| IN | Minutes in which the criteria for AW, AS, and QS are not fulfilled, or minutes in which these criteria are fulfilled for less than 30 consecutive seconds (state transitions) |

## Time and Length of Monitoring Sessions

Physiologic functioning during nocturnal hours cannot be considered identical to functioning during daytime hours. In adults, a circadian modulation of many autonomic functions, including respiration, has been documented *(114)* with mostly nadirs during the nocturnal portion of the 24-hour day. In infants, a circadian influence upon heart rate, temperature, and urinary sodium and potassium levels was described by Hellbrügge *(115)*. These manifestations appeared between six weeks and three months of age. We recently extended these observations by presenting evidence for the emergence of a circadian influence upon respiratory rates (Figure 2–4, *a, b,* and *c*). In addition, this circadian modulation appeared at one month of age in AS and at three months of age in QS respiratory and cardiac rates (Figure 2–4, *b* and *c* ) *(116)*. Normative values obtained during the night will therefore differ from those during the day from one

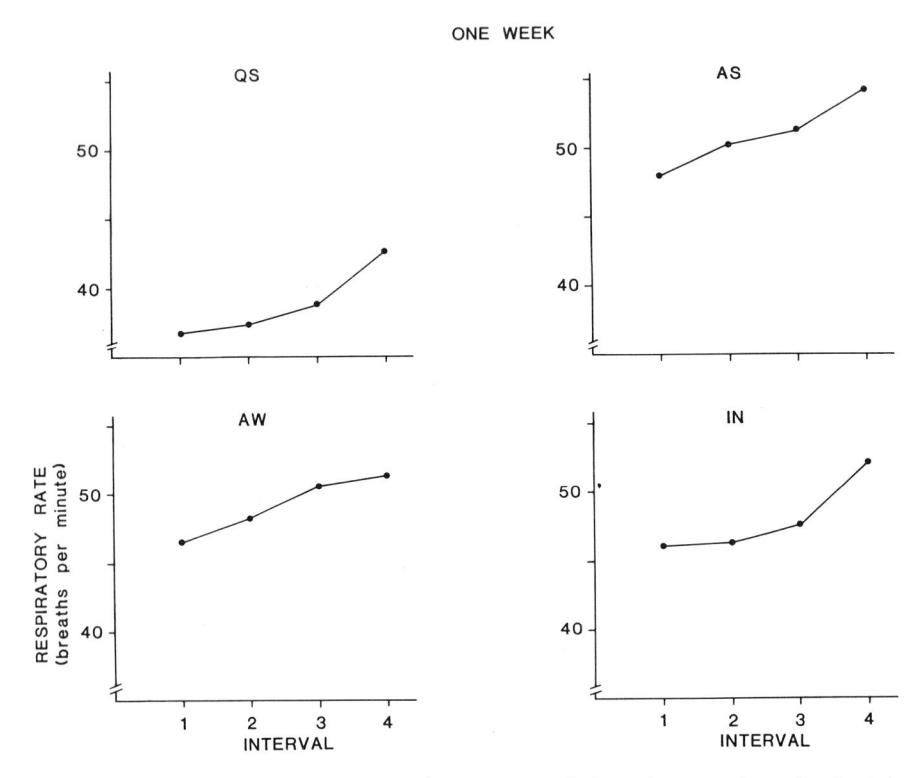

*Sleeping and waking disorders: indications and techniques*

**Figure 2–4a.** Graphs of the mean respiratory rate in breaths per minute (ordinate) as a function of the interval during the night (abscissa). A significant linear increase characterized the respiratory rates across sequential intervals in one-week-old infants. This was true for every state.

month of age on. With respect to premature infants, de Kraker *(117)* obtained evidence suggesting that conceptual rather than postnatal age determines the time of appearance of circadian influences, an observation first made by Hellbrügge *(115)*. In addition to this nonequivalence of daytime and nighttime functioning, two reasons can be advanced for favoring nighttime over daytime monitoring in the infant. First, Tammeling et al. *(118)* found no differences in esophageal pressure in normal healthy adults. Subjects with colds, however, exhibited increased levels during the early morning hours. Abnormal physiologic conditions can apparently transiently reveal circadian influences. Other clinical disease entities also followed a temporal distribution with an elevated incidence in the early morning *(119)*. In the newborn period, the infant exhibits a polyphasic sleep-wakefulness cycle that is gradually replaced by a monophasic pattern of sustained wakefulness during the daytime and sustained sleep through the night *(120)*. Although the newborn infant will sleep a good portion of the 24-hour day, the older infant will

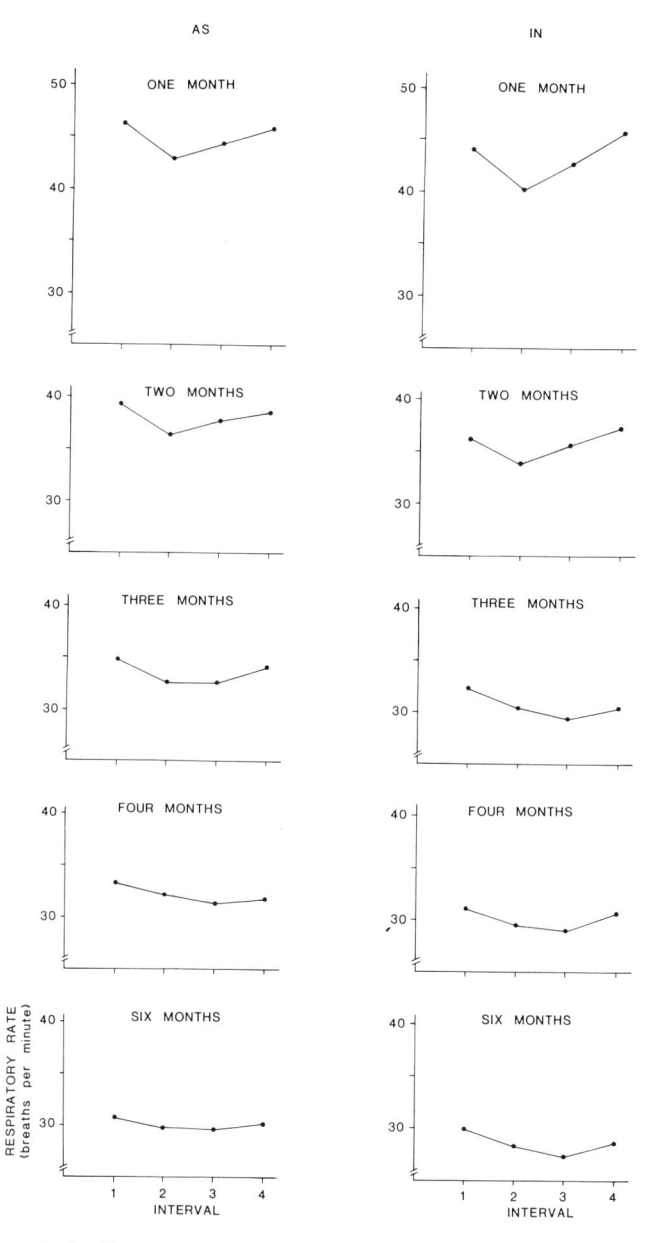

*Electronic monitoring in the newborn and young infant*

**Figure 2–4b.** A significant quadratic trend emerged at one month of age in AS and IN, with a decrease in respiratory rates between approximately 2200 and 0100 hours. Minimum rates were sustained for two intervals at three months of age.

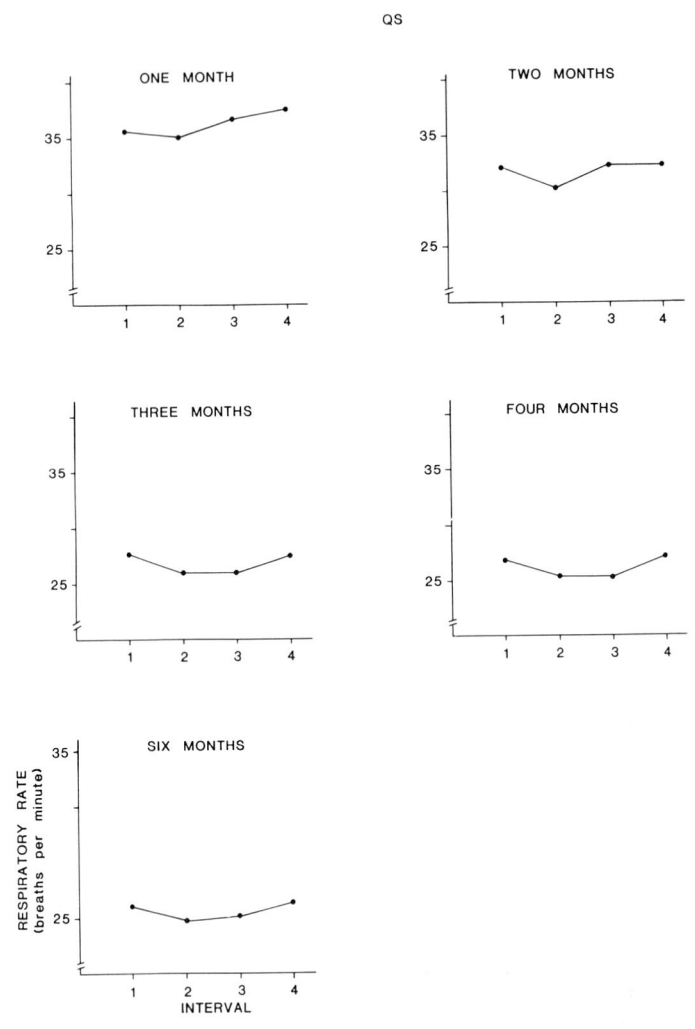

*Sleeping and waking disorders: indications and techniques*

**Figure 2–4c.** Mean respiratory rates in QS across sequential intervals of the night. Note the significant linear increase at one month of age. At three months of age and beyond, respiratory rates declined and remained lower between approximately 2200 and 0400 before increasing again.

simply refuse to sleep except at nighttime and will therefore frustrate our efforts to obtain a good sample of both AS and QS. What is a good sample of both AS and QS? Figures 2–5 and 2–6 are plots of all-night laboratory sleep recordings. Figure 2–5 shows both the worst and the best sleepers, judged primarily by number and length of awakenings. Figure 2–6 represents normal laboratory sleep as exhibited by the majority of infants. The variability discussed previously is quite obvious. Infants were fed on a demand schedule and the number of awakenings for feedings varied greatly among and within infants across ages. As can be seen, eight AS-QS cycles were not uncommon. Sleep latency varied among infants and was not systematically studied. The effect of recording length was examined in the case of apnea. Apnea densities were greatly reduced if they were only based on the first two hours of monitoring, compared to the entire night *(82)*. Since respiratory rate declined between 2200 and 0200 *(116)*, and respiratory rates were correlated with short apnea *(82)*, this finding is entirely expected and in agreement with observations made by Guilleminault et al. *(121)*.

Therefore, variables purporting to measure CNS integrity as well as ventilatory and cardiac measures, if obtained between 2200 and 0200, will be representative of a nadir of functioning, whereas measures obtained prior to 2200 and after 0200 will be more representative of functioning during daytime sleep. Both estimates are necessary for a complete description of infant functioning. In addition, the duration of recording affects apnea counts. Nighttime monitoring sessions of at least five hours will therefore allow sampling of nadirs and peaks of functioning. An average of at least four AS-QS cycles can be expected. The longer the session is extended, the higher the probability that such anomalies as nocturnal seizures will be detected. In the older infant, this is likely to be the only time such estimates can be obtained. Finally, in most hospitals there is less commotion around the crib at night, so conditions are more favorable for obtaining valid and reliable measurements.

## Infant Observation

Electronic monitoring cannot substitute for frequent observation of the infant. At the beginning of a monitoring session, we need to assure ourselves that signals reliably represent the infant's behavior. During the session, repeated close inspection of the infant and the polygraphic record is essential to interpret the signals and aid in the state scoring. Interesting or deviant-looking patterns need to be reliably discriminated from artifacts in the tracings. Transducers and electrodes must be checked periodically. The infant's color, posture, and breathing sounds must be noted, as well as interventions for feeding or treatment. Episodes of crying or gross body movements can dislodge the electrodes. Finally, other infant needs, such as those for warmth and contact comfort, must be detected and satisfied.

# Summary and Conclusion

Can some useful suggestions be offered to prevent redundancy and to keep the variables to a minimum without losing our ability to gain essential information? Three guidelines may be helpful in the clinical setting. (In a purely research setting, decisions will be based on other factors.) First, under some conditions it may be desirable to be able to

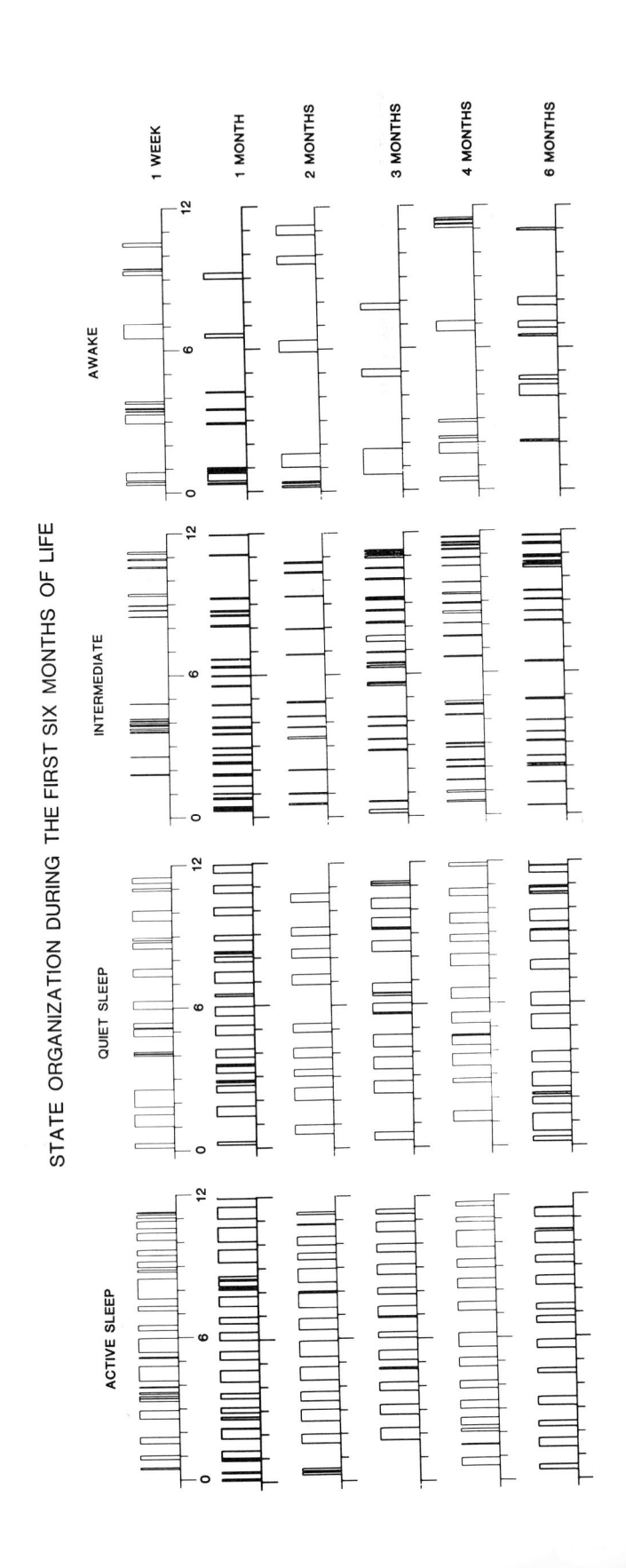

STATE ORGANIZATION DURING THE FIRST SIX MONTHS OF LIFE

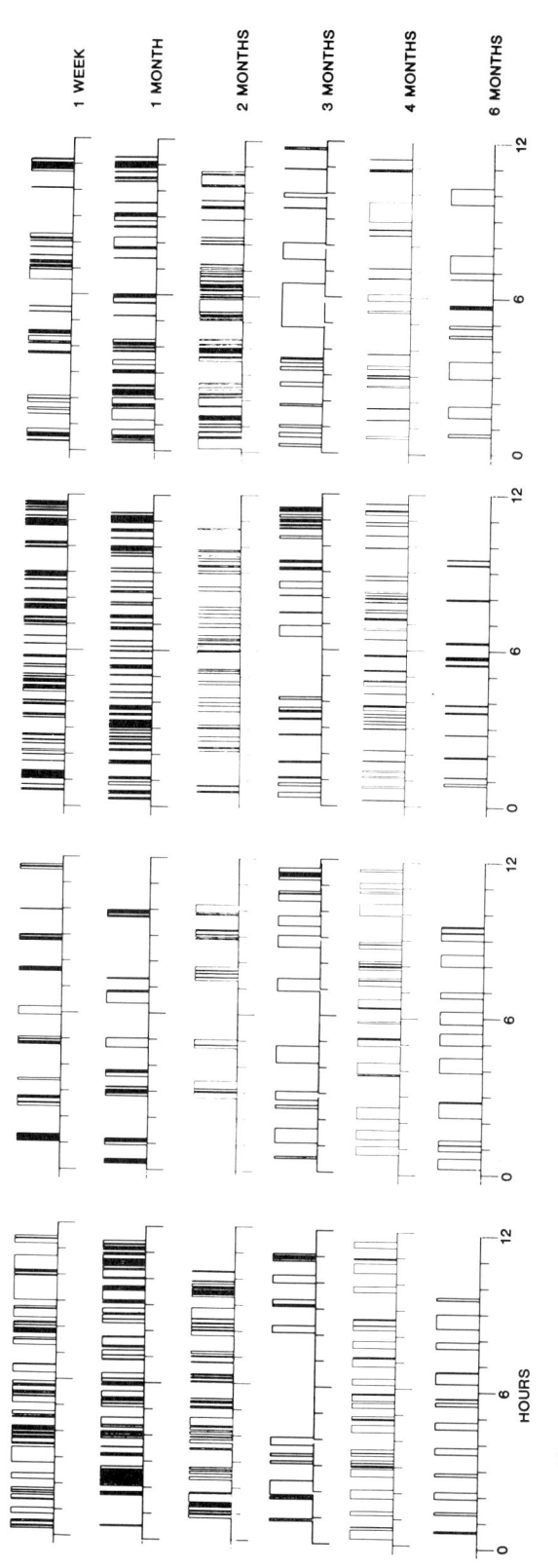

**Figure 2–5.** Computer state plots derived from 12-hour polygraphic recordings between one and six months of age. The top six tracings were selected from the 25% "best" sleepers as judged by the number of awakenings and the time awake. The bottom six tracings represent the "worst" sleepers. Note how poor sleep tends to affect cyclicity of AS and QS during the first three months of life, but to a lesser extent in older infants.

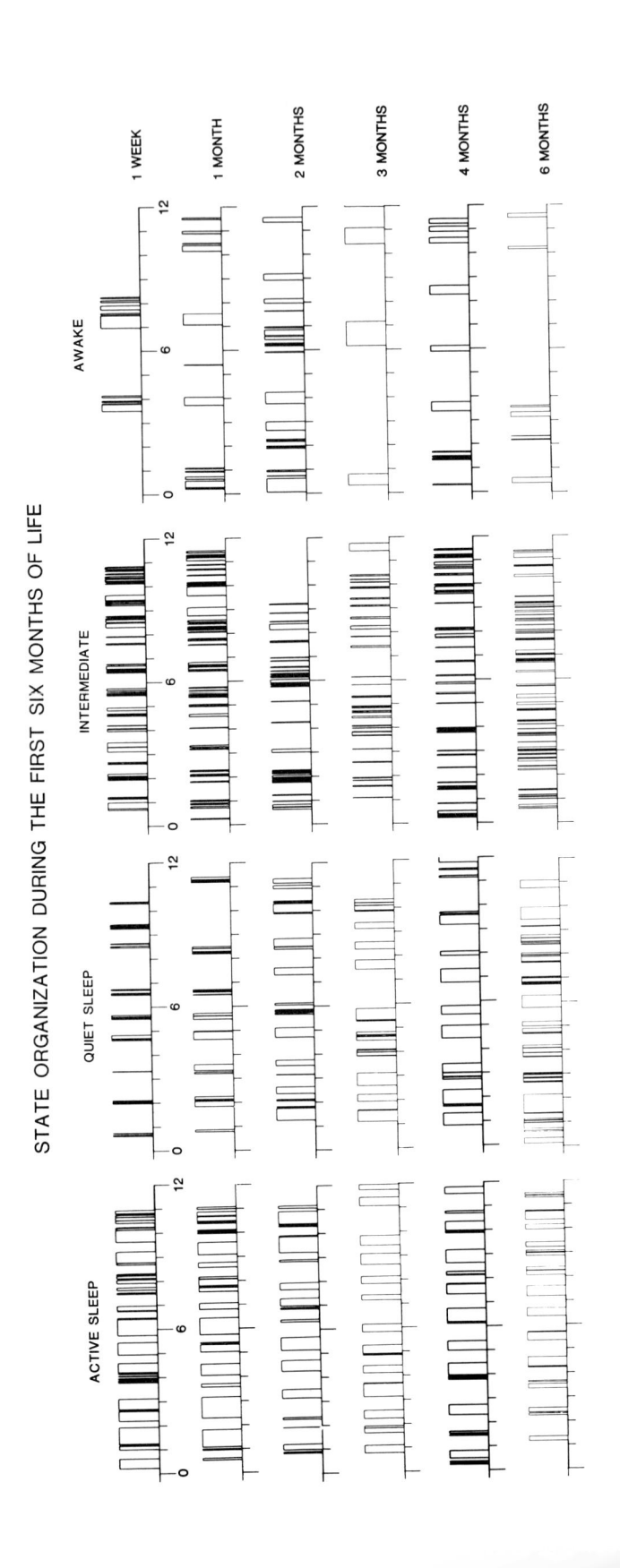

STATE ORGANIZATION DURING THE FIRST SIX MONTHS OF LIFE

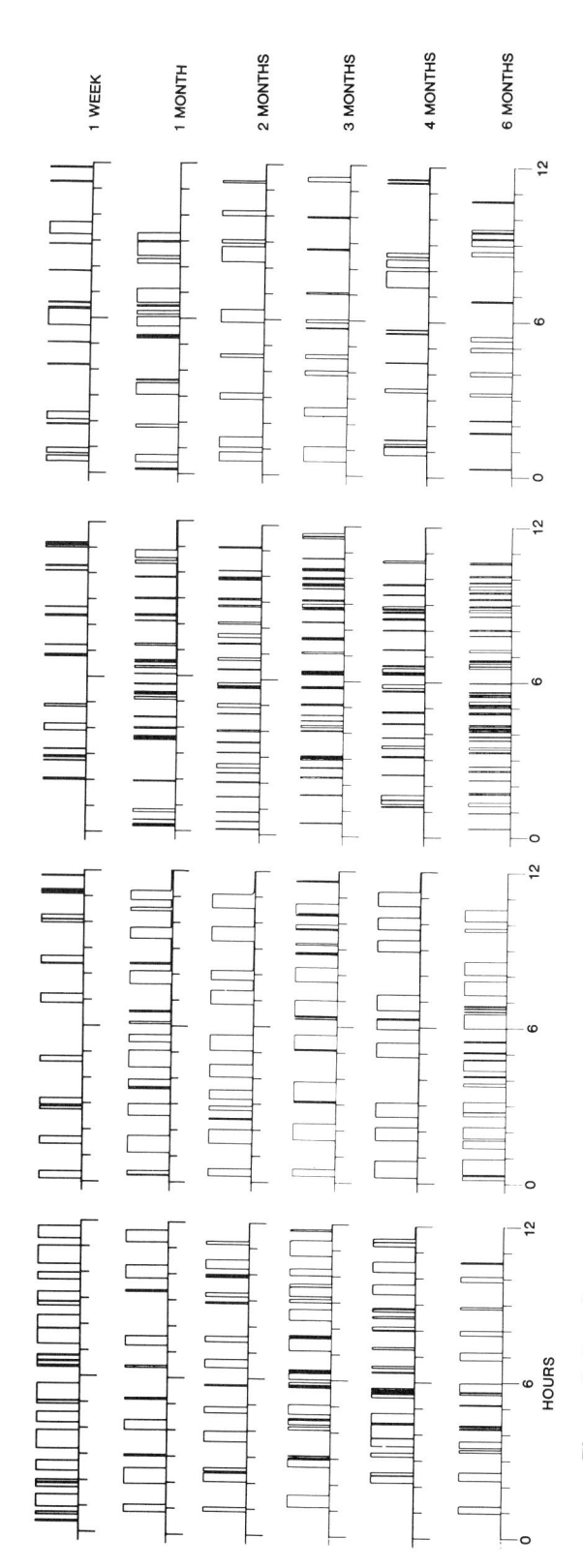

**Figure 2-6.** Computer state plots from infants between one week and six months of age. These traces represent the average sleep-state organization. Although more wakefulness characterized the recordings of the bottom six infants during the first three months of life, their QS cycles appeared more mature than those of the top six infants.

code every minute of a recording into either AW, QS, AS, or IN. In that case, all criteria outlined in Tables 2–5 and 2–6 are essential, For clinical purposes, the identification of several sustained and unequivocal episodes of QS and AS is often sufficient. This can be accomplished by monitoring three variables. First, respiratory regularity, preferably as measured by a well-functioning respiratory tachometer, will under most circumstances (except tachypnea) quite accurately identify episodes of QS. The addition of a somatic activity sensor under the mattress helps to discriminate between AW and AS, whereas cardiac rate (in particular, tachycardia) can provide additional information. An eye-movement sensor may be necessary to differentiate episodes of AS from both AW and QS in the premature infant with tachypnea and periodic breathing. Second, some parameters do display a rather strong correlation. Short, medium, and long apnea, as well as AS and QS apnea, constitute such an example. Respiratory rates also show a significant correlation with short and medium apnea. Identification of short apnea (2–5 seconds) is frequently unreliable (especially in QS), costly, and unnecessary, given the strong correlation with other respiratory events. In the older infant (beyond two months of age), these short pauses become identical to normal respiratory intervals. Therefore, the judicious choice of variables for analysis can produce savings. A third and last issue becomes crucial here. Are there alternate and cheaper ways to gather the same information? I was once asked to monitor an infant whose polygraphic pattern exhibited a remarkable lack of concordance between variables. In that respect she resembled the physiologic behavior of a thalamic cat. Although this constituted an interesting theoretical observation, a light against the skull had already told the physician the extent of her brain abnormality, a hydrocephaly. Surely this was a fast, cheap, and accurate diagnosis to which the polygraphic recording did not add significant clinical detail.

The general objectives of surveillance, diagnosis, treatment, and evaluation of the efficacy of treatment plans must influence the choice of monitored parameters. In the neonate, including the premature infant, measuring tcPo$_2$ is essential to determining the clinical significance of apnea and bradycardia and to detecting and treating hypoxemia. This combination is likely to be profitable for ongoing surveillance. Selection of variables for clinical diagnostic purposes will be partially determined by the availability of normative data for each age group. Because of the variable development of a number of parameters, values at one age cannot be conveniently extrapolated from those at other ages (66). Simultaneous monitoring of sleep and waking states will reduce the variance of the data and aid interpretation. A nighttime recording session lasting at least five to six hours will contribute to a complete assessment of functioning, further reduce the variance in the data, and optimize the probability of detecting physiologic anomalies.

---

Research reported here was funded by NICHD Contracts Nos. N01-HD-2-2777 and HD-4-2810, and Grant No. 1 R01-HD-13689-01. I wish to thank Dr. J. E. Hodgman for her continuous support and her valuable contribution. I thank Mrs. Helen Dosik for her editorial advice.

# REFERENCES

1. Cabal LA, Goldberg RN, Hodgman JE, Siassi B, Plajstek CE. A primer of neonatal intensive care monitoring. Book I: Neonatal heart rate. New Haven, Connecticut: William J Mack Co, 1977.
2. Huch A, Huch R, Lübbers DW. Quantitative polarographische Sauerstoffdruckmessung auf der Kopfhaut des Neugeborenen. Arch Gynaekol 1969; 207:443–51.
3. Peabody JL, Neese AL, Philip AGS, Lucey JF, Soyka LF. Transcutaneous oxygen monitoring in aminophylline-treated apneic infants. Pediatrics 1978; 62:698–701.
4. Bucher H, Arbenz U, Bucher A. tcPO$_2$ in pediatric cardiology: Application during balloon septostomy, tolazoline administration, and in children with right-to-left shunt. In: Huch A, Huch R, Lucey JF, eds. Continuous transcutaneous blood gas monitoring. Birth defects: original article series, Volume XV, Number 4. New York: Alan R Liss, Inc, 1979:355–63.
5. Dangman B, Indyk L, Hegyi T, Hiatt IM, Caceres F, James LS. The variability of PO$_2$ in newborn infants in response to routine care. In: Rooth G, Bratteby L, eds. Proceedings of the 5th European Conference on Perinatal Medicine. Stockholm: Almqvist and Wiksell, 1976:137–40.
6. Rice RD. The effects of the Rice infant sensorimotor stimulation treatment on the development of high-risk infants. In: Anderson GC, Raff B, eds. Birth defects: original article series, Volume XV, Number 7. New York: Alan R Liss, Inc, 1979:7–26.
7. Kattwinkel J, Nearman JS, Fanaroff AA, Katona PG, Klaus MH. Apnea of prematurity. J Pediatr 1975; 86:588–92.
8. Kennell JH, Jerauld R, Wolfe H, et al. Maternal behavior one year after early and extended postpartum contact. Dev Med Child Neurol 1974; 16:172–9.
9. Lambesis CC, Vidyasagar D, Anderson GC. Effects of surrogate mothering on physiologic stabilization in transitional newborns. In: Anderson GC, Raff B, eds. Birth defects: original article series, Volume XV, Number 7. New York: Alan R Liss, Inc, 1979:201–23.
10. Lucey JF, Peabody JL, Philip AGS. Recurrent undetected hypoxia and hyperoxia, a newly recognized iatrogenic problem of "intensive care." In: Schmidt E, Dudenhausen GW, Saling E, eds. Perinatale Medizin. Stuttgart: Thieme, 1978:524–7.
11. Pörksen C, Larsen H, Hürter P. Evaluation of tcPO$_2$, beat-to-beat heart rate and respiration in neonates with episodes of cyanosis, bradycardia, or apnea. In: Huch A, Huch R, Lucey JF, eds. Continuous transcutaneous blood gas monitoring. Birth defects: original article series, Volume XV, Number 4. New York: Alan R Liss, Inc, 1979:447–59.

12. Bödefeld E, Schachinger H, Huch A, Huch R, Lucey JF. Continuous tcPO$_2$ monitoring in healthy and sick newborn infants during and after feeding. In: Huch A, Huch R, Lucey JF, eds. Continuous transcutaneous blood gas monitoring. Birth defects: original article series, Volume XV, Number 4. New York: Alan R Liss, Inc, 1979:503–8.
13. Hohenauer L. Transcutaneous monitoring of PO$_2$ (tcPO$_2$) in sick newborn babies: three years of clinical experience. In: Huch A, Huch R, Lucey JF, eds. Continuous transcutaneous blood gas monitoring. Birth defects: original article series, Volume XV, Number 4. New York: Alan R Liss, Inc, 1979:375–6.
14. Peabody JL, Willis MM, Gregory GA, Severinghaus JW. Reliability of skin (tc)PO$_2$ electrode heating power as a continuous noninvasive monitor of mean arterial pressure in sick newborns. In: Huch A, Huch R, Lucey JF, eds. Continuous transcutaneous blood gas monitoring. Birth defects: original article series, Volume XV, Number 4. New York: Alan R Liss, Inc, 1979: 127–33.
15. Dreyfus-Brisac C, Fischgold H, Samson-Dollfus D, Saint-Anne-Dargassies S, Monod N, Blanc C. Veille, sommeil, réactivité sensorielle chez le prématuré, le nouveau-né et le nourrisson. Electroencephalogr Clin Neurophysiol 1956; [Suppl 6] 417–40.
16. Parmelee AH Jr, Schulte FJ, Akiyama Y, Wenner WH, Schultz MA, Stern E. Maturation of EEG activity during sleep in premature infants. Electroencephalogr Clin Neurophysiol 1968; 24:319–29.
17. Metcalf DR. The effect of extrauterine experience on the ontogenesis of EEG sleep spindles. Psychosom Med 1969; 31:393–9.
18. Lenard HG. The development of sleep spindles in the EEG during the first two years of life. Neuropaediatrie 1970; 1:264–76.
19. Lenard H, Schulte F. Sleep studies in hormonal and metabolic diseases of infancy and childhood. In: Petre-Quadens O, Schlag JB, eds. Basic sleep mechanisms. New York: Academic Press, 1974:381–403.
20. Schulte FJ, Bell EF. Bioelectric brain development, an atlas of EEG power spectra in infants and young children. Neuropaediatrie 1973; 4:30–45.
21. Haas GH, Prechtl HFR. Normal and abnormal EEG maturation in newborn infants. Early Hum Dev 1977; 1:69–90.
22. Sterman MB, Harper RM, Havens B, Hoppenbrouwers T, McGinty DJ, Hodgman JE. Quantitative analysis of infant EEG development during quiet sleep. Electroencephalogr Clin Neurophysiol 1977; 43:371–85.
23. Varner JL, Peters JF, Ellingson RJ. Interhemispheric synchrony in the EEGs of full-term newborns. Electroencephalogr Clin Neurophysiol 1978; 45:641–7.
24. Ornitz EM, Ritvo ER, Lee YH, Panman LM, Walter RD, Mason A. The auditory evoked response in babies during REM sleep. Electroencephalogr Clin Neurophysiol 1969; 27:195–8.

25. Salamy A, Fenn CB, Bronshvag M. Ontogenesis of human brainstem evoked potential amplitude. Dev Psychobiol 1979; 12:519–26.
26. Ohlrich ES, Barnet AB, Weiss IP, Shanks BL. Auditory evoked potential development in early childhood: a longitudinal study. Electroencephalogr Clin Neurophysiol 1978; 44:411–23.
27. Barnet AB, Weiss IP, Sotillo MV, Ohlrich ES, Shkurovich ZM, Cravioto J. Abnormal auditory evoked potentials in early infancy malnutrition. Science 1978; 201:450–1.
28. Orlowski JP, Nodar RH, Lonsdale D. Abnormal brainstem auditory evoked potentials in infants with threatened sudden infant death syndrome. Cleve Clin Q 1979; 46:77–81.
29. Despland PA, Galambos R. Use of the auditory brainstem responses by prematures and newborn infants. Neuropaediatrie 1980; 11:99–107.
30. O'Brien MJ, van Eykern LA, Prechtl HFR. Diaphragmatic, intercostal and abdominal muscle tonic EMG activity in normal and hypotonic newborns. In: Ontogenesis of the brain. Proceedings of the International Symposium Neuroontogeneticumterium. Charles University, 1979, Volume 3.
31. Dreyfus-Brisac C. The electroencephalogram of the premature infant and full-term newborn: normal and abnormal development of waking and sleeping patterns. In: Kellaway P, Peterson I, eds. Neurological and electroencephalographic correlative studies in infants. New York: Grune and Stratton, 1964:186–207.
32. Parmelee AH, Schulte FJ, Akiyama Y, Wenner WH, Schultz MA, Stern E. Maturation of EEG activity during sleep in premature infants. Electroencephalogr Clin Neurophysiol 1968; 24:319–29.
33. Cabal LA, Devaskar V, Siassi B, Hodgman JE, Emmanouilides G. Cardiogenic shock associated with perinatal asphyxia in preterm infants. J Pediatr 1980; 97:705–10.
34. Minton SD, Herbst JJ, Book LS. Respiratory changes induced by gastroesophageal reflux (GER). Clin Res 1979; 27:127A.
35. Fenner A, Schalk V, Hoenicke H, Wendenburg A, Roehling T. Periodic breathing in premature and neonatal babies: incidence, breathing pattern, respiratory gas tensions, response to changes in the composition of ambient air. Pediatr Res 1973; 7:174–83.
36. Davi M, Sankaran K, MacCallum M, Cates D, Rigatto H. Effect of sleep state on chest distortion and on the ventilatory response to $CO_2$ in neonates. Pediatr Res 1979; 13:982–6.
37. Dittrichová J, Paul K. Respiratory rate during quiet sleep in high-risk infants during the first six months of life. In: Levin P, Koella W, eds. Sleep 1974: Second European Congress on Sleep Research, Rome 1974. Basel: Karger, 1975.
38. Curzi-Dascalova L. Thoracico-abdominal respiratory correlations in infants: constancy and variability in different sleep states. Early Hum Dev 1978; 2:25–38.

39. Prechtl HFR, O'Brien MJ, van Eykern LA. Neonatal breathing in different states of sleep and wakefulness. In: von Euler C, Lagercrantz H, eds. Central nervous control mechanisms in breathing. Elmsford, New York: Pergamon Press, 1979:443–55.
40. Peabody JL, Philip AGS, Lucey JF. 'Disorganized breathing'—an important form of apnea and cause of hypoxia. Pediatr Res 1977; 11:540.
41. Huch R, Fallenstein F, Seiler D, Lübbers D, Huch A. tcPo$_2$—state of development. In: Huch A, Huch R, Lucey JF, eds. Continuous transcutaneous blood gas monitoring. Birth defects: original article series, Volume XV, Number 4. New York: Alan R Liss, Inc, 1979:413–9.
42. Stothers JK, Warner RM. Oxygen consumption and sleep state in the newborn. J Physiol 1977; 269:57P–58P.
43. Stabell U, Junge M, Fenner A. Metabolic rate and O$_2$ consumption in newborns during different states of vigilance. Biol Neonate 1977; 31:27–31.
44. de Geeter B, Messer J, Benoit M, Willard D. Right-to-left shunt and transcutaneous Po$_2$. In: Huch A, Huch R, Lucey JF, eds. Continuous transcutaneous blood gas monitoring. Birth defects: original article series, Volume XV, Number 4. New York: Alan R Liss, Inc, 1979:387–92.
45. Yamanouchi I, Igarashi I. Ductal shunt in premature infants observed by tcPo$_2$ measurements. In: Huch A, Huch R, Lucey JF, eds. Continuous transcutaneous blood gas monitoring. Birth defects: original article series, Volume XV, Number 4. New York: Alan R Liss, Inc, 1979:323–40.
46. Rooth G. Transcutaneous oxygen tension measurements in newborn infants. Pediatrics 1975; 55:232–5.
47. Huch R, Huch A, Bucher HU. Experience with the oxygen-cardiorespirogram in newborn infants. Presented at the 5th European Congress of Perinatal Medicine, Uppsala, Sweden, June 9–12, 1976.
48. Huch R, Lübbers DW, Huch A. Reliability of transcutaneous monitoring of arterial Po$_2$ in newborn infants. Arch Dis Child 1974; 49:213.
49. Versmold HT, Linderkamp O, Holzmann M, Strohhacker I, Riegel K. Transcutaneous monitoring of Po$_2$ in newborn infants: Where are the limits? Influence of blood pressure, blood volume, blood flow, viscosity, and acid base state. In: Huch A, Huch R, Lucey JF, eds. Continuous transcutaneous blood gas monitoring. Birth defects: original article series, Volume XV, Number 4. New York: Alan R Liss, Inc, 1979:285–94.
50. Bellée H, Schwarze R, Schönjahn V, Krause W. Continuous determination of oxygen partial pressure in the field of neonatology. In: Huch A, Huch R, Lucey JF, eds. Continuous transcutaneous blood gas monitoring. Birth defects: original article series, Volume XV, Number 4. New York: Alan R Liss, Inc, 1979:407–9.
51. Leraillez J, Iannascoli F, Brioude R, Canet J. Cutaneous Po$_2$: value of analysis of the tracings of neonatal cardiorespiratory pathology. In: Huch

A, Huch R, Lucey JF, eds. Continuous transcutaneous blood gas monitoring. Birth defects: original article series, Volume XV, Number 4. New York: Alan R Liss, Inc, 1979:399–406.
52. Bompard Y, Beaufils F, Azancot A, Asensi D. Continuous transcutaneous Po$_2$ monitoring in vital distress of children. In: Huch A, Huch R, Lucey JF, eds. Continuous transcutaneous blood gas monitoring. Birth defects: original article series, Volume XV, Number 4. New York: Alan R Liss, Inc, 1979:383–6.
53. Hoppenbrouwers T. Personal observation.
54. Duc G, Frei H, Klar H, Tuchschmid P. Reliability of continuous transcutaneous Po$_2$ (Hellige) in respiratory distress syndrome of the newborn. In: Huch A, Huch R, Lucey JF, eds. Continuous transcutaneous blood gas monitoring. Birth defects: original article series, Volume XV, Number 4. New York: Alan R Liss, Inc, 1979:305–13.
55. Haddad GG, Leistner HL, Lai TL, Mellins RB. Ventilation and ventilatory pattern during sleep in aborted sudden infant death syndrome. Pediatr Res 1981; 15:879–83.
56. Sorkin B, Rapoport DM, Falk DB, Goldring RM. Canopy ventilation monitor for quantitative measurement of ventilation during sleep. J Appl Physiol 1980; 48:724–30.
57. Cabal LS. Personal communication.
58. Epstein RA, Reznik AM, Epstein MAF. Determinants of distortions in CO$_2$ catheter sampling systems: a mathematical model. Respir Physiol 1980; 41:127–36.
59. Ellingson RJ. Electroencephalograms of normal, full term newborns immediately after birth with observations on arousal and visual evoked responses. Electroencephalogr Clin Neurophysiol 1958; 10:31–50.
60. Stockard J, Sharbrough F. Non-pathologic factors influencing brainstem auditory evoked potentials. Am J EEG Technol 1978; 18:172–209.
61. Ellingson RJ, Danahy T, Nelson B, Lathrop G. Variability of auditory evoked potentials in human newborns. Electroencephalogr Clin Neurophysiol 1974; 36:155–62.
62. Monod N, Guidasci S. Sleep and brain malformation in the neonatal period. Neuropaediatrie 1976; 7:229–49.
63. Ashton R, Connolly K. The relation of respiration rate and heart rate to sleep states in the human newborn. Dev Med Child Neurol 1971; 13:180–7.
64. Bolton DPG, Herman S. Ventilation and sleep state in the new-born. J Physiol 1974; 240:67–77.
65. Thoman EB, Miano VN, Freese MP. The rôle of respiratory instability in the sudden infant death syndrome. Dev Med Child Neurol 1977; 19:729–38.
66. Hoppenbrouwers T, Harper RM, Hodgman JE, Sterman MB, McGinty

DJ. Polygraphic studies of normal infants during the first six months of life. II. Respiratory rate and variability as a function of state. Pediatr Res 1978; 12:120–5.
67. Hoppenbrouwers T, Hodgman JE, McGinty D, Harper RM, Sterman MB. Sudden infant death syndrome: sleep apnea and respiration in subsequent siblings. Pediatrics 1980; 66:205–14.
68. Siassi B, Hodgman JE, Cabal L, Hon E. Cardiac and respiratory activity in relation to gestation and sleep states in newborn infants. Pediatr Res 1979; 13:1163–6.
69. Katona PG, Frasz A, Egbert J. Maturation of cardiac control in full-term and preterm infants during sleep. Early Hum Dev 1980; 4:145–59.
70. Watanabe K, Iwase K, Hara K. Heart rate variability during sleep and wakefulness in low-birthweight infants. Biol Neonate 1973; 22:87–98.
71. Harper RM, Hoppenbrouwers T, Sterman MB, McGinty DJ, Hodgman J. Polygraphic studies of normal infants during the first six months of life. I. Heart rate and variability as a function of state. Pediatr Res 1976; 10:945–51.
72. Cabal LA, Siassi B, Zanini B, Hodgman JE, Hon E. Factors affecting heart rate variability in preterm infants. Pediatrics 1980; 65:50–6.
73. Mazza NM, Epstein MAF, Haddad GG, Law HS, Mellins RB, Epstein RA. Relation of beat to beat variability to heart rate in normal sleeping infants. Pediatr Res 1980; 14:232–5.
74. Parmelee AH, Stern E, Harris MA. Maturation of respiration in prematures and young infants. Neuropaediatrie 1972; 3:294–304.
75. Gabriel M, Albani M, Schulte FJ. Apneic spells and sleep states in preterm infants. Pediatrics 1976; 57:142–7.
76. Monod N, Curzi-Dascalova L, Guidasci S, Valenzuela S. Pauses respiratoires et sommeil chez le nouveau-né et le nourrisson. Rev Electroencephalogr Neurophysiol Clin 1976; 6:105–10.
77. Krauss AN, Solomon GE, Auld PAM. Sleep state, apnea and bradycardia in pre-term infants. Dev Med Child Neurol 1977; 19:160–8.
78. Hoppenbrouwers T, Hodgman JE, Harper RM, Hofmann E, Sterman MB, McGinty DJ. Polygraphic studies of normal infants during the first six months of life. III. Incidence of apnea and periodic breathing. Pediatrics 1977; 60:418–25.
79. Gould JB, Lee AFS, James O, Sander L, Teager H, Fineberg N. The sleep state characteristics of apnea during infancy. Pediatrics 1976; 59:182–94.
80. Kelly DH, Shannon DC. Periodic breathing in infants with near-miss sudden infant death syndrome. Pediatrics 1979; 63:355–8.
81. Guilleminault C, Ariagno R, Korobkin R, et al. Mixed and obstructive sleep apnea and near miss for sudden infant death syndrome. 2. Comparison of near miss and normal control infants by age. Pediatrics 1979; 64:882–91.
82. Hoppenbrouwers T, Hodgman JE, Arakawa K, Harper R, Sterman MB.

Respiration during the first six months of life in normal infants. III. Computer identification of breathing pauses. Pediatr Res 1980; 14:1230–3.
83. Curzi-Dascalova L. E.E.G. de veille et de sommeil du nourrisson normal avant 6 mois d'age. Rev Electroencephalogr Neurophysiol Clin 1977; 7:316–26.
84. Havlicek V, Childiaeva R, Chernick V. EEG frequency spectrum characteristics of sleep states in infants of alcoholic mothers. Neuropaediatrie 1977; 8:360–73.
85. Nolte R, Haas G. A polygraphic study of bioelectrical brain maturation in preterm infants. Dev Med Child Neurol 1978; 20:167–82.
86. Wu H, Gould JB, Lee AFS, Fineberg N. Factors affecting sleep spindle activity during infancy. Dev Med Child Neurol 1980; 22:344–51.
87. Hecox K, Galambos R. Brain stem auditory evoked responses in human infants and adults. Arch Otolaryngol 1974; 99:30–3.
88. Schulman-Galambos C, Galambos R. Brain stem auditory-evoked responses in premature infants. J Speech Hear Res 1975; 18:456–65.
89. Martin RJ, Okken A, Ruben D. Arterial oxygen tension during active and quiet sleep in the normal neonate. J Pediatr 1979; 64:271–4.
90. Hanson N, Okken A. Transcutaneous oxygen tension of newborn infants in different behavioral states. Pediatr Res 1980; 14:911–5.
91. Shannon DC, Kelly DH, O'Connell K. Abnormal regulation of ventilation in infants at risk for sudden-infant-death syndrome. N Engl J Med 1977; 297:747–50.
92. Rigatto H, Kalapesi Z, Leahy FN, Durand M, MacCallum M, Cates D. Chemical control of respiratory frequency and tidal volume during sleep in preterm infants. Respir Physiol 1980; 41:117–25.
93. Dahl M, Välimäki I. Postural effect on respiration and heart rate of newborn infants: an impedance pneumographic study. Biol Neonate 1972; 20:161–9.
94. Hutchinson AA, Ross KR, Russell G. The effect of posture on ventilation and lung mechanics in preterm and light-for-date infants. Pediatrics 1979; 64:429–32.
95. Thoman EB, Freese MP, Becker PT, Acebo C, Morin VN, Tynan WD. Sex differences in the ontogeny of sleep apnea during the first year of life. Physiol Behav 1978; 20:699–707.
96. Hoppenbrouwers T, Hodgman JE, Harper RM, Sterman MB. Respiration during the first six months of life in normal infants. IV. Gender differences. Early Hum Dev 1980; 4:167–77.
97. Avery ME, Fletcher BD. The lung and its disorders in the newborn infant. 3rd ed. Philadelphia: WB Saunders, 1974.
98. Askanazi J, Silverberg PA, Foster RJ, Hyman AI, Milic-Emili J, Kinney JM. Effects of respiratory apparatus on breathing pattern. J Appl Physiol 1980; 48:577–80.
99. SAS User's Guide, Statistical Analysis System. SAS Institute, Inc, 1979.

100. Hoppenbrouwers T. Infant state development. In: Hodgman JE, Sterman MB, Hoffman H, Stark R, eds. Ontogeny of sleep in cardiopulmonary regulation: factors related to risk for the sudden infant death syndrome. In press.
101. Guilleminault C, Ariagno RL, Forno LS, Nagel L, Baldwin R, Owen M. Obstructive sleep apnea and near miss for SIDS. I. Report of an infant with sudden death. Pediatrics 1979; 63:837–43.
102. Hoppenbrouwers T, Hodgman JE, Arakawa K, et al. Sleep apnea as part of a sequence of events: a comparison of three month old infants at low and increased risk for sudden infant death syndrome (SIDS). Neuropaediatrie 1978; 9:320–37.
103. Rigatto H. Apnea and periodic breathing. Semin Perinatol 1977; 1:375–81.
104. Gibbs EL, Gibbs FA. Clinical correlates of various types of extreme spindles. Clin Electroencephalogr 1973; 4:89–100.
105. Cronje RE, Human GP, Simson IW. Hypoxaemic pulmonary hypertension in children. S Afr Med J 1966; 1:2–7.
106. Brady JP, Donovan M, Dumpit FM. Absence of abnormal control of ventilation in infants with aborted sudden infant death syndrome (SIDS). Clin Res 1980; 28:128A.
107. Brady JP, Ariagno RL, Watts JL, Goldman SL, Dumpit FM. Apnea, hypoxemia and aborted sudden infant death syndrome. Pediatrics 1978; 62:686–91.
108. Jacky JP. Ventilatory responses to inhaled $CO_2$ during sleep in the infant primate. Diss Abstr B Sci Eng 1977; 1:122.
109. James LS, Row RD. The pattern of response of pulmonary and systemic arterial pressures in newborn and older infants to short periods of hypoxia. J Pediatr 1957; 51:4–11.
110. Prechtl HFR. Patterns of reflex behavior related to sleep in the human infant. In: Clemente CD, Purpura DP, Mayer FE, eds. Sleep and the maturing nervous system. New York: Academic Press, 1972:287.
111. Vakhrameeva A, Finkel ML. Changes in reflex excitability of spinal motor neurons during day sleep in newborn infants. *Translated from* Zhurnal Evolyutsionnoi Biokhimii i Fiziologii 1976; 12:161–8.
112. Parmelee AH, Stern E. Development of states in infants. In: Clemente CD, Purpura DP, Mayer FE, eds. Sleep and the maturing nervous system. New York: Academic Press, 1972:199–215.
113. Prechtl HFR, Beintema D. The neurological examination of the fullterm newborn infant. In: Clinics in Developmental Medicine, No. 12, Spastics International Medical Publication. London: William Heineman Medical Books Ltd. Philadelphia: JB Lippincott Co, 1964:74.
114. Reinberg A, Gervais P. Circadian rhythms in respiratory functions with specific reference to human chronophysiology and chronopharmacology. Bull Physiopathol Resp 1972; 8:663–75.

115. Hellbrügge T. The development of circadian rhythms in infants. Quant Biol 1960; 25:311–23.
116. Hoppenbrouwers T, Jensen D, Hodgman J, Harper R, Sterman M. Respiration during the first six months of life in normal infants. II. The emergence of a circadian pattern. Neuropaediatrie 1979; 10:264–80.
117. de Kraker J. Het 24-uurs ritme bij vroeggeborenen. Thesis, Amsterdam (in press).
118. Tammeling GJ, Kruyt EW, Oliver CN, Sluiter HJ. Circadian pattern of the ventilatory function in healthy subjects and patients with obstructive lung disease. Int J Chronobiol 1976; 3:155–69.
119. MacWilliams JA. Blood pressure and heart action in sleep and dreams. Br Med J 1923; 22:1195–1200.
120. Kleitman N, Engelman I. Sleep characteristics of infants. J Appl Physiol 1953; 6:269–82.
121. Guilleminault C, Ariagno R, Korobkin R, Coons S, Owen-Boeddiker M, Baldwin R. Sleep parameters and respiratory variables in "near miss SIDS" infants. Pediatrics (in press).

# THREE

# ELECTRONIC MONITORING IN THE NEWBORN AND YOUNG INFANT: TECHNICAL GUIDELINES

TOKE HOPPENBROUWERS
SUE GEIDEL
MARIA ELENA RUIZ
LORIE JUDSON

## Introduction

The objective of this chapter is to provide technical information about electronic monitoring of one or more physiologic variables in newborns and young infants.

This introduction will provide some general guidelines about preparation for monitoring and procedures to increase the probability of obtaining high-quality recordings. The second section will discuss in detail the necessary supplies and application of transducers to monitor the variables listed in Table 3–1. With the discussion of some parameters, known advantages will be mentioned and, when appropriate, another technique will be introduced. Essential procedures, such as observation and charting, will be found in the third section along with some examples of good tracings. The fourth and final section is devoted to technical aspects of the monitoring system, such as recording speed and analysis strategies. The need for special equipment will be briefly touched upon so that a preliminary cost-benefit estimate can be reached.

Although the techniques described were developed for use with full-term newborns and infants up to the age of six months, they can also be used with premature infants. Since skin surface is reduced in the premature infant and the skin is more sensitive, some special care in application is required. Transducers and other supply items mentioned here have been shown to yield good results. Some have been chosen because they can be readily gas-sterilized, and others because they are disposable.

*Sleeping and waking disorders: indications and techniques*

**Table 3–1** Variables, Transducers, and Interface Circuitry

| Variable | Transducer/Electrode | Equipment* |
|---|---|---|
| ECG **1** | Pregelled chest electrode **1** | Preamplifier **13** |
| Skin temperature<br>Room temperature | Temperature probe **2** | Temperature coupler **14**<br>Multiplexer |
| Abdominal or chest breathing movements | Pregelled electrodes **1**<br>Strain gauge **3** | Impedance coupler **15**<br>Strain gauge coupler **16** |
| $tcPo_2$, $tcPco_2$ | Manufacturer's heated electrodes **4** | Transcutaneous gas monitor **17** |
| EMG | Silver chloride electrodes **5** | Preamplifier **13** |
| EEG | Silver chloride electrodes **5** | Preamplifier **13** |
| Brainstem auditory-evoked potential (BAEP) | Silver chloride electrodes **5**<br>Ear clip **6** | Evoked-potential averager **18** |
| Eye movements **2** | Eye-movement sensor **7**<br>Silver chloride disc electrode **5** | Coupler **19**<br>Preamplifier **13** |
| Expired $CO_2$ **1** | Cannula **8**<br>Soft rubber catheter **9** | Carbon dioxide sensor and analyzer **20** |
| Nasal airflow | Thermistor **10** | Thermistor coupler **21** |
| Respiratory sounds | Microphone **11** | |
| Somatic activity **1** | Somatic activity electrodes **12** | |

*In addition to Grass 16-channel polygraph with differential amplifiers and integrators.
Boldface numbers throughout this chapter refer to equipment and suppliers given in Appendix 3–A (pages 94–95).

Inclusion of items does not mean that other adequate substitutes are not available. In small premature infants, smaller electrode sizes than the ones indicated here may be desirable. The incidence of blisters has been minimal, but reddening of the skin under the electrode is a common occurrence. This is mentioned in our consent forms. Some infants with fair skin are particularly prone to reddening and skin lesions. We have kept salves in stock to send home with the mother. With the use of the $tcPo_2$ and $tcPco_2$ electrodes, the danger of blisters is not imaginary. Prevention will be discussed below.

The key to high-quality recordings is careful preparation. This includes readying the facility prior to the infant's arrival. Some electrodes must be soaked for better performance, others heated. Supplies should be set out in the order that they are needed. If identical-looking electrodes are used for different purposes, they should be labeled in advance.

In our laboratory, we set aside approximately one hour prior to preparation of the baby for an unhurried talk with the infant's parent or caretaker. This is reassuring and reduces tension in both parent and infant. Whereas monitoring procedures are discussed and appropriate consent forms signed during a prior home visit, mothers are shown the facility at this time and are permitted to stay overnight. This can be especially useful if the baby is breast-fed. The mother's presence is often desirable, both for the benefit of the infant and for the parent's continued satisfaction with monitoring participation. A relaxed mother may calm the infant during set-up and waking periods. Information about the infant's current health status, diet, schedules, and idiosyncratic sleep habits (most comfortable position, use of pacifier, etc.) is obtained before the parent leaves. Rectal temperature is taken and the general health and skin condition is assessed. Systematic physical and neurologic examinations are also performed at this time. Infants may be hungry on arrival, so solid foods are given before preparation begins, with bottle or breast-feeding in all age groups given during application of head electrodes.

We have obtained the best results using the following sequence for the application of electrodes: ECG, impedance electrodes or strain gauges, skin-temperature probe, EEG, EMG, $tcPO_2$ and $tcPCO_2$ electrodes, microphone, cannula, and eye-movement sensor. After application of chest and abdominal electrodes, the infant is dressed for the night. (A one-piece terrycloth stretch suit is ideal because it provides warmth during the night and eliminates the need to intervene if the infant kicks off the blanket. It is also manageable for diapering.) The leads are joined and brought over the shoulder. At this time, elbow restraints are applied to young infants, and newborns may be swaddled in a blanket (Figure 3–1).

We have found it necessary to use some arm restraints so that the infant's movements do not inadvertently dislodge the electrodes. Six tongue blades placed side by side are covered with cotton and secured with one-inch tape. These are then covered with $4'' \times 4''$ gauze and wrapped around the extended arm. This method allows the infant arm movements while restricting elbow movement (Figure 3–2).

Upon completion of preparation, the infant can be positioned in the crib and quieted for sleep. The supine position is preferable because interference with chest and facial electrodes is minimal. Placing a young infant in the supine position necessitates constant surveillance, in case the infant spits up. The side-lying position (infant's back propped with a blanket) is adequate, though the chest impedance and ECG signal may be affected more readily by movement. The prone position, though often the position preferred by the infant, is least satisfactory because the facial electrodes are readily disturbed. Thus the infant is never placed in the prone position. If, however, the infant turns over onto his stomach during sleep, as an older infant is inclined to do, no

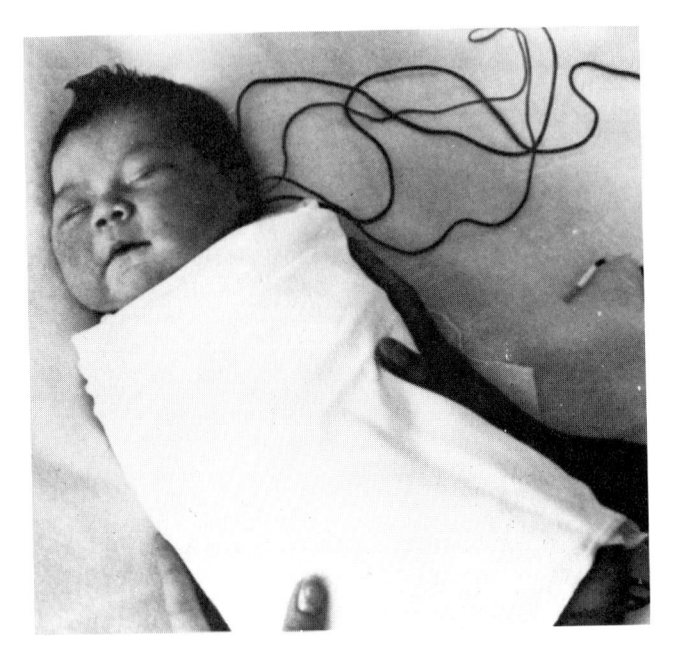

*Sleeping and waking disorders: indications and techniques*

**Figure 3–1.** Newborn infant swaddled to limit arm movements.

intervention is made as long as the signals remain adequate. While one of the staff members positions and quiets the infant, the assistant can make all connections to the pin board and straighten the room for the night's recording.

Infant needs during monitoring include feeding, diapering, and comforting. In our unit, infants are fed on a demand schedule. Although the infant cannot be removed from the crib at any time during the monitoring, his upper body can be held upright and supported during the feeding and burping. The length of the electrodes should allow for a seated position. The child is diapered in a supine position before or after the feeding. We have found disposable diapers to be convenient.

A crib of at least waist height is optimal for the breast-feeding mother. She leans over the crib and holds the infant to her breast and is able to cuddle the child. Initially, the procedure is often uncomfortable for the mother, and help with the positioning as well as encouragement may be needed.

Fussiness may continue in spite of meeting the infant's feeding and diapering needs. If an infant is accustomed to being held at home, he may need extra tactile contact. The older infant, used to being awake and active at a particular time, may require company and verbal stimulation. Sometimes the infant merely needs to have a "fussy period." Signal quality will return after the "fussy period."

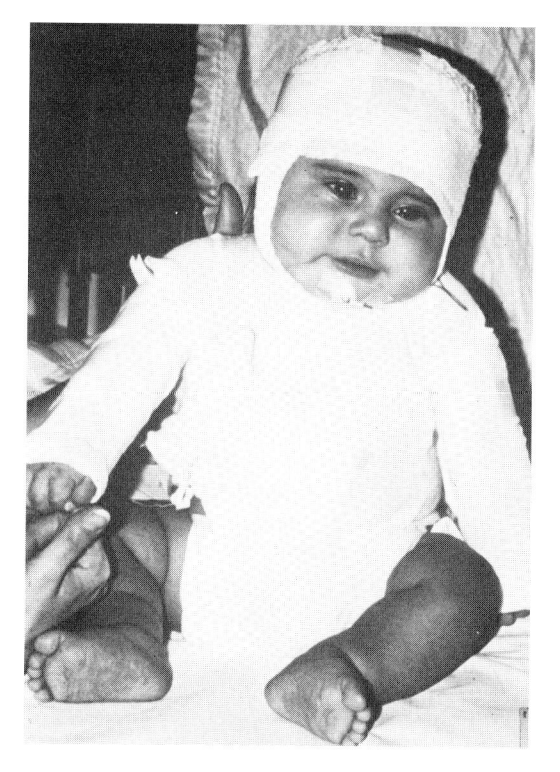

**Figure 3–2.** Arm restraints applied to older infants.

# Application of Electrodes and Transducers

### ECG

Supplies: Three pregelled chest electrodes **1**
Three extension connectors **22**
Alcohol wipes
Benzoin
Electrode jelly **23**

Label electrodes as follows: two ECG, one ground. Good application sites for ECG electrodes are indicated in Figure 3–3. In small infants, a site far enough beneath the clavicles should be selected so that head motion does not interfere. Equidistance from the midline is essential. The application site for the *ground* electrode is exactly at the midline immediately above the umbilicus. Thorough cleansing of this area will assure good contact (Figure 3–4).

65

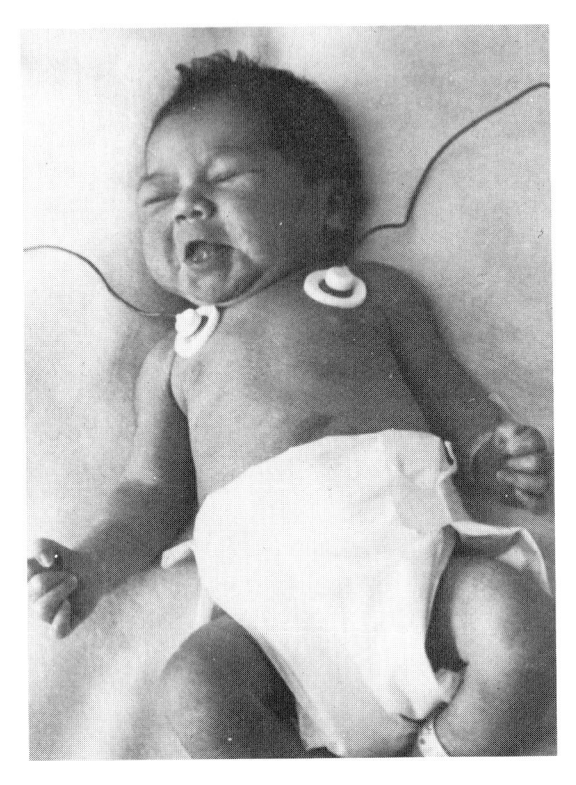

*Sleeping and waking disorders: indications and techniques*

**Figure 3–3.** Location of ECG electrodes. An area beneath the clavicles was chosen so that head motion does not introduce artifact; equidistance from the midline is necessary.

To apply electrodes, examine the chosen sites for irritation. If the baby is perspiring heavily or has fragile skin, the use of benzoin applied to the adhesive portion of the electrodes is desirable. Also, if the active part of the eye of the electrode is dry, supplement with jelly. Otherwise, cleanse the areas thoroughly with an alcohol wipe and vigorously rub a small amount of electrode jelly into each place until the skin is again dry to the touch. Apply labeled electrodes as indicated. Check and record skin resistances of each set of electrodes with an ohmmeter. Make sure electrodes and jellies are used before the expiration date.

Other electrode placements are sometimes preferred, in particular when the $tcPO_2$ and $tcPCO_2$ electrodes are used. The latter are best applied to the skin of the upper chest. The second ECG electrode can be applied in the intercostal margin below the rib cage on the ipsilateral side as the first ECG electrode. One ECG is usually obtained in sleep recordings. The R-wave polarity chosen is arbitrary, but analysis is facilitated if one polarity can be adhered to across recordings.

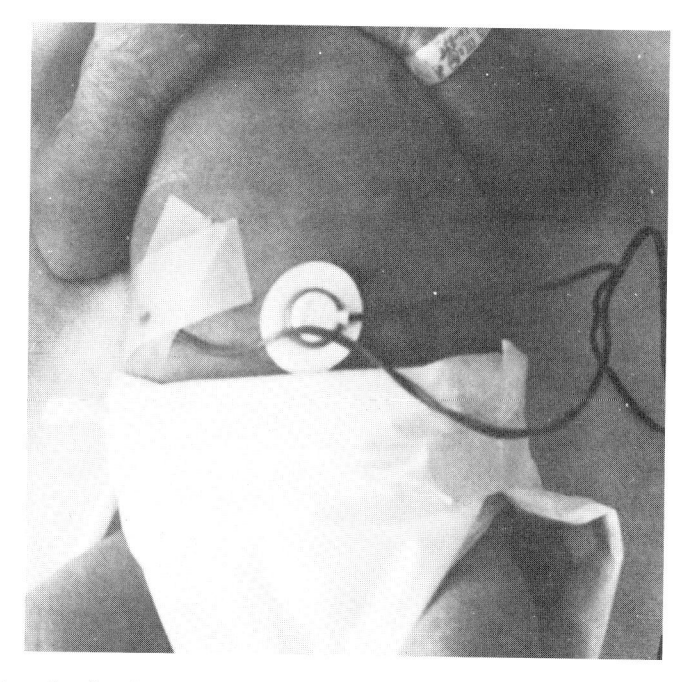

**Figure 3–4.** Application site of the ground electrode on the midline above the umbilicus. The temperature sensor has been applied to the skin over the liver with hypoallergenic tape.

## Skin Temperature

    Supplies:    One skin temperature probe **2**
                     Hypoallergenic tape **24**
                     Alcohol wipes
                     Benzoin

The skin temperature sensor **3** should be taped over the liver with the shiny side of the disk against the skin (Figure 3–4).

## Abdominal and Chest Excursions

    1. Impedance technique

    Supplies:    Two to four pregelled chest electrodes **1**
                     Two to four extension connectors **22**
                     Alcohol wipes
                     Benzoin
                     Electrode jelly **23**

*Sleeping and waking disorders: indications and techniques*

Label electrodes as follows: Two chest, two abdominal

While the infant is undressed, observe the breathing pattern. The optimal locations of *impedance electrodes* are over the areas of greatest excursion. Figure 3–5 shows the electrode placement to record thoracic respiratory motion. It is important that the sites are equidistant from the midline and at the same level; maximal separation of electrodes and symmetric placement are essential for a good recording. Figure 3–6 shows the desirable application sites when abdominal respirations are recorded. We utilize both methods when monitoring and change, by means of manual switch box, from one mode of recording to another as necessary throughout the night. The monitor measures the respiratory movements through changes in impedance across the thorax or abdomen. A minimal, safe current is applied to the skin sites. The equipment must be in perfect operating condition and balanced to prevent electrical interference with other signals. This is a disadvantage of this method.

2. Strain gauges

This method is easy and allows identification of paradoxical breathing.

Supplies: Two strain gauges; these can be ordered in any chosen length; the area filled with mercury should cover the width of the chest **3**
Alcohol wipes
Benzoin
One-inch hypoallergenic tape **24**

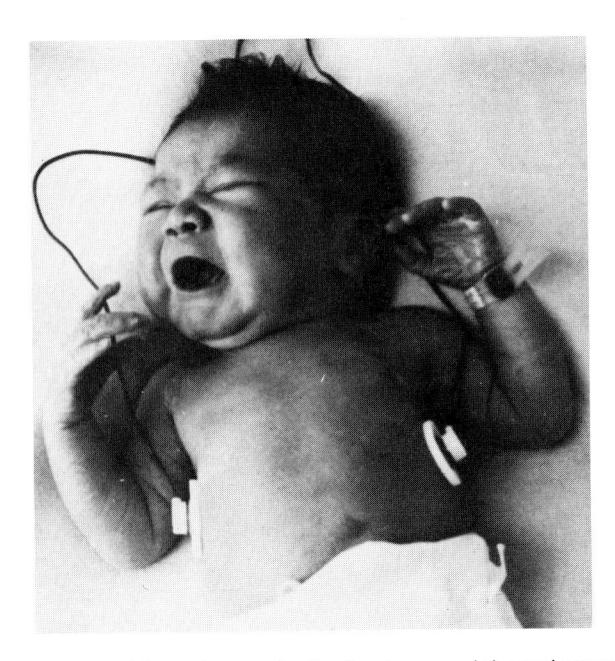

**Figure 3–5.** Location of impedance electrodes to record thoracic respiratory motion. Note the symmetric placement on the axillary line.

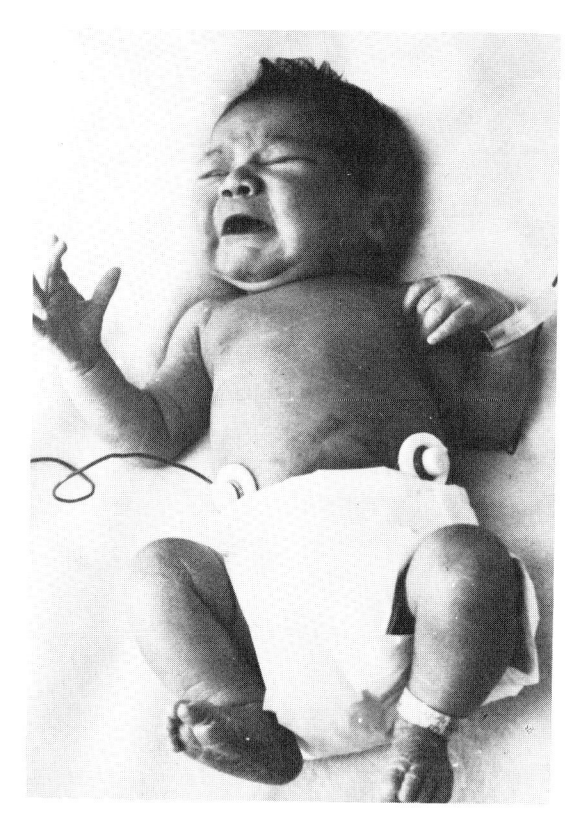

*Electronic monitoring in the newborn and young infant: technical guidelines*

**Figure 3–6.** Location of impedance electrodes to record abdominal respiratory motion. Note again the symmetric placement.

The top strain gauge, intended to measure chest excursions, can be applied 1 cm above or below the nipple line. The strain gauge should be lightly stretched prior to securing with one-inch hypoallergenic tape. Prior cleansing of the area will improve tape attachment. The second strain gauge is placed on the site of the greatest abdominal excursion, usually in the vicinity of the diaphragm.

With adequate amplification, these combined traces will reveal incidence of paradoxical breathing. This is further facilitated by adding a third strain gauge at the lower margin of the rib cage.

## tc$Po_2$ and tc$Pco_2$

Measurement of tc$Po_2$ in our unit is performed with a Novametrics monitor **17**, which simultaneously supplies a tc$Pco_2$ electrode and reading. Both electrodes are heated to obtain accurate values and to reduce calibration time, although reliability and validity data on the unheated tc$Pco_2$ unit suggest its usefulness *(3)*. Unlike the other transducers

69

*Sleeping and waking disorders: indications and techniques*

discussed, the tcPO₂ and tcPCO₂ electrodes and tracings require considerable attention prior to and during prolonged continuous recordings. The electrodes are heated to between 42.5 and 44 C, depending on the age of the infant, and should be rotated at least every four hours in order to prevent blisters and burns (Figure 3–7). In our laboratory, rotation of electrode placement is performed according to the schedule outlined in Table 3–2. We prefer to change electrodes during feedings or other spontaneous awakenings. At each time, electrodes require recalibration.

*Equipment Preparation*   If the transcutaneous monitor (TCOM) is used only weekly, electrode membranes should be changed every seven to ten days. If used continuously, the membranes require changing every three days. Indications for membrane change include (a) membrane appears dark and dry; (b) air bubbles appear under the membrane; (c) inability to calibrate properly. To facilitate stabilization of the electrodes, membrane exchange should be performed one day prior to the monitoring session. On the day of monitoring, we prefer to turn on this equipment one hour prior to the infant's arrival. The equipment is calibrated prior to and after electrode application.

## TCQM™
### O₂ & CO₂ ELECTRODE PLACEMENT

**NEONATE**

| O₂ | CO₂ |
|---|---|
| BEST<br>1, 2 | BEST<br>1, 2, 16 |
| GOOD<br>3, 4 | GOOD<br>3, 4, 14, 15 |
| FAIR TO GOOD<br>6, 7, 12, 13 | FAIR TO GOOD<br>6, 7, 12, 13 |
| TRY<br>5, 8, 9, 10, 11 | TRY<br>5, 8, 9, 10, 11 |

**SUGGESTED TEMPERATURE SETTINGS**

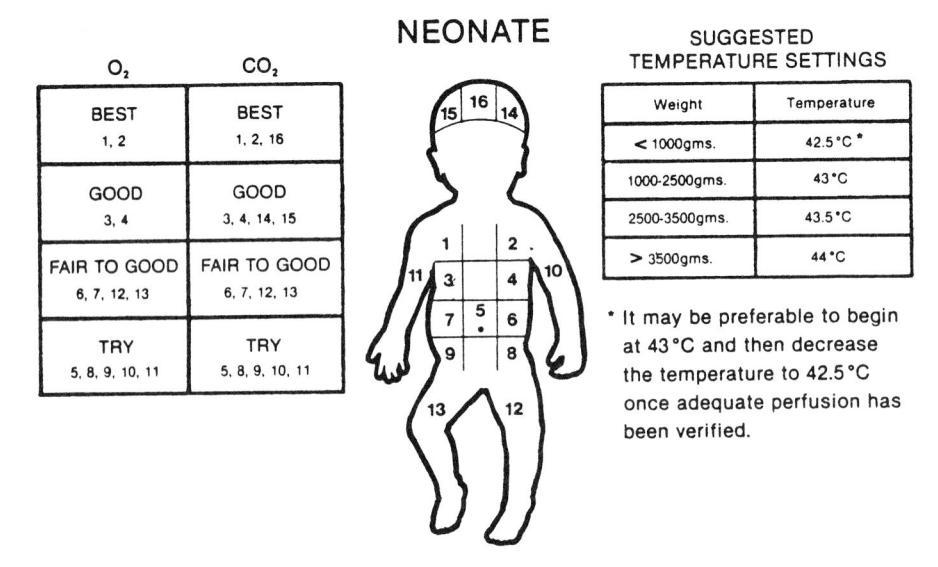

| Weight | Temperature |
|---|---|
| < 1000gms. | 42.5 °C * |
| 1000-2500gms. | 43 °C |
| 2500-3500gms. | 43.5 °C |
| > 3500gms. | 44 °C |

\* It may be preferable to begin at 43 °C and then decrease the temperature to 42.5 °C once adequate perfusion has been verified.

**Figure 3–7.**   Placement and suggested temperature settings of the transcutaneous O₂ and CO₂ electrodes. Reprinted with permission from Novametrix Medical Systems, Inc.

*Electronic monitoring in the newborn and young infant: technical guidelines*

**Table 3-2**  TCOM Placement of Electrodes During 12-Hour Monitoring Session

|       | $O_2$ |  |  | $CO_2$ |  |  |
|-------|-------|-------|--------|--------|--------|--------|
| Time  | 5–10 pm | 10–2 am | 2–6 am | 5–10 pm | 10–2 am | 2–6 am |
| Site* | #1 | #1 | #2 | #3 | #3 | #4 |

*Refer to Figure 3–7.

Supplies:   tcPo$_2$ electrode
            tcPco$_2$ electrode **4**
            Electrode preparation kit and contact gel **25**
            Adhesive rings **25**
            One-inch hypoallergenic tape **24**

Sites are selected according to the diagram in Figure 3–7. The skin should be cleansed with alcohol to ensure good contact. Before the electrodes are secured to the skin with the adhesive rings, one drop of contact gel is placed in the center of each electrode. We use, in addition, one to two inches of one-inch tape to further secure the electrode leads. A round heat shield approximately one inch in diameter is placed on top of the tcPo$_2$ electrode to protect the electrode from environmental temperature changes. Upon electrode removal, the skin must be carefully examined for irritation blisters and burns.

## EEG

Supplies:   Four silver chloride cup electrodes soaked in normal saline for a minimum of one-half hour **5**
            Transpore tape, one-inch **27**
            One roll of 4½-inch, six-ply gauze (Kerlix) **28**
            Electrode paste **26**
            Modified compass and/or tape measure
            Acetone-alcohol
            Cotton swabs
            Cotton balls

The application is best performed while the infant is quiet; a bottle- or breast-feeding at this time provides both a method of calming an active infant and a preparation for later sleep. The infant should be held in a comfortable position by an assistant.

Assess the condition of hair and scalp. Hair treated with pomades and oils, or a scalp with cradle cap, should be thoroughly shampooed and rinsed prior to electrode application. Hair must be allowed to dry.

*Sleeping and waking disorders: indications and techniques*

To mark the sites for EEG electrode application, begin by locating the midpoint on the skull using ears and nose as reference points. Measuring 1.5 cm to either side of the midline, mark the scalp for site #1. Similarly, measure 6.0 cm to either side of the midline as site #2 (Figure 3–8).

Now, evaluate these sites. If you find them on a fontanel, or on sutures that are separated or overriding, then slightly alter the sites bilaterally to a firm, intact cranial surface. Note also that the distances from the midline may vary slightly with infant age or head size; such changes, however, should be bilaterally equal for that infant. Using cotton swabs, separate the hair on one side and thoroughly cleanse the scalp with acetone-alcohol. Use a firm back-and-forth stroke and enough pressure to abrade the skin (Figure 3–9). Severe cradle cap or hyperkeratotic newborn skin is a problem, and several dry layers may have to be removed. For a good application, some abrasion is necessary, but care must be taken not to scrub so vigorously that the scalp is injured.

Maintain the hair separation and site location with one hand, and with the other rub a small amount of paste into the prepared site. Dry the electrode cup and fill to slightly overflowing with paste. Push it firmly onto the prepared skin, covering electrode and paste with a small cotton ball (Figure 3–10). Push firmly on the electrode for about one minute to ensure good contact. Prepare the other sites in a similar manner. Throughout this period, it is essential to apply firm pressure periodically to each electrode so that good contact is maintained during drying. Note, for future reference, the location of your electrodes, either by color coding or direct labeling of each lead.

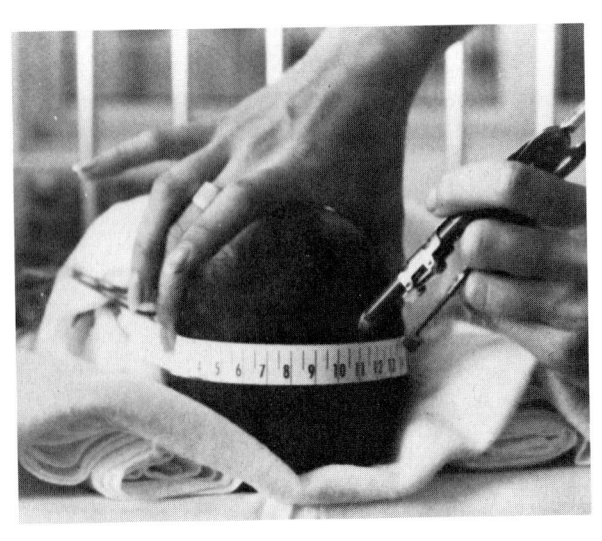

**Figure 3–8.** Determination of EEG electrode sites with a modified compass and tape measure.

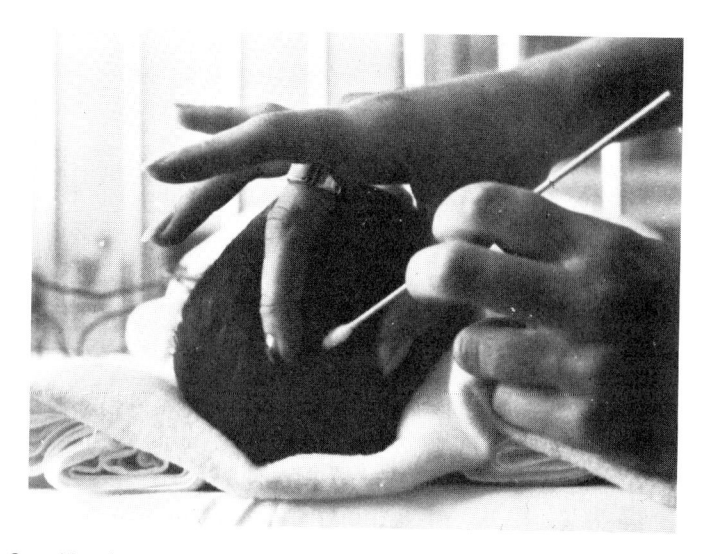

*Electronic monitoring in the newborn and young infant: technical guidelines*

**Figure 3-9.** Hand position while abrading the skin sites with a cotton swab dipped in acetone-alcohol.

## BAEP

Supplies: Three silver chloride cup electrodes soaked in normal saline
Ear clips **5,6**
See EEG for remainder of supplies

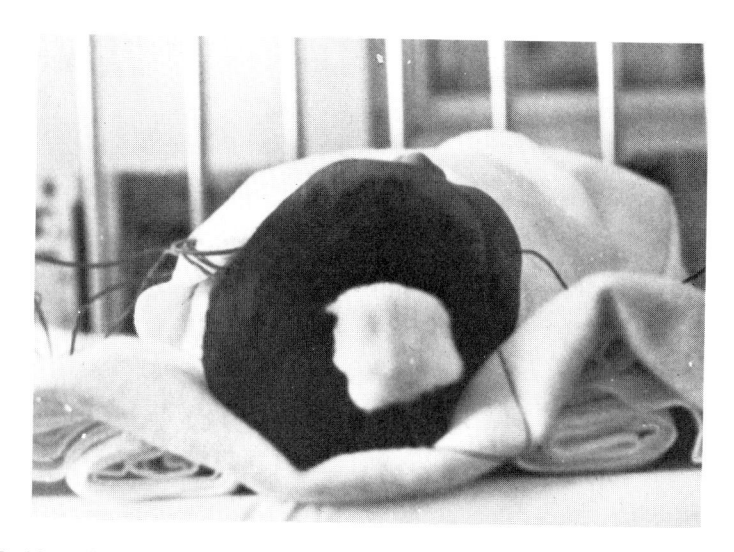

**Figure 3-10.** An EEG electrode covered with a small cotton ball.

*Sleeping and waking disorders: indications and techniques*

Begin by locating the vertex. The application of BAEP electrodes is identical to that of EEG electrodes. Electrodes on earlobes or mastoids can be used as reference. After appropriate preparation of the skin, the electrode surface of a Grass ear clip can be covered with electrode paste and the ear clip attached to the lobe. Extra tape will provide for a more secure hold. Because the ear clips are sometimes irritating, a cup electrode can also be used and taped over the ear lobe. In this case, and if the mastoids are selected as reference, the electrodes are applied in the same way as the EMG electrodes.

## EMG

Supplies:   Two silver chloride cup electrodes soaked in normal saline
Five alcohol swabs
Transpore tape **27**
Electrode paste **26**

Begin by locating the two sites for electrode application. Site #1 is at the point of the chin (Figure 3–11). Site #2 is located on the belly of the digastric muscle just to the left of the infant's trachea. It is easiest to find this spot by encouraging the infant to suck and simultaneously palpating the area of greatest muscle reaction (Figure 3–12).

Cleanse both sites with acetone-alcohol swabs, again abrading the skin lightly.

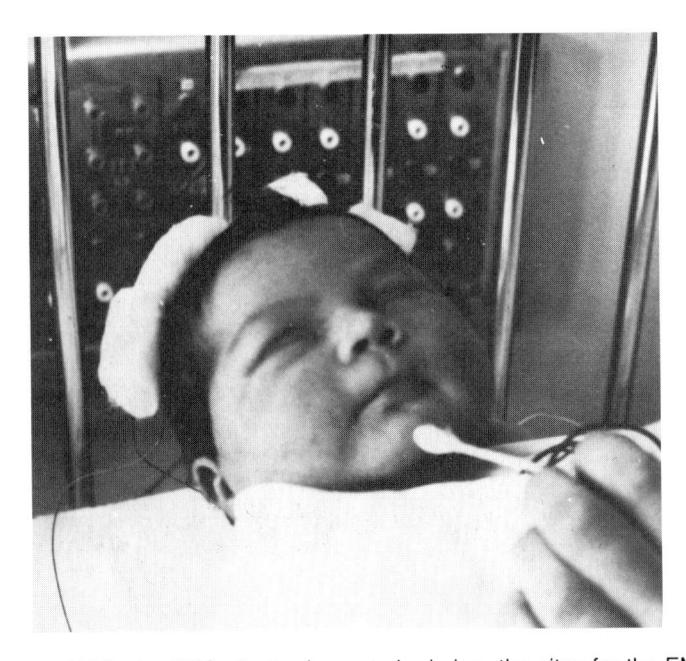

**Figure 3–11.**   While the EEG electrode paste is drying, the sites for the EMG electrodes can be prepared. This photograph shows the abrasion of site #1, the tip of the chin or mental protuberance.

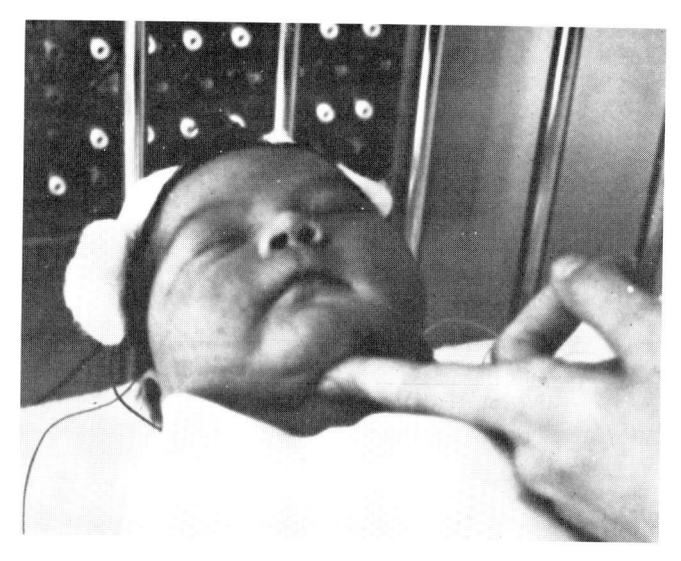

*Electronic monitoring in the newborn and young infant: technical guidelines*

**Figure 3–12.** Palpation of the digastric muscle to locate EMG site #2.

Allow the skin to dry thoroughly. While the skin is drying, the electrodes can be prepared. Tear off a two-inch-long strip of one-inch-wide tape and thread the electrode cup through it for increased stability (Figure 3–13).

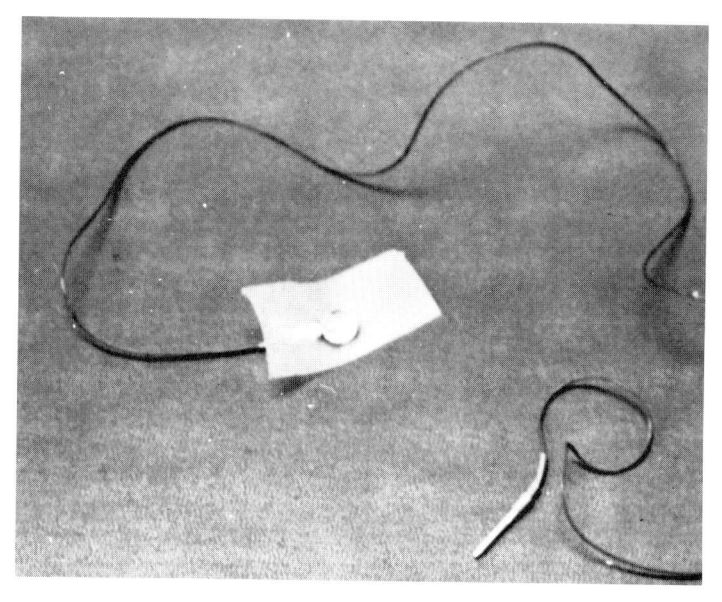

**Figure 3–13.** Demonstration of electrode threaded through a two-inch-long strip of one-inch hypoallergenic tape.

*Sleeping and waking disorders: indications and techniques*

Fill the electrode cup with paste to the rim only (too much paste will spill over and weaken the application) and apply to site #1. Pleat the tape as you press it to the skin to achieve good conformity with the chin contours. Reinforce these pleats with one-half-inch-wide tape strips.

The electrode at site #2 is applied most easily with the infant's neck slightly extended. Observe the infant carefully during this period for cyanosis or respiratory difficulty. Apply the electrode at site #2 in a similar manner and reinforce it with a second strip of one-inch tape (Figure 3–14).

## Head Wrapping

To ensure even pressure on the head electrodes and to protect them throughout the night, the head is wrapped in a roll of 4½-inch, six-ply gauze. Begin by pressing firmly on each scalp electrode. It is important that at least fifteen minutes' drying time has elapsed since their initial application and that the paste has begun to harden. If wrapping is done too soon, electrodes may slide and bilateral symmetry will be lost. Be certain that electrodes remain separate; that is, the paste in one electrode must not be in contact with that in any other, forming a bridge. Small bridges can be eliminated by cleaning the space between electrodes with cotton swabs saturated with acetone-alcohol. If this is not effective, a total reapplication of that side is necessary. Check and record resistances of electrode pairs with an ohmmeter or other appropriate measuring device.

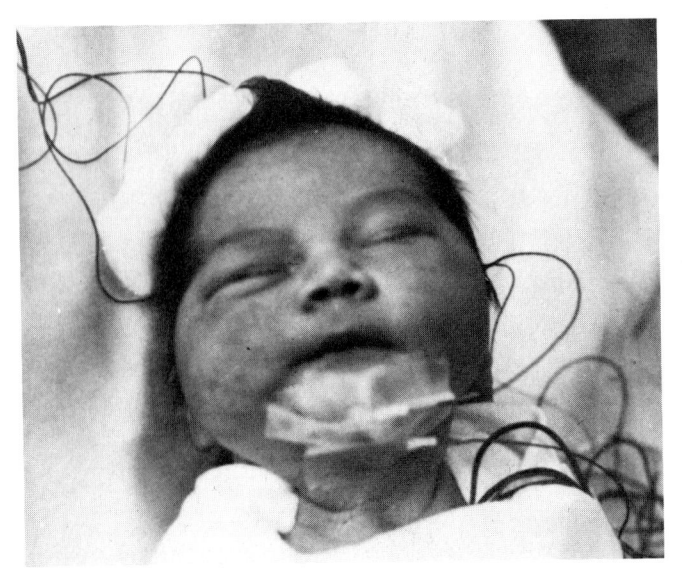

**Figure 3–14.** An infant instrumented with EMG electrodes.

*Electronic monitoring in the newborn and young infant: technical guidelines*

For easiest wrapping, place the infant in a supported sitting position. Begin with a firm lateral wrap extending over the electrodes and under the chin. Repeat this for two to three circles (Figure 3–15). Now, wrap in an anterior-posterior plane, being sure to bring the roll of gauze (Kerlix) down under the back of the head each time for a secure hold (Figure 3–16). This wrap usually takes about one-half roll of standard-width Kerlix. For exceptionally small infants, it may be necessary to split the Kerlix longitudinally.

Be sure to wrap with a firm and even pressure. This can be a most important step in achieving a high-quality, long-lasting signal. Secure the Kerlix ends with tape. Similarly, attach EEG and EMG leads to the left side of the head with short tape strips (Figure 3–17). Return the infant to the crib.

## Airflow

*$P_{CO_2}$ and Thermistor*   A sample of expired air is continuously obtained through the nasal cannula and analyzed for $CO_2$ concentration. A temperature-sensitive bead in the nasal cannula discriminates between expired air (higher temperature) and inspired air (lower temperature) through the nose.

Supplies:   $Po_2$ cannula with thermistor **8,10**
Two strips of one-half-inch-wide tape, each approximately one inch in length **27**

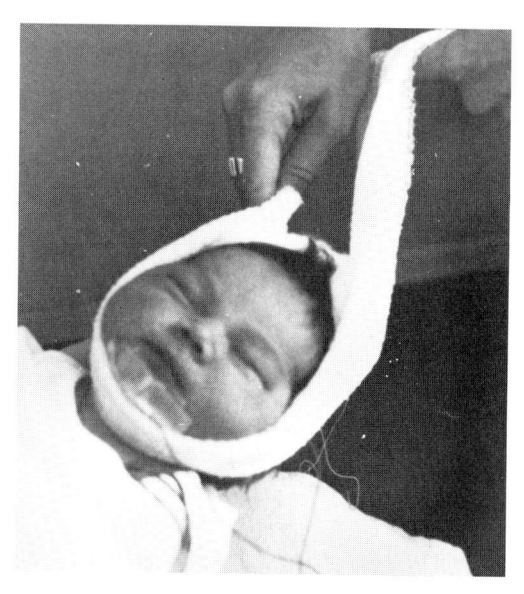

**Figure 3–15.**   Initial lateral wrap over the electrodes and under the chin.

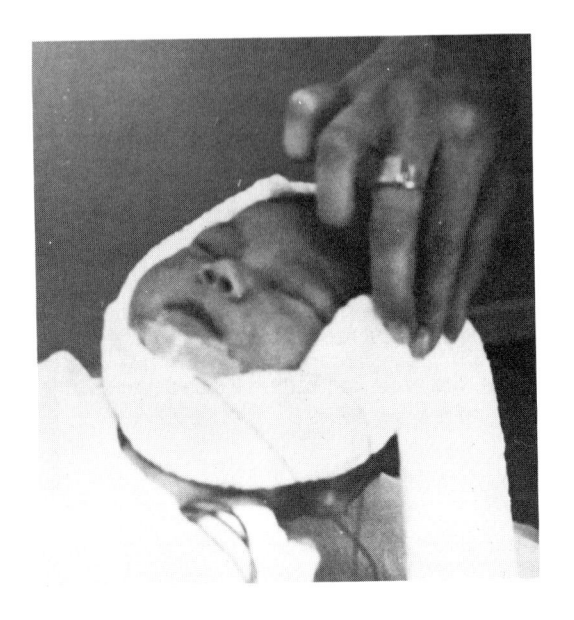

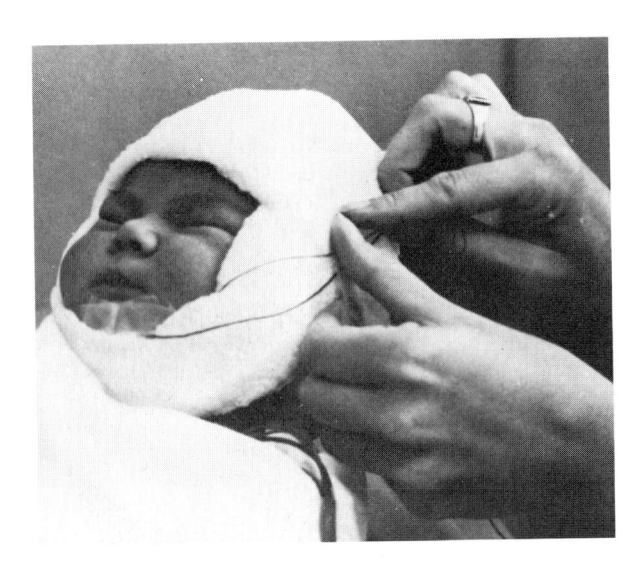

*Sleeping and waking disorders: indications and techniques*

**Figures 3–16 & 3–17.** Continuation of head wrapping to the anterior-posterior plane. After completion of the head wrapping, both EEG and EMG electrode leads are secured to the Kerlix on the left side of the head with tape strips.

*Electronic monitoring in the newborn and young infant: technical guidelines*

When the infant is on his back in the crib, and an assistant is stabilizing his head, insert cannula tips into the nostrils and tape the tubing to each cheek. Pinch the tape firmly around the tubing and check its adherence to the skin (Figure 3–18). If it fits too loosely, it will be dislodged by activity. Be careful not to bend or stretch the cannula during this application. The thermistor bead is small, fragile, and easily broken.

*Microphone*

    Supplies:    Miniature microphone **11**
                   Hypoallergenic tape **24**

With the infant on his back, the microphone is taped to the skin overlying the trachea. Prior cleansing of the area with alcohol assures good contact.

## Eye Movements

Conventional procedures utilize disk electrodes lateral (superior and inferior) to the eye with a reference electrode placed on the ears (Figure 3–19b). A number of problems are associated with this technique *(4)*.

(a) To assure good contact, the sensitive facial skin is abraded to break down surface oil and to reduce impedance between the electrode-skin interface. The electrolyte used to maintain good electrical contact further affects the abraded skin.

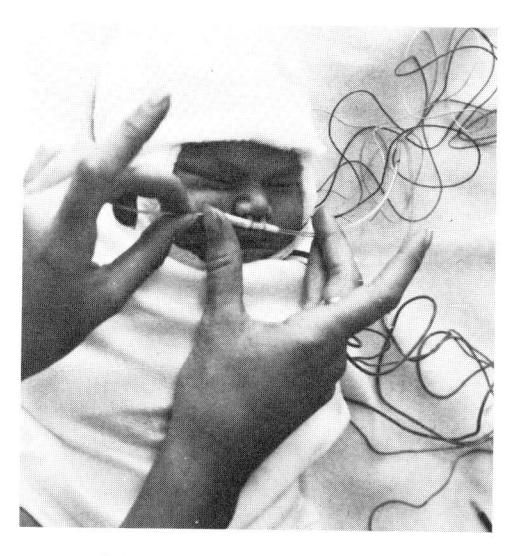

**Figure 3–18.**   Placement of the nasal cannula in the nostrils.

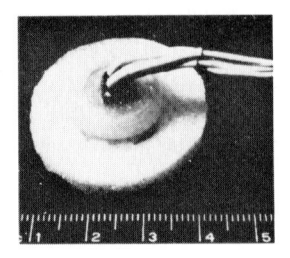

*Sleeping and waking disorders: indications and techniques*

**Figure 3–19a.** Photograph of eyepiece.

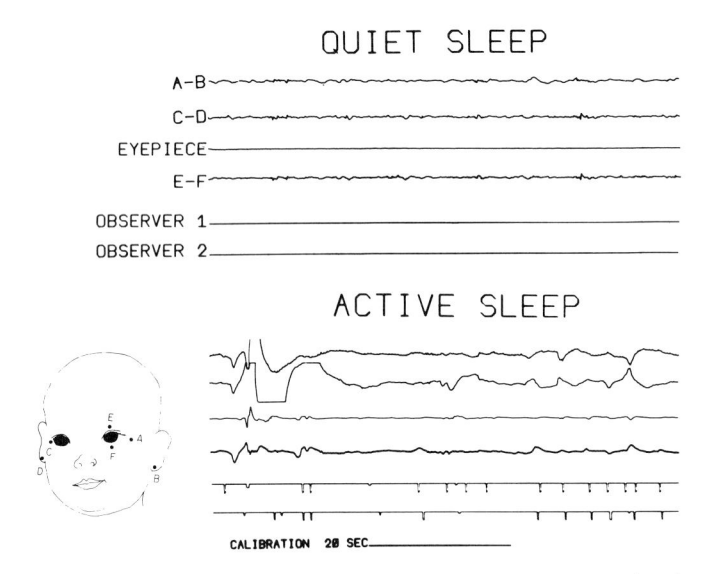

**Figure 3–19b.** Polygraphic traces from conventional eye-movement leads and from the output of the eyepiece during two stages of sleep. Note the large-amplitude EEG waves on the conventional eye-movement electrodes during quiet sleep and the absence of such waves on the eyepiece leads. The large deflections by the observers indicate visually detected eye movements; the small deflections indicate gross body movements.

(b) It is difficult to find adequate surface area on a small face.
(c) The electro-oculogram (EOG) is often contaminated by EEG signals, especially during quiet sleep (QS). When computer detection of eye movements is the objective, this contamination poses severe problems.

*EOG*

Supplies: Three Grass disk electrodes **5**
One Grass ear clip **6**
Electrode paste **26**
Hypoallergenic tape **24**

Prepare sites A, B, and C with alcohol (Figure 3–19*b*). Some abrasion is necessary, but care must be taken to avoid scrubbing too vigorously or getting alcohol in the eye. Rub a small amount of paste into the prepared site. Apply paste lightly to the disk electrode and secure it with tape to the skin. This application should be performed prior to head wrapping, so that the leads can be buried under the Kerlix and brought out together with the EEG leads. Careful labeling is essential. These two channels do not allow differentiation between horizontal and vertical eye movements. The derivations E-B and F-B can be added for this purpose.

*Infrared Method*   We have developed a new technique for recording eye movements in infants that avoids many of the disadvantages of the conventional electrodes *(2)*. This technique consists of measuring reflected infrared light from an open or closed eye, which is illuminated by an external infrared source. The transducer is mounted on a package 2.5 cm in diameter (Figure 3–19*a*), which is taped, using hypoallergenic tape, over one eye so that the photodevice is directly over the eye, and soft edges of the package rest on the bony orbit and nose. This procedure has several advantages.

(a) The application is extremely easy, obviating the need for abrasion of the infant's skin.
(b) Recovery from movement artifacts is rapid.
(c) Output signals are unaffected by ECG, EMG, or EEG activity.
(d) High-quality recordings are maintained for at least 12 hours.

The technique does suffer from some of the same faults as use of conventional electrodes, i.e., the signal is affected by movements other than eye movements, such as gross body motility, facial movements, and sucking.

The device was developed for sleeping infants. When the eyes are open, signal amplitudes tend to increase, thus allowing for a differentiation between active sleep and wakefulness. Eyelid flutters during active sleep, however, cannot be differentiated from rapid eye movements.

Supplies: One eyepiece **7**
One-half-inch-wide tape (four strips, each about four inches long) **27**

With the infant on his back, apply the eyepiece over the left eye with its inner edge resting on the lateral surface of the nose. Secure on four sides with tape strips. It is usually easiest at this point for an assistant to hold the eyepiece and the infant's head, while another person tapes it (Figure 3–20).

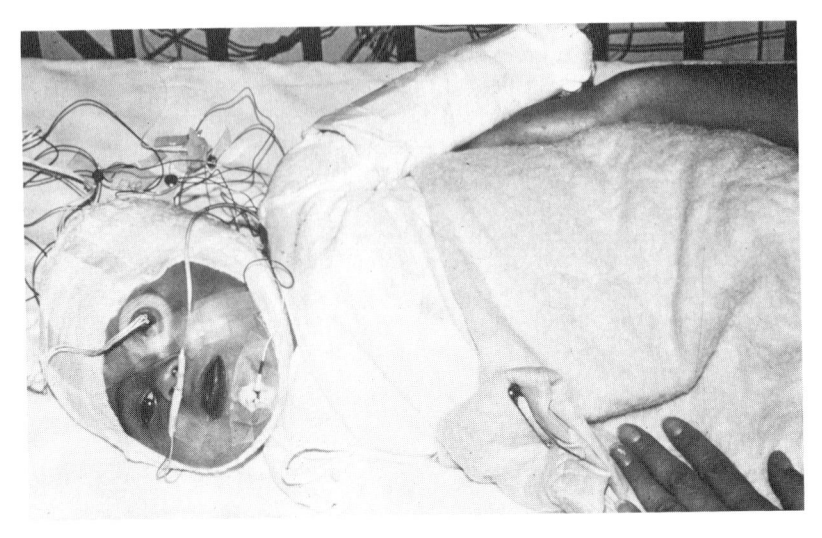

*Sleeping and waking disorders: indications and techniques*

**Figure 3-20.** Application of eye-movement sensor and completion of preparation for long-term monitoring.

# Guidelines for Monitoring

Uninterrupted monitoring can rarely be obtained. Infants are irritated to a varying degree by the monitoring process and will show a larger number of sleep interruptions than if they were sleeping at home. Meticulous preparation reduces the number of induced awakenings for the purpose of electrode reapplication. The number of spontaneous awakenings will depend on the infant's health status, age, and home sleeping patterns.

It is advisable to write a protocol for the monitoring staff specifying which equipment adjustments are allowed. Data reduction strategies dictate which signals should or should not be adjusted on the polygraph during the monitoring. The decision to interrupt sleep to adjust or reapply an electrode should be made on the basis of signal importance. Such a protocol will vary with the purpose of each study.

To interpret the data later, a system of charting must be followed. Behavioral observations are made on the chart with both pencil and coded keys. The behaviors to be charted include: eyes open or closed, feeding or sucking, awake or asleep, gross movements, vocalizations. A video monitor is helpful for this task **29.** A signal log is kept to record the quality of channel output hourly and to facilitate communication between monitoring shifts and engineering staff (Appendix 3-B). Feeding and infant-care information can also be incorporated. In addition, incidences of infant manipulations and machine interventions must be noted on the polygraph paper.

*Electronic monitoring in the newborn and young infant: technical guidelines*

An oscilloscope 30 is essential for monitoring the quality of the signals being taped, especially if the order of data acquisition consists of infant-polygraph amplifiers and subsequently, in parallel, polygraph pens and tape recorders. An alternate way to monitor the quality of the taped signals is to alter this order to: infant-polygraph amplifiers and then, in series, first tape recorders, then polygraph pens.

When a monitoring unit is located within a hospital, interference from surrounding electromagnetic fields is sometimes encountered. This problem can be controlled by completely shielding monitoring units; the tracings shown throughout these chapters were obtained in an unshielded environment.

Sufficient time should be allowed for initial signal evaluation and adjustment. It is essential for the infant to be in a quiet state, though not necessarily sleeping. It should be noted that several of the signals change as a function of behavioral state and are in fact included in the array to allow for discrimination between sleep and waking states. Notable among these are EEG, EMG, eye movements, and respiration. Figure 3–21 summarizes the salient characteristics of three of these signals as a function of behavioral state.

The EEG reflects electrical activity of the brain and characteristically varies with sleep state and age. A good signal is preserved without artifacts during at least portions

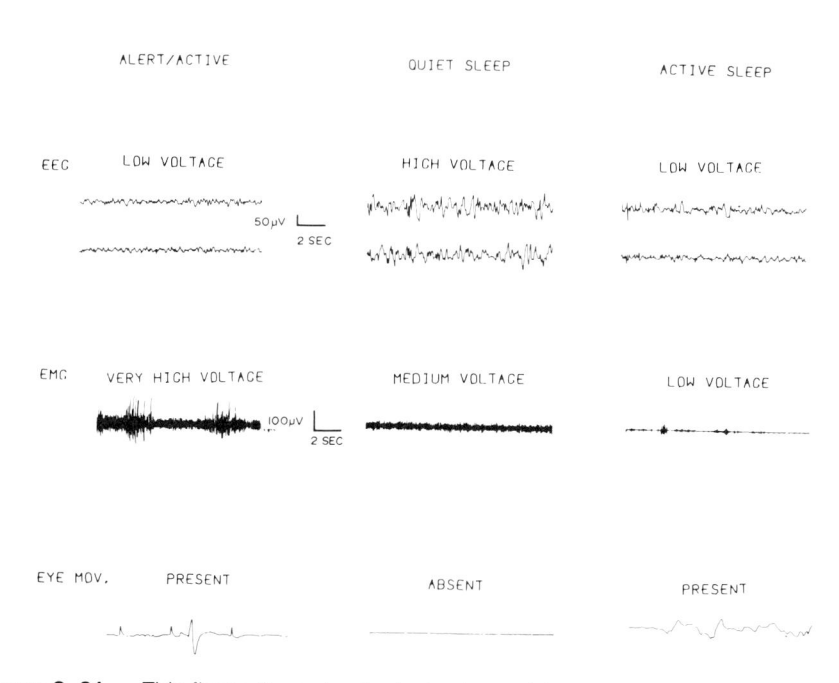

**Figure 3–21.** This figure illustrates typical polygraphic tracings obtained from the same infant during different behavioral states. Note differing patterns of low- and high-voltage EEG and EMG and absence or presence of eye movements.

of wakefulness. The EMG represents fluctuations in body muscle tone as reflected by changes in the digastric muscle. In the initial evaluation of the signal, sleep state must be considered. A high enough setting must be used to differentiate changes in muscle tone corresponding to state changes. An optimal setting on the eyepiece provides a baseline of slight ripples or low-amplitude deflections during quiet sleep, with no false-positive deflections. The eyepiece output should be validated during active sleep (AS). Changes in ambient light, the use of infrared lighting for closed-circuit television monitoring, or position changes of the infant's head may necessitate further adjustments while monitoring.

In general, when a signal shows considerable or unusual artifact, several checks can be made before a decision is reached to reapply the electrodes or make drastic departures from usual polygraph settings.

(a) Impedances for EEG, BAEP, EMG, and EOG electrodes are routinely checked and should not exceed 5000 ohms.
(b) The position of the infant can affect such signals as the impedance respiration, the configuration of the ECG, and the EEG.
(c) Overhead fluorescent lights may introduce 60 cycles. In addition, a dimmed room is optimal for eye-movement recordings and sleep.
(d) The impedance respiration leads must be correctly applied and the signal balanced, otherwise this channel will interfere with other signals. It can, for instance, produce 60 cycles or an offset in one or both EEG channels.

Occasionally, if the humidity in the room is very low ($< 20\%$), the quality of a recording may decrease. In an uncontrolled environment, this must be tolerated. Also, the behavior of newborns is marked by a great deal of active sleep and concomitant phasic activity, such as twitches, jerks, and head movements. These tend to transiently introduce artifacts, especially in the EEG. Two means can be employed to reduce movement artifacts. Miniature amplifiers can be affixed to the EEG electrodes applied to the infant's head. Such units are not yet commercially available. Small preamplifiers 13 can also be mounted as an assembly to the bed; we have used this solution in our unit. Neither system, however, eliminates movement artifacts generated by the friction between the electrode and the scalp.

Continuous, long-term monitoring is feasible, but requires vigilance. The presence of two staff members is considered necessary, and rotation of the monitoring staff every one to two hours has proven to be helpful in maintaining good-quality recordings and charting.

Polygraphic signals are shown in Figures 3–22 to 3–28. The tracé alternant of the newborn (Figure 3–22) is a discontinuous EEG pattern of QS, which usually disappears by one month of age (5). An example of AS in the newborn is shown in Figure 3–23. Sleep spindles (12–14 cps) tend to appear by five to seven weeks of age (6, Figure 3–24). Sometimes, adult sleep stages 3 and 4 can be recognized at three to four months of age in the infant (5,7). Ocular patterns based on both methods described here are shown in Figure 3–19a. With the infrared method, eyes opening and closing and eye movements during wakefulness can be differentiated from rapid eye movements by the amplitude of the signal (Figure 3–25).

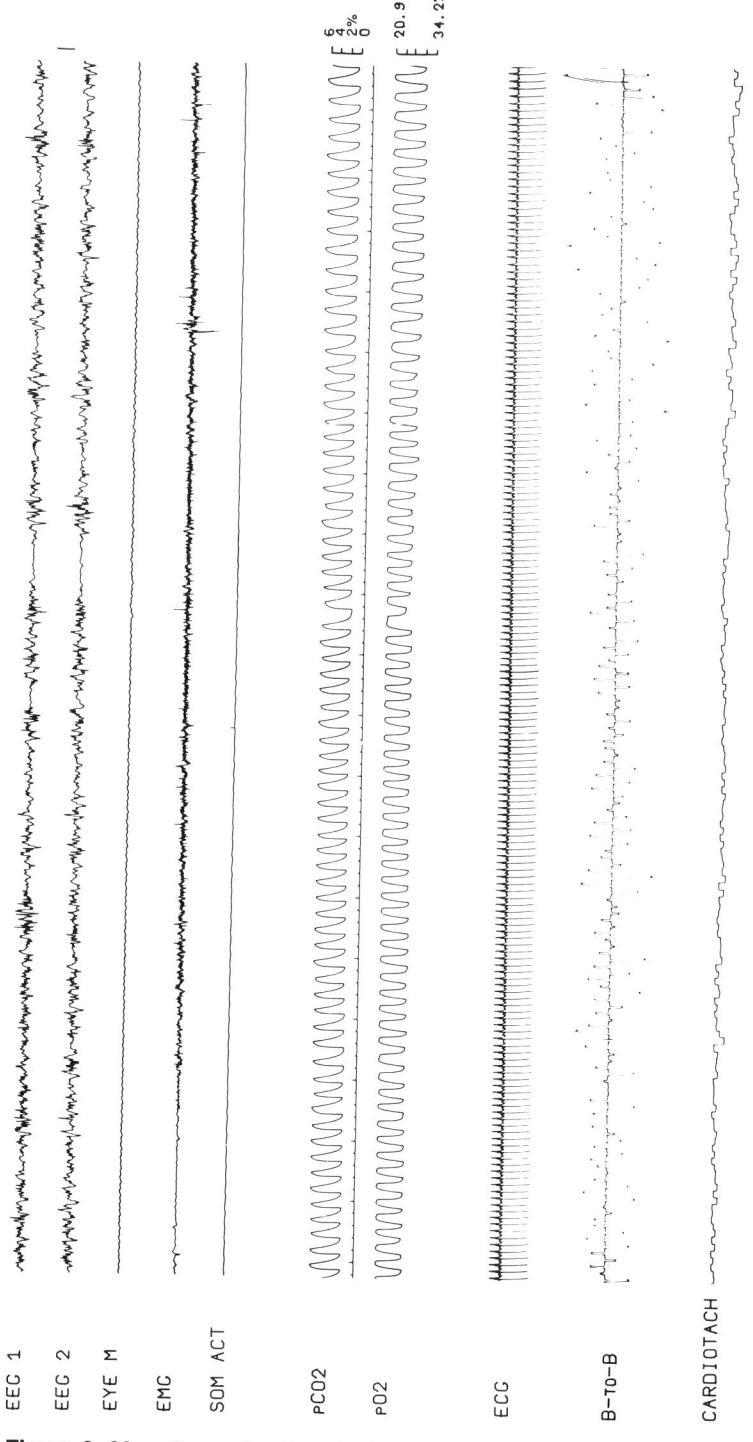

**Figure 3–22.** Example of tracé alternant from a newborn infant. Vertical line next to EEG tracings ($C_3/T_3$, $C_4/T_4$) represents 100 μV.

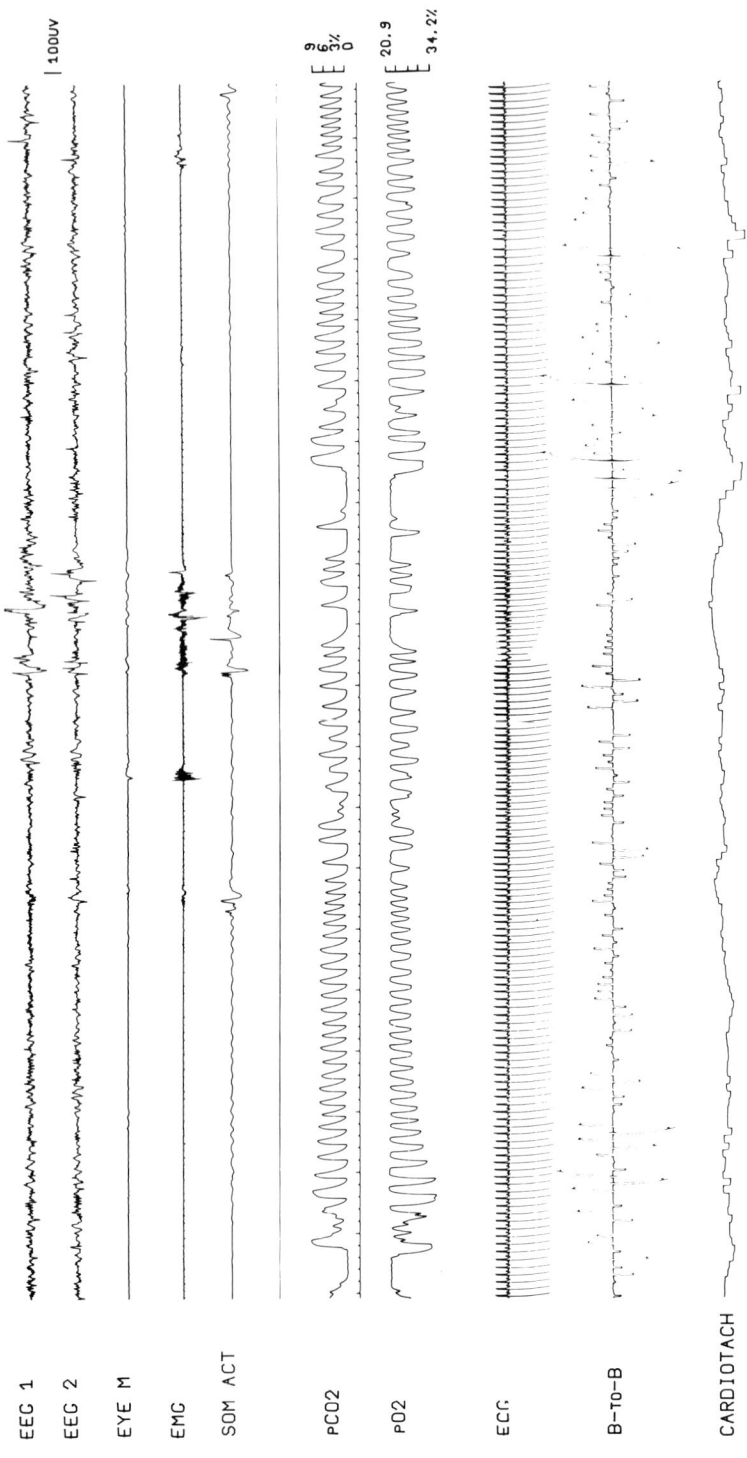

**Figure 3–23.** AS episode in a newborn infant. Note the absence of EMG muscle tone and the irregularity in breathing.

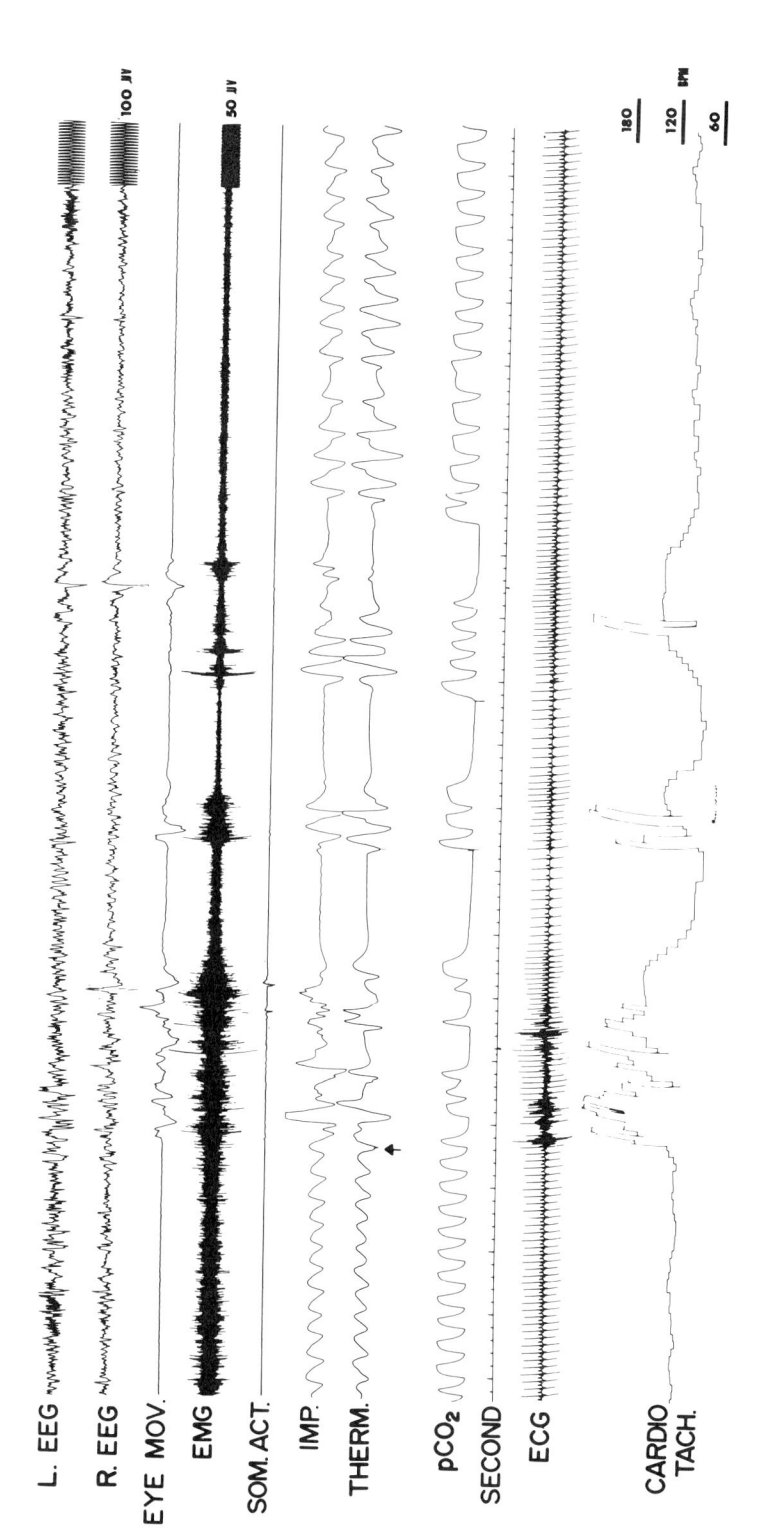

**Figure 3-24.** Sleep spindles (black) in the QS EEG tracings of a three-month-old infant. Same derivations as Figure 3-22. Two central apneas with HR decelerations are followed by a mixed apnea.

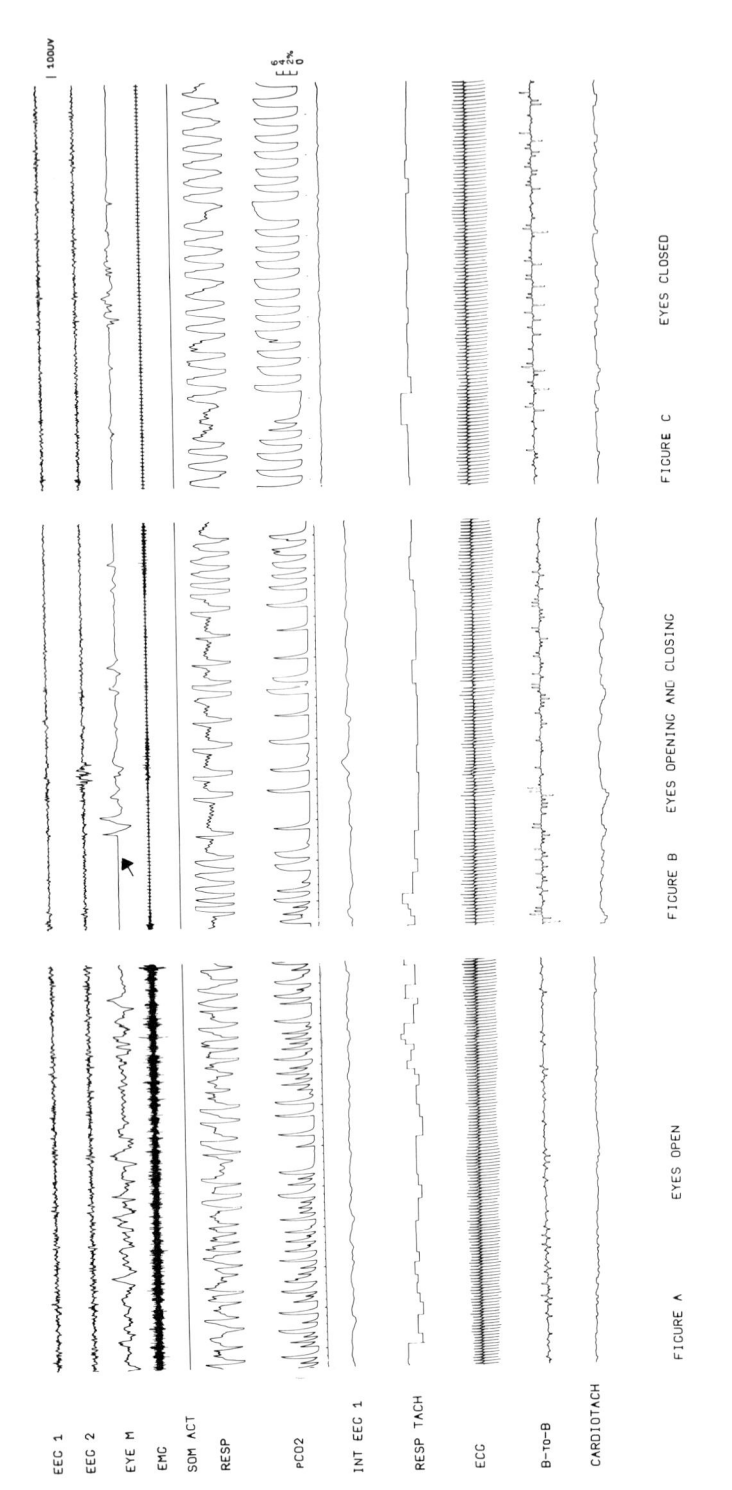

**Figure 3–25.** Ocular patterns during wakefulness, drowsiness, and AS. Eyes open, and opening/closing can be differentiated from rapid eye movements by the amplitude of the signal.

*Electronic monitoring in the newborn and young infant: technical guidelines*

Respiratory tracings based on the impedance technique, thermistor, and expiratory $CO_2$ are shown in Figure 3–26. Because of room air contamination, the $CO_2$-sampling technique cannot provide an accurate level of end-expiratory $P_{CO_2}$. The airflow measured through a thermistor bead is instantaneous, whereas the $CO_2$-sampling technique shows a lag of approximately one second. The main advantage of the latter technique, however, for measurement of respiratory rates and apnea, is resistance to movement artifacts. During periods of crying, when mouth breathing dominates, this method becomes unreliable. A set of respiratory traces, including strain gauges and a microphone, is presented in Figure 3–27. Notice the ability to identify in-phase and out-of-phase respiratory movements, as well as short episodes of obstructions.

Tracings of $tcPO_2$ and $tcPCO_2$ are shown in Figure 3–28. Automatic temperature, an estimate of local perfusion, was found to correlate with mean arterial blood pressure *(8)*. A decrease in local perfusion preceded a 19-second apnea in the tracing of this three-month-old, near-miss infant. Her tissue oxygen levels were within the normal range. The apnea induced a perceptible but nonsignificant drop in $tcPO_2$. Because of inadequate scaling, the increase in $tcPCO_2$, prior to the apnea, cannot be seen.

Several BAEPs from a newborn infant are depicted in Figure 3–29 *(9)*. A number of nonpathologic factors influence the latencies of these potentials, including stimulation, intensity and rate, reference site, temperature, and gender. Relative amplitudes tend to be more variable and are affected by a slightly different set of conditions, including stimulus mode, signal-to-noise ratio, and filter settings *(10)*.

# Technical Aspects of the Monitoring System

Ambient temperatures affect physiologic parameters *(11)*. Many instruments generate heat and noise. A controlled environment can be more readily achieved when the infant's room is separated from the equipment room. A detailed description of calibra-

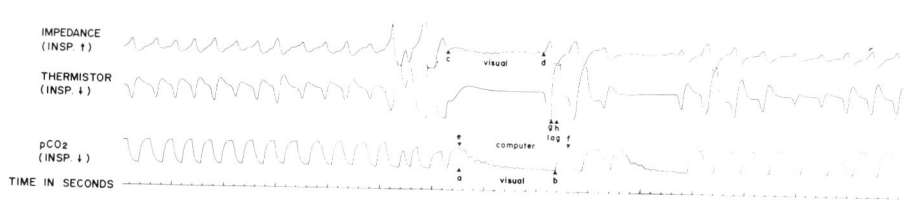

**Figure 3–26.** Computer identification of breathing pauses involves measurement between points *e* and *f*. Note that this interval is approximately one second longer than *a–b*, and *c–d*, used for visual analysis. The interval *g–h* reflects the lag time between the respiratory cycle from a nasal thermistor and the $P_{CO_2}$ signal.

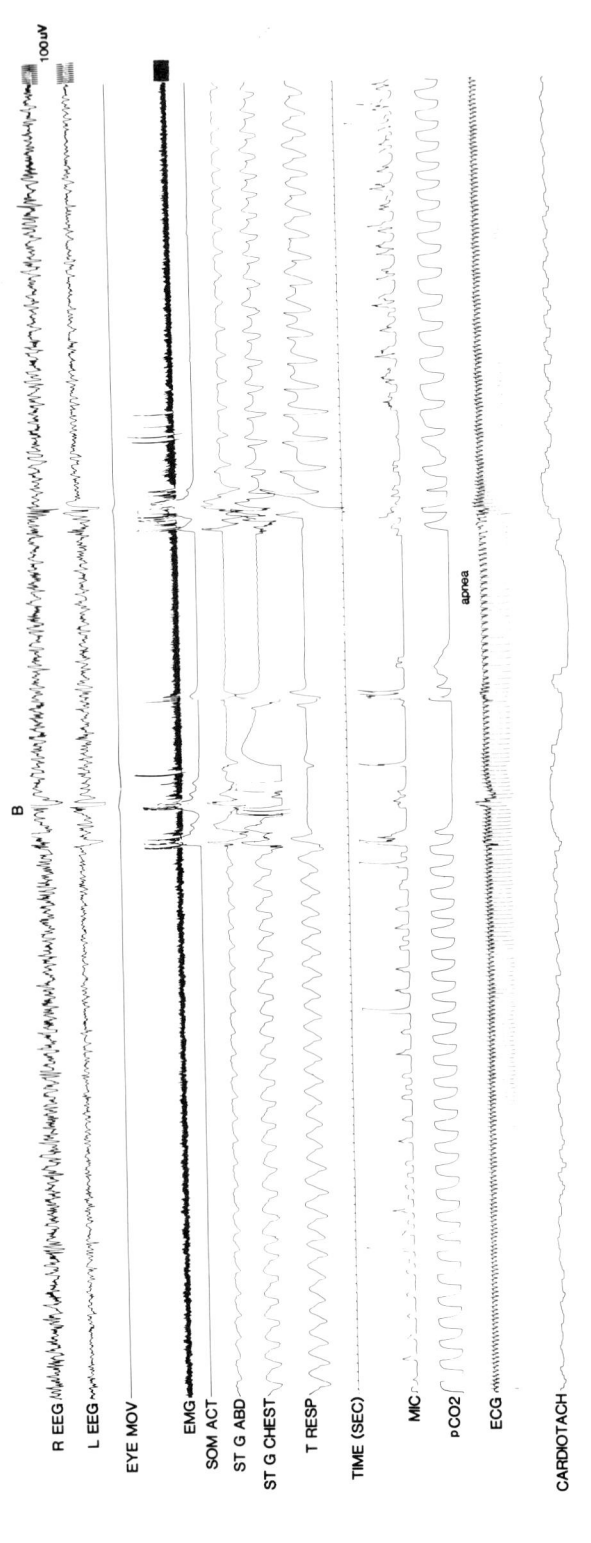

**Figure 3—27.** Polygraphic tracing from a three-month-old, near-miss infant in QS. Notice the relative absence of EEG sleep spindles. Use of a microphone aided in the identification of breathing pauses. During body movements, mouth breathing took place followed by a six-second central apnea. The infant took a deep breath and a prolonged central apnea (19 seconds) ensued. For calibration of the cardiotachometer see Figure 3–28.

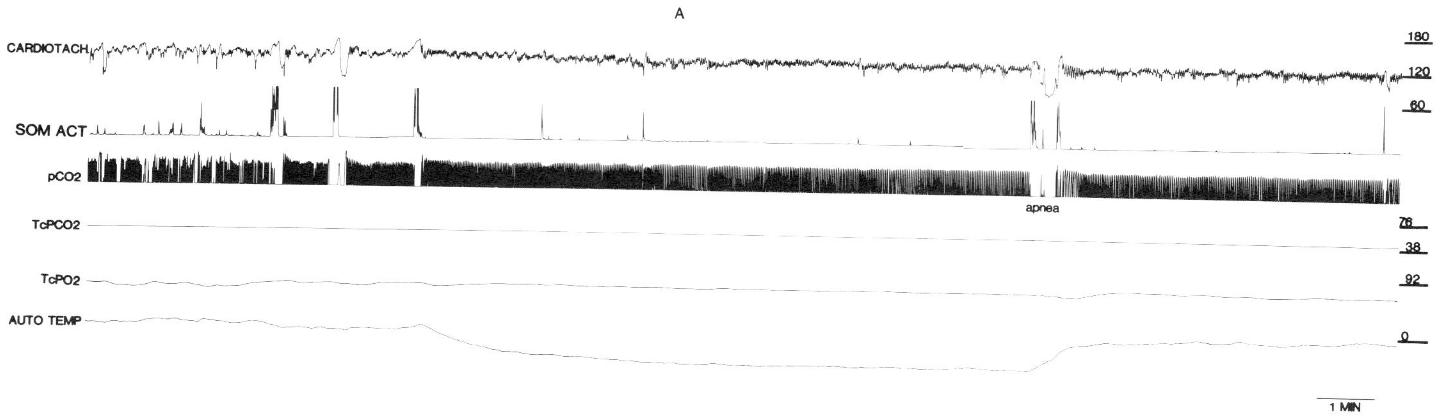

**Figure 3–28.** Polygraphic recording using a slow paper speed (0.5 mm/sec). The apnea shown here is identical to the one in Figure 3–27. TcP$co_2$ values ranged between 38 and 76 mm/Hg and the tcP$o_2$ was normal, approximately 70 mm/Hg. Calibration values for tcP$o_2$ are 0 and 92 mm/Hg. Notice the distinction between AS and QS by respiratory and cardiac rate regularity and somatic activity. Respiratory sinus arrhythmia tends to have a larger amplitude during QS.

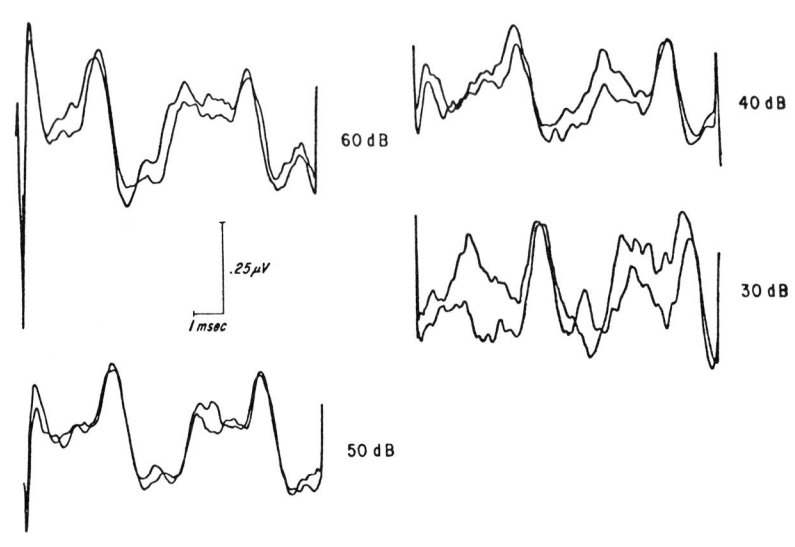

*Sleeping and waking disorders: indications and techniques*

**Figure 3-29.** Brainstem-evoked responses from a newborn infant (39 weeks gestational age). Each trace sums the response of 4096 clicks presented at 33⅓ per second. Superimposed traces are replications. Reprinted with permission *(9)*.

tion procedures is beyond the scope of this chapter. In our unit, we adhere to a calibration sequence that is performed prior to, and at the termination of, a monitoring session. The EEG and EMG are calibrated with a series of sine waves of various amplitudes and frequencies (Figure 3-24). Cardio tachometers and respiratory tachometers are calibrated as well. When the end expiratory $CO_2$ monitor is adapted to measure valid levels of $CO_2$, known gas concentrations must be used to calibrate this signal. Before and after four hours of transcutaneous monitoring, both electrodes are calibrated in vitro using gas mixtures at two levels of oxygen (0 and 92 mm/Hg) and $CO_2$ (38 and 76 mm/Hg) **31**. A small signal drift will sometimes be observed. An adjustment for this error has been proposed by Löfgren *(12)*.

Our data are recorded at two different paper speeds. Although a speed of at least 10 mm/sec has been recommended for EEG recordings, we have reduced this to 6 mm/sec (Figures 3-22 through 3-27). The rate of change in $tcPO_2$ and $tcPCO_2$ is low, and reduced paper speed facilitates the identification of patterns. The relationship between heart rate, respiration, somatic activity, and blood gases is therefore examined separately at a paper speed of 0.5 mm/sec.

Both computer and visual analyses are performed in our research unit. Every tracing is first scanned to identify aberrant physiologic patterns and artifacts. This information is used for immediate feedback to the clinical, monitoring, and engineering staff. State coding is then accomplished through visual analysis of the tracings. Identification of central, mixed, or obstructive apnea ($\geq$ 6 sec) and disorganized breathing is based on visual scanning as well. Conventions of state coding vary among investigators, both in terms of the number of variables used and the time frame for analysis. Anders et al. *(4)* recommend a 20–30 second epoch approach. We have used a one-minute epoch without regard to the duration of the episode *(13)*. Prechtl *(14)* disregards a state change of less than three minutes' duration, a convention derived from adult sleep recordings *(15)*.

Our data are taped for off-line analysis 32. Some preliminary analysis, however, is performed through preprocessing, such as signal integration and conversion to cardiac and respiratory rates. This is followed by on-line digitization and disk storage on a microcomputer. An elegant on- and off-line analysis system is reported in detail by Prechtl's group *(14,16–18)*. Extensive experience with off-line computer analysis of data *(6,19–22)* has revealed a need for vigorous quality control, strict adherence to protocol, and reliable recognition of artifacts. Many of the software packages developed contain an interactive component, so that the operator can select portions of the data for analysis *(21,22)*.

# Summary

Techniques for obtaining long-term polygraphic recordings in newborns and young infants have been described. Careful preparation and meticulous electrode application are key factors in successful monitoring. Variables such as apnea and paradoxical breathing require a special set of transducers for accurate identification. Determination of the factors that contribute to the apnea and the consequences of the apnea can be facilitated by transcutaneous measurement of blood gases. Decisions about data collection and analysis strategies such as paper speed, preprocessing, and visual versus computer analysis will be predicated on the objectives of each project. Whether in a clinical or research setting, the involvement of one or more trained research specialists backed by an electronic technician and engineer are essential for reliable and valid collection of data. In our unit, specially trained nurses function successfully in that role.

We acknowledge the contributions of Elvira Hoffman and Beverly Havens, who helped develop many of the techniques described here. We also thank Jiri Jilek, Don Lewis, and George Park for valuable technical feedback. Work described here was supported under NICHD Contracts Nos. NO1-HD-2-2777 and HD 4-2810 and Grant No. 1 RO1-HD-13689-01.

*Sleeping and waking disorders: indications and techniques*

# APPENDIX 3–A

## Equipment and Suppliers

1. Chest electrodes, pregelled and disposable, no. 65375–100, American Hospital Supply, Santa Ana, California 92705.
2. Skin temperature sensor, VWR Scientific, Yellow Springs, Ohio 45387.
3. Strain gauge, Parks Laboratory, Beaverton, Oregon 97005.
4. TcPO$_2$ and tcPCO$_2$ electrodes, Novametrix Medical Systems, Inc., Wallingford, Connecticut 06492.
5. Silver cup electrodes (E5S), Grass Instrument Company, Quincy, Massachusetts 02169.
6. Ear clips, Grass Instrument Company, Quincy, Massachusetts 02169.
7. Eye movement sensor, American Hospital Supply, Santa Ana, California 92705.
8. Cannula, American Hospital Supply, Santa Ana, California 92705.
9. CPAP nasal cannula, Novametrix Medical Systems, Inc., Wallingford, Connecticut 06492.
10. Thermistor bead (Tenwal GB 32J2), Newark Electronics Company, Inglewood, Californnia 90304.
11. Microphone, ASC apnea monitor, Japan.
12. Somatic activity electrodes, American Hospital Supply, Santa Ana, California 92705.
13. Preamplifier, no. 3621, Burr-Brown Research Corporation, Tucson, Arizona 85706.
14. Temperature coupler.*
15. Brush impedance, no. 11–4307–06, Gould, Inc., Instrument System Division, Cleveland, Ohio 44114.
16. Strain gauge coupler.*
17. Transcutaneous gas monitor, Novametrix T Com, Novametrix Medical Systems, Inc., Wallingford, Connecticut 06492.
18. Evoked potential averager, Nicolet Instruments, Madison, Wisconsin 53711.
19. Eye movement coupler.*
20. CO$_2$ analyzer, no. LB-2, Beckman Instruments, Inc., Fullerton, California 92634.

*Items designed and assembled by our engineer, Mr. J. Jilek.

*Electronic monitoring in the newborn and young infant: technical guidelines*

21. Thermistor coupler.*
22. Extension connectors, KDC connecting wires, no. 65356, American Hospital Supply, Santa Ana, California 92705.
23. Electrode jelly, Beckman Instruments, Inc., Electronic Instrument Division, Schiller Park, Illinois 60176.
24. Hypoallergenic tape, no. 1533 (Micropore skin tone surgical tape), 3M Company, St. Paul, Minnesota 55101.
25. Contact gel adhesive rings, Novametrix Medical Systems, Inc., Wallingford, Connecticut 06492.
26. Electrode cream, Grass Instrument Company Quincy, Massachusetts 02169.
27. Surgical tape (Transpore), American Hospital Supply, Santa Ana, California 92705.
28. Gauze roll (Kerlix), no. 6715, Kendall Hospital Products Division, Chicago, Illinois 60607.
29. Video monitor and Shibaden CCTV camera HV-166, Pelco Sales, Inc., Gardena, California 90247.
30. Oscilloscope, no. 5103N, Tektronix, Beaverton, Oregon 97005.
31. Gas calibrator, no. 804, Novametrix Medical Systems, Inc., Wallingford, Connecticut 06492.
32. Tape recorder, Honeywell Test Instrument Division, Denver, Colorado 80217.

# APPENDIX 3–B

## SIGNAL LOG for INFANT RUN

Please write down any problems, otherwise OK it.
Please enter set number being used.

Starting (time) _____ (footage) _____

Patient's Name _____
Shift 1. _____ and _____
Shift 2. _____ and _____
End (time) _____ (footage) _____

| TIME | Time Code | EEG | EOG | S.A. | #1 St. Gauge | #2 St. Gauge | THER | $P_{CO_2}$ | MIC | RTAC | CTAC | $tcP_{O_2}$ | tc $P_{CO_2}$ | Auto Temp | Beh Code | ECG | Temp /Hum | COMMENTS |
|---|---|---|---|---|---|---|---|---|---|---|---|---|---|---|---|---|---|---|
| 1700 | | | | | | | | | | | | | | | | | | |
| 1800 | | | | | | | | | | | | | | | | | | |
| 1900 | | | | | | | | | | | | | | | | | | |
| 2000 | | | | | | | | | | | | | | | | | | |
| 2100 | | | | | | | | | | | | | | | | | | |
| 2200 | | | | | | | | | | | | | | | | | | |
| 2300 | | | | | | | | | | | | | | | | | | |
| 2400 | | | | | | | | | | | | | | | | | | |
| 0100 | | | | | | | | | | | | | | | | | | |
| 0200 | | | | | | | | | | | | | | | | | | |
| 0300 | | | | | | | | | | | | | | | | | | |
| 0400 | | | | | | | | | | | | | | | | | | |
| 0500 | | | | | | | | | | | | | | | | | | |
| 0600 | | | | | | | | | | | | | | | | | | |
| 0700 | | | | | | | | | | | | | | | | | | |
| 0800 | | | | | | | | | | | | | | | | | | |

Impedance Reading   LEEG _____   EMG _____   RESP. _____
                    REEG _____   ECG _____

# REFERENCES

1. Hofmann E, Havens B, Geidel S, Hoppenbrouwers T, Hodgman JE. Long-term, continuous monitoring of multiple physiological parameters in newborn and young infants. Acta Paediatr Scand 1977 [Suppl 266].
2. Harper RM, Hoppenbrouwers, T, and Ross SA. A New technique for long-term recording of eye movements in iinfants. Electroencephalogr Clin Neurophysiol 1976; 40:109–12.
3. Cabal L, Cruz H, Plajstek C, Yeh S, Siassi B, Hodgman J. Factors affecting heated transcutaneous $Po_2$ and unheated transcutaneous $Pco_2$ in preterm infants. Crit Care Med J 1980 (in press).
4. Anders T, Emde R, Parmelee A, eds. A manual of standardized terminology, techniques and criteria for scoring of states of sleep and wakefulness in newborn infants. Los Angeles: UCLA Brain Information Service: BRI Publications Office, 1971.
5. Metcalf DR. Some critical points in normal EEG ontogenesis. Electroencephalogr Clin Neurophysiol 1971; 30:163.
6. Sterman MB, Harper RM, Havens B, Hoppenbrouwers T, McGinty DJ, Hodgman JE. Quantitative analysis of infant EEG development during quiet sleep. Electroencephalogr Clin Neurophysiol 1977; 43:371–85.
7. Crowell D. Personal communication.
8. Peabody JL, Willis MM, Gregory GA, Severinghaus JW. Reliability of skin (tc)$Po_2$ electrode heating power as a continuous noninvasive monitor of mean arterial pressure in sick newborns. In: Huch A, Huch R, Lucey JF, eds. Continuous transcutaneous blood gas monitoring. Birth defects: original article series, Volume XV, Number 4. New York: Alan R Liss, Inc, 1979:127–33..
9. Schulman-Galambos C, Galambos R. Brain stem auditory-evoked responses in premature infants. J Speech Hear Res 1975; 18:456–65.
10. Stockard JJ, Stockard JE, Sharbrough FW. Nonpathologic factors influencing brainstem auditory evoked potentials. Am J EEG Technol 1978; 18:177–209.
11. Avery ME, Fletcher BD. The lung and its disorders in the newborn infant. 3rd ed. Philadelphia: WB Saunders, 1974.
12. Löfgren O. On transcutaneous $Po_2$ measurements in humans, some methodological, physiological and clinical studies. Litos Reprotryck i Malmö AB, 1978.
13. Hoppenbrouwers T, Hodgman JE, Harper RM, Hofmann E, Sterman MB, McGinty DJ. Polygraphic studies of normal infants during the first six months of life. III. Incidence of apnea and periodic breathing. Pediatrics 1977; 60:418–25.

14. Prechtl HFR. Clinical neurophysiology of early life. Contemporary clinical neurophysiology. Electroencephalogr Clin Neurophysiol 1972 [Suppl 34] 57–66.
15. Rechtschaffen A, Kales A, eds. A manual of standardized terminology, techniques and scoring system for sleep stages of human subjects. Los Angeles: UCLA Brain Information Service/Brain Research Institute, 1968.
16. Vos JE. Representation in the frequency domain of nonstationary EEG's. In: Dolce G, Künkel H, eds. CEAN—computerized EEG analysis. Stuttgart: Fischer, 1975: 41–50.
17. Scholten CA. Computer-Analyse van Polygrammen een Methodologisch Onderzoek. Groningen: Veenstra-Visser Offset, 1976.
18. O'Brien MJ, van Eykern LA. Monitoring the newborn's breathing by surface electromyography—research and clinical aspects. Presented at the International Conference on Foetal and Neonatal Physiological Measurements. Oxford: September 1979.
19. Harper RM, Hoppenbrouwers T, Sterman MB, McGinty DJ, Hodgman J. Polygraphic studies of normal infants during the first six months of life. I. Heart rate and variability as a function of state. Pediatr Res 1976; 10:945–51.
20. Hoppenbrouwers T, Harper RM, Hodgman JE, Sterman MB, McGinty DJ. Polygraphic studies of normal infants during the first six months of life. II. Respiratory rate and variability as a function of state. Pediatr Res 1978; 12:120–5.
21. Hoppenbrouwers T, Hodgman JE, Arakawa K, et al. Sleep apnea as part of a sequence of events: a comparison of three month old infants at low and increased risk for sudden infant death syndrome (SIDS). Neuropaediatrie 1978; 9:320–37.
22. Harper RM, Mason J. Computer analysis procedures. In: Hodgman JE, Sterman MB, Hoffman H, Stark R, eds. Ontogeny of sleep in cardiopulmonary regulation: Factors related to risk for the sudden infant death syndrome. In progress.

# FOUR
# THE SECOND DECADE

MARY A. CARSKADON

## Introduction

The second decade includes the time of life with the most rapid body growth and development beyond infancy. Accompanying the overt physical changes of puberty are the prodigious changes in hormonal secretion, psychological growth and development, and marked alterations in the social milieu. Thus the childlike 10-year-old, secure in the bosom of his family, becomes the awkward, rebellious, peer-oriented teenager who later transforms into a mature, independent young adult. The scope of this transformation is an important factor to be reckoned with in assessing sleep and sleep disorders of the second decade.

This period of life has often been cited as critical in a number of specific sleep disorders. Chief among these is narcolepsy, for which the typical age of onset has been specified within the second decade *(1–3)*. Periodic disorders of excessive sleepiness associated with psychological disturbance *(4,5)* or the menstrual cycle *(6)* have also been related to the adolescent years. In addition, recent reports suggest that insomnia complaints may also be frequent in teenagers *(7,8)*.

This chapter will review findings regarding sleep habits in the second decade. In addition, normative data will be presented for sleep and multiple sleep latency tests in subjects grouped using a simple pubertal-staging schema *(9)* who were recorded in a standard setting. A final section will offer suggestions for evaluating sleep in this age group and a brief appraisal of narcolepsy in adolescents.

## Surveys of Sleep Habits

### Early Adolescents

We have performed an evaluation of sleep habits in a small group of early adolescents using a 68-item sleep-habits questionnaire designed for this age group *(10,11)*. The forms were completed by 218 children, 120 girls (mean age = 11.7 years) and 98 boys (mean age = 11.6 years). In addition to items relating to specific sleep events (e.g., sleepwalking, bed-wetting, snoring), the questionnaire contained items relating to bedtimes, arising times, and the child's perceived reasons for going to bed or arising at specific times. An analysis of the children's responses was performed for chronological age: 10-year-olds, N = 35; 11-year-olds, N = 58; 12-year-olds, N = 78; 13-year-olds, N = 47.

Table 4–1 summarizes bedtime, arising time, and total sleep time (nocturnal) from these questionnaires. Several interesting trends were apparent. Children in each age group tended to go to bed and arise later on nonschool nights than on school nights, and these differences were greater in older children than in younger children. In the older children (12- and 13-year-olds), these trends were reflected by a significant difference between school and nonschool night total sleep times. Thus, although average total sleep time on school and nonschool nights in the 10-year-olds was 587 minutes, the 13-year-olds reported an average sleep time of 522 minutes on school nights and 562 minutes on nonschool nights.

The reasons children gave for going to bed or arising at specific times showed several interesting patterns. For example, over 50% of 10-year-old children had schoolnight bedtimes that were set by their parents, whereas only 19% of 13-year-olds gave that response. A similar trend, though involving fewer children, was apparent on nonschool nights. In terms of morning arousals, about 60% of the children were awakened by alarm or parent on school mornings, compared to about 4% on nonschool days. On the other hand, 70% of children reported that they "just wake up" on nonschool mornings, compared to 30% on school mornings. Age played a significant role in the reasons children gave for getting up on school mornings. That is, the 12- and 13-year-olds tended to be awakened by alarm or by parents on school mornings more frequently than the younger children; the younger children tended to awake spontaneously on school mornings more frequently than the older children.

We feel that these data suggest that sleep and nonschool nights is less controlled by outside influences and more naturalistic than on school nights in these young adolescents. At each age, more children reported going to bed when "sleepy" and "just waking up" on nonschool nights. In the younger children, school-night bedtime was controlled primarily by parents, and a substantial number reported spontaneous arousals even on school mornings. Older children, however, reported more social control of school night bedtimes (homework, television), and well over half of the 12- and 13-year-olds relied on an external agency (alarm, parents) to wake them on school mornings. Thus younger children appeared to sleep roughly the same amount on school and nonschool nights. But the older children appeared to use nonschool-night sleep to recover from losing sleep during the week. These data lead to the speculation that the need for sleep may not be changing across this span of years, but that school and social pressures on older children may decrease the amount of time they have available for sleep.

These young adolescents reported relatively few sleep complaints. On a global questionnaire item, approximately 10% responded that they have a "sleep problem." Whether or not it was perceived as a problem, 19% said that it usually takes them 30

**Table 4-1** Reported Sleep Habits in Early Adolescents (24-Hour Clock Time, SD in Minutes)

| Parameter | 10-yr-olds Mean | SD | 11-yr-olds Mean | SD | 12-yr-olds Mean | SD | 13-yr-olds Mean | SD |
|---|---|---|---|---|---|---|---|---|
| *Bedtime* | | | | | | | | |
| School | 2122 | (34) | 2137 | (39) | 2146 | (34) | 2214 | (40) |
| Nonschool | 2222* | (46) | 2239* | (60) | 2300* | (49) | 2332* | (74) |
| *Arising time* | | | | | | | | |
| School | 0704 | (71) | 0705 | (26) | 0703 | (28) | 0656 | (26) |
| Nonschool | 0807* | (70) | 0808* | (73) | 0840* | (65) | 0855* | (64) |
| *Sleep Time* | | | | | | | | |
| School | 587 | (30) | 569 | (38) | 557 | (47) | 522 | (49) |
| Nonschool | 587 | (84) | 566 | (82) | 580† | (68) | 562† | (88) |

NOTE: Significant differences between school and nonschool nights (*t* test for related means) are indicated as follows:
*p < .001
†p < .02

minutes or longer to fall asleep; 5% reported three or more arousals per night; and fewer than 1% stated that they have trouble (greater than 30 minutes) returning to sleep if they wake up during the night. Napping at least once per week was reported by 10% of the children, and 13% reported having fallen asleep in school at least once in the present school year.

## Older Adolescents

Table 4–2 lists the reported sleep times of 4424 entry-level university students surveyed by Webb and Agnew *(12)*. We assume that this group was heavily weighted in favor of older adolescents. Over three-quarters of the group reported sleeping from 6.5 to 8.5 hours each night. A rough extrapolation from these data suggest an average sleep time very close to 7.5 hours for the entire group. Data from Williams's group *(13)*, who set laboratory recording times according to "each person's usual bedtime until his usual time of arising," showed an average time in bed of 502 minutes for girls and 511 minutes for boys who were 13 to 15 years old. In the group aged 16 to 19 years, the girls were in bed for 480 minutes and the boys for 475 minutes. Thus, there appears to be an overall reduction of reported sleep time across the second decade that amounts to a total of approximately two hours. In the older adolescents, as in the younger children, however, there remains a question of the factors that underlie this reduction. For example, Webb and Agnew *(14)* have reported a study of students whose weekends and weekdays showed a pattern similar to our findings in younger adolescents. In the sleep-diary study reported by Webb and Agnew *(14)*, weekday sleep averaged 7.4 hours, whereas weekend sleep averaged 8.3 hours. Thus it appears that older adolescents have a tendency to restrict sleep on school nights and compensate by sleeping longer on the weekends.

Along with these changes in reported sleep time, older adolescents report greater difficulty with daytime sleepiness and nocturnal sleep than early adolescents. In an unpublished survey that we made of 311 college students (196 men, 114 women, mean

**Table 4–2** Sleep Length Report in 4424 University Students

| Reported Sleep Time | Men (N = 2389) | Women (N = 2035) |
|---|---|---|
| < 5.5 hours | 1.3% | 0.8% |
| 5.5 to < 6.5 hours | 6.6 | 9.7 |
| 6.5 to < 7.5 hours | 27.8 | 31.0 |
| 7.5 to < 8.5 hours | 48.6 | 44.2 |
| 8.5 to < 9.5 hours | 12.4 | 11.3 |
| > 9.5 hours | 3.4 | 3.0 |

SOURCE: Webb WB and Agnew HW Jr. *Sleep and Dreams*. Dubuque, Iowa: Wm. C. Brown Company, 1973, p. 8.

age = 19.7 years), 48% of the group responded "yes" to the question, "Are you sleepy during the day?" At least one nap per week was reported by 39% of the students. Thirty-six percent said that they had difficulty staying awake in afternoon classes (compared to 11% of 10- to 13-year-olds in our previous survey *(11)*; and 24% reported actually having fallen asleep in class (compared to 13% of 10- to 13-year-olds).

In a survey of 219 students (109 males, 110 females) aged 16 to 19 years, White and his colleagues *(8)* reported a sleep latency greater than 45 minutes in 24%. Price et al. *(7)*, who surveyed 627 eleventh and twelfth graders aged 15 to 18 years, found that 32% reported difficulty falling asleep. By way of comparison, 19% of the 10- to 13-year-olds in our previous survey *(11)* reported a sleep latency of greater than 30 minutes. The Price et al. *(7)* subjects reported numerous nighttime arousals in 20% of the cases, compared to 5% (three or more wakes per night) in the younger children *(11)*. Thirty-three percent of the eleventh- and twelfth-grade students said they experienced problems returning to sleep when they awakened in the night. Fewer than 1% of 10- to 13-year-olds reported a similar difficulty.

One final, very interesting finding reported by Price et al. *(7)* was the number of students who reported that they "enjoy staying up at night." Overall, approximately 64% of the students reported that they enjoyed staying up. In a group of "chronic poor sleepers," this report was given by 79.5%. This finding suggests the possibility that a certain number of cases of adolescent insomnia may be related to the delayed sleep phase syndrome *(15)*.

The extent to which reported difficulties with sleep and daytime sleepiness in older adolescents interact with the reduction in reported nocturnal sleep is unclear. One may speculate that the increasing daytime sleepiness reported by older adolescents is related to the declining nocturnal sleep time. Sleep and daytime-sleepiness findings reported below suggest that a maturational augmentation of daytime sleepiness may also influence the rise in reported daytime sleepiness that occurs during the adolescent years.

# Normative Values—Nocturnal Sleep

## Background

The normal development of sleep patterns, particularly in the first year of life, has been given much attention in recent years. Many studies have also described the typical nocturnal patterns of the young child, emphasizing the large amounts of NREM slow-wave (stages 3 and 4) sleep that is present in the early part of the night. These patterns are present as the child enters the second decade and change to the typical adult patterns over the course of the adolescent period. Previous studies have included an examination of daytime naps in children between seven and nine years of age *(16)* and an evaluation of nocturnal sleep patterns in preadolescent children *(17)*. Perhaps the most ambitious work in this area is the "atlas" of Williams et al. *(13)*. Other studies of sleep in adolescents include the 1972 study of the Williams group *(18)* and the longitudinal study of Karacan et al. *(19)*. Significant findings from these studies include a reduction in total sleep time across the four years of active puberty *(19)*; a slight increase in stage 4 sleep from preadolescence to midpuberty, with a subsequent decline in young adulthood, although the proportionate amount of REM sleep remained constant *(13,18)*; and two to five hours less sleep in preadolescent male children than in adults *(17)*. Certain of these findings are not substantiated in the data presented below.

A significant difficulty that accrues to research on adolescents concerns the basis for grouping data. Clearly, gender is often a significant factor and is one that must be assessed. Grouping data by age, however, is a more complex problem. Many of the changes one might expect to see in adolescents are more likely to be related to pubertal/hormonal changes than strictly to age, although age is certainly correlated with these variables. The Williams group *(13)* acknowledged this problem by selecting premenstrual girls for their 10- to 12-year-old group and postmenstrual girls for older groups. Even so, many maturational changes take place well before menarche. On the average, for example, menarche does not occur until Tanner stage 4 is reached *(20)*. In addition, it has been shown that nocturnal augmentation of luteinizing hormone can occur in children at Tanner stages 2 and 3 *(21)*.

The data presented below (and in the section on multiple sleep latency tests) are included in an attempt to provide normative values from the second decade that can be more useful in a clinical setting than past compilations. Several factors should facilitate clinical use of these data. First, standard data-gathering procedures have been used throughout. Thus, for example, bedtimes are known and have been standardized across subject groups. Second, data are grouped according to a simple, but clinically relevant, system of maturational staging. Third, data are presented for each of three consecutive nights that subjects were recorded. Thus clinics that record only a single night can utilize the norms without extrapolating for first-night effects. Finally, data for older adolescents have been gathered in two groups. In one group, the data were gathered in a manner identical to that used in younger adolescents, facilitating direct comparisons across the second decade. In a second group, data were collected in a similar manner, but with a shorter nocturnal bedtime that may be more comparable to actual clinical practice in older adolescents.

## Subjects

Subjects in the younger groups (ages 10 to 16) were recorded at the Stanford Summer Sleep Camp *(11,22)* as part of a longitudinal study of sleep and daytime sleepiness. A total of 52 three-day sessions were recorded in 24 children who had no personal or family history of sleep disorders. Several children included in this presentation have been evaluated on multiple occasions. In these cases, the recording sessions were separated by 11 to 13 months. The data have been grouped according to pubertal status using Tanner staging of secondary sexual development *(9)*. (Tanner staging will be more fully described later in this chapter. To preview briefly, Tanner stages range from a score of 1, which indicates prepubertal development, to 5, which indicates adult maturity.) Tanner staging was performed by a pediatrician during each Sleep Camp session, except in the first year of the study. Children recorded in the first year were excluded from the group unless subsequent Tanner staging was performed within one year. In the latter cases, the first-year Tanner stage was determined using norms for the duration of intervals between pubertal stages *(23)*.

The Tanner stage 1 group included 15 sessions recorded in 11 subjects (four girls, seven boys), with repeat sessions in four children. The children in this group ranged in age from 10.1 to 14.6 years, with a mean age of 11.6. At Tanner stage 2, one session was recorded in each of 12 individuals, including six girls and six boys. Ages ranged from 11.2 to 13.5, with a mean age of 12.5. Ten sessions were recorded at Tanner stage 3 in nine individual subjects (five girls, four boys). The mean age was 13.4 (range = 12.2 to 15.2). Six children (two girls, four boys) were recorded in eight sessions at Tanner stage 4. The group ranged in age from 13 to 15.7 (mean = 14.1). In the Tanner stage 5 group, six children (four girls, two boys) were recorded in seven sessions. The Tanner stage 5 subjects ranged in age from 14 to 16 years, with a mean age of 15 years.

Data from two groups of older adolescents recorded under similar circumstances (but for other studies) will also be presented. The first group of older adolescents was recorded with a ten-hour bedtime, as were the younger subjects. This group included eight subjects (five women and three men). The ages of this group ranged from 17 to 20 years, with a mean age of 18.9. The second group of older adolescents was recorded with an eight-hour time in bed. This group of 14 subjects included eight women and six men whose ages ranged from 18 to 20 years. The mean age of these subjects was 19 years.

## Data-Gathering Methods

All data presented below are taken from the first three consecutive days that subjects were in the laboratory. The first recording session of these three days was always Night 1. (Day 1 in the next section on the multiple sleep latency tests always followed this first recording night.) All subjects were recorded in individual, darkened bedrooms using a standard sleep-recording montage. This montage included EEG from $C_3$ or $C_4$ referred to the opposite $A_1$ or $A_2$ placement (on the earlobe or mastoid). $O_1$ and $O_2$ were also applied and were used to assist in visualizing sleep onset for subjects with poorly defined central alpha. EOG was recorded on two channels from the right (ROC) and left (LOC) outer canthi, referenced to the opposite $A_1$ or $A_2$. EMG was recorded from any two of three electrodes placed on the surface of the chin. All sleep periods were recorded on Grass model 7 polygraphs at a paper speed of 10 mm/sec. EEG and EOG channels were calibrated at 50 μV/cm. In subjects aged 17 or older, EEG was recorded with a low-frequency cutoff of 0.3 cps and a high-frequency filter of 35 cps. In younger adolescents, the EEG was recorded using a low-frequency cutoff of 1.0 cps and a high-frequency filter of 35 cps. All sleep records were scored in 30-second epochs according to the standard criteria of Rechtschaffen and Kales *(24)*.

In the younger adolescents (Tanner stage 1 to Tanner stage 5 groups) and one group of older adolescents, bedtime was 2200 on each night, with minor variations from night to night. (In four of the younger subjects, the bedtime was 2300.) In the second group of older subjects, bedtime was midnight. All subjects remained in bed until 0800 (except for brief excursions to the bathroom). This arising time did not vary by more than one minute in any study.

Much of the data recorded in the Tanner stage 1 through Tanner stage 5 subjects was compared directly to gender- and age-matched subjects from the Williams et al. study *(13)* in a previous report *(11)*. These comparisons showed that the subjects were roughly comparable and that significant differences in the two studies were largely attributable to methodological differences between the studies, including recording variables (Williams et al. did not record EMG), scoring-epoch length (Williams et al. used a one-minute scoring epoch), and variations in the length of the recording period.

## Nocturnal Sleep Parameters

The most useful format for presenting the nocturnal sleep parameters was felt to be a presentation of the mean values (and standard deviations) for the absolute minutes. These data can then be readily converted by those who prefer percentages using the total dark time (time in bed) or total sleep-period time (total sleep time plus wake after sleep onset) as the denominator. A brief description of the sleep parameters may be helpful.

- *Total dark time:* elapsed minutes from lights-out to the end of the recording session (end of night).
- *Total wake time:* includes all wakefulness recorded within the dark period.
- *Wake after sleep onset:* includes all wakefulness recorded after the onset of sleep, except periods of wakefulness contiguous with the end of the night.
- Thus final arousals are not included in this parameter.
- *Latency to stage 1 sleep:* elapsed minutes from lights-out to the first 30-second epoch scored as stage 1 sleep.
- *Latency to stage 2 sleep:* elapsed minutes from lights-out to the first 30-second epoch scored as stage 2 sleep.
- *Stages 1, 2, 3, 4, and REM time:* all minutes of these sleep stages scored using standard criteria *(24)*.
- *Total sleep time:* all minutes of sleep recorded during the dark period.
- *Latency to REM:* elapsed minutes from sleep onset to the first 30-second epoch scored as REM sleep.
- *Spontaneous arousals:* number of subjects who were awake for one minute or longer immediately before the end of night.

Tables 4A 1–6 present the nocturnal sleep data from subjects recorded with a ten-hour time in bed. The values in each group are listed for each of three consecutive nights. Gender comparisons (*t* test) were made for each parameter in each group; this analysis showed no consistent effect of gender within or across subject groups. Because there was an absence of gender effects, the data were pooled across gender within each group.

These data were also analyzed using analysis of variance for day and group effects. Significant findings and mean values are listed in Tables 4-3 and 4-4. The night-to-night changes were consistent with "first-night effects" (25), showing increased total wake time, wake after sleep onset, latency to REM sleep, and reduced total sleep and REM sleep on the first night. Conspicuously absent from significant days effect was latency to stage 1 or stage 2 sleep. One might expect, however, that youngsters in a clinical setting would have a longer first-night delay to sleep onset if anxiety levels were high.

Table 4-4 shows an interesting pattern of changes in nocturnal sleep across the second decade. Given the stable bedtimes and arising times in the six subject groups, slow-wave sleep stages (3 and 4) tended to decline and stage 2 sleep to increase across the second decade. Of interest was the apparent plateau of these changes in the Tanner stage 5 subjects and the older adolescents. The group effect on REM latency appeared to be due primarily to the high average REM latency in the Tanner stage 1 group. It should be noted that REM latency had the highest variance of virtually all sleep parameters in each group. It should also be emphasized that total sleep time was not significantly affected by group. Thus, when each individual from age 10 to age 20 was given an equal opportunity to sleep at night, the average total sleep time was unchanged.

Table 4-5 lists the sleep parameters for older adolescents who were given an eight-hour time in bed (midnight to 0800). Gender comparisons ($t$ test) for this group showed no significant differences on any parameter. No significant days effects were apparent from analysis of variance, although inspection of the mean values showed trends similar to those seen in the other groups. A comparison of the two older adolescent groups showed that the chief effect of the eight-hour bedtime was an overall reduction in stage 2 sleep time. REM and slow-wave sleep were apparently unaffected by the shorter time in bed.

**Table 4-3** Significant Effects of Days on Nocturnal Sleep (Time in Minutes)

|  | Mean Values |  |  |  |
| --- | --- | --- | --- | --- |
|  | Day 1 | Day 2 | Day 3 | $p <$ |
| Total wake time | 63 | 38 | 44 | .001 |
| Wake after sleep onset | 28 | 11 | 16 | .001 |
| REM sleep time | 99 | 118 | 115 | .001 |
| Total sleep time | 512 | 546 | 542 | .005 |
| Latency to REM | 145 | 116 | 109 | .002 |

**Table 4-4** Significant Effects of Groups on Nocturnal Sleep (Time in Minutes)

|  | Tanner 1 | Tanner 2 | Tanner 3 | Tanner 4 | Tanner 5 | Older Adolescents* | $p <$ |
|---|---|---|---|---|---|---|---|
| Stage 2 time | 248 | 255 | 264 | 280 | 288 | 293 | .001 |
| Stage 3 time | 35 | 34 | 34 | 26 | 20 | 26 | .001 |
| Stage 4 time | 94 | 84 | 78 | 76 | 59 | 62 | .001 |
| Latency to REM | 150 | 110 | 102 | 125 | 124 | 119 | .01 |

*Older adolescents in the group with a bedtime of 2200 to 0800.

*The second decade*

**Table 4–5** Nocturnal Sleep in Older Adolescents
(Time in Minutes, Bedtime = Midnight to 0800, N = 14)

|  | Night 1 |  | Night 2 |  | Night 3 |  |
|---|---|---|---|---|---|---|
|  | Mean | SD | Mean | SD | Mean | SD |
| Total dark time | 476 | 4 | 478 | 3 | 478 | 2 |
| Total wake time | 44 | 34 | 34 | 34 | 25 | 18 |
| Wake after sleep onset | 17 | 17 | 17 | 30 | 5 | 6 |
| Latency to stage 1 | 24 | 27 | 17 | 18 | 18 | 16 |
| Latency to stage 2 | 31 | 28 | 21 | 19 | 23 | 18 |
| Stage 1 time | 34 | 9 | 31 | 14 | 26 | 5 |
| Stage 2 time | 231 | 35 | 221 | 39 | 225 | 26 |
| Stage 3 time | 23 | 7 | 28 | 11 | 29 | 16 |
| Stage 4 time | 56 | 22 | 56 | 23 | 68 | 18 |
| REM time | 82 | 18 | 92 | 33 | 99 | 24 |
| Total sleep time | 426 | 33 | 437 | 34 | 447 | 22 |
| Latency to REM | 120 | 52 | 85 | 52 | 83 | 35 |
| Number with spontaneous arousal | 1 | ... | 1 | ... | 2 | ... |

# Normative Values—Multiple Sleep Latency Test

## Background

Compilations of sleep data in adolescents have not attempted to evaluate the night and the day in the same subjects. Thus, as regards daytime function in children and adolescents, one must rely on anecdotal information. During waking hours, a prepubertal child is generally thought of as consistently alert and energetic. Often in the teenage years, however, the child who had exhibited this abundant exuberance begins to prefer to sleep late in the mornings and perhaps to take an afternoon nap. This stereotypic view of adolescence is familiar to most of us, and most parents consider it to be "just another phase" their child is passing through. Others, however, may worry about the child's health or wonder if he is taking drugs.

Of clinical interest, and of special interest to parents with narcolepsy, is the significance of these changes in children who may be at risk for developing excessive daytime sleepiness. At what point do these "typical adolescent patterns" reach a pathologic level, and when should there be clinical intervention?

This section outlines our normative multiple sleep latency test findings in control subjects. These data should provide a useful guide for clinical assessment of daytime sleepiness in the second decade.

## Subjects

Normative multiple sleep latency test findings are presented for subjects included in the previous section.

## Data-Gathering Methods

As described previously, subjects were recorded during three-day sessions in the laboratory. Bedtimes were set at 2200 to 0800 for Tanner stage 1–5 subjects and one group of older adolescents, and midnight to 0800 in the second group of older adolescents. The multiple sleep latency testing procedures used in these studies differed somewhat from the usual clinical testing procedures and will therefore be described in detail.

On each day, the first sleep latency test (SLT) was started at 0930. Thus, in each case, testing was begun at 90 minutes after the end of the night. The test was repeated at two-hour intervals until 1930. Each subject, therefore, received six sleep latency tests per day. (That six SLTs were given daily is important to note when one considers the daily mean SLT values.) Subjects were continuously observed to ensure that no sleep occurred between SLTs. Meals were served before the 0930 SLT and after the 1130 and 1730 SLTs. Sedentary activities (performance testing) were scheduled for 60–75 minutes at 1000, 1400, and 2000.

For each sleep latency test, the following standard procedures were used. All vigorous activity was suspended 15 minutes before the test. Subjects were requested to use the bathroom facilities at this time if necessary. Five minutes before the test, subjects were asked to lie in bed and perform several simple calibrating maneuvers (open eyes, close eyes, look right, look left, etc.). Subjects usually wore their street clothes, with shoes off, during the SLTs. Subjects were instucted to "Please lie quietly, keep your eyes closed, and try to fall asleep," and the bedroom lights were extinguished and door closed to mark the beginning of the test.

The recording montage and filter settings were as described for nocturnal recordings, with the exception that chin EMG was usually not recorded during the SLTs after the first day. On the first day of each session, the SLTs lasted 20 minutes, whether or not subjects fell asleep. On subsequent days, the SLT was terminated at 20 minutes if there was no sleep or after three consecutive epochs of sleep (usually stage 1) if sleep occurred. The SLTs were later scored in 30-second epochs according to the Rechtschaffen and Kales [24] sleep-stage scoring criteria, and the elapsed time from lights-out to the first epoch of sleep was obtained as the SLT score. (The use of this sleep-onset criterion is fully described in other reports [11,26]). Because of the procedures used in obtaining these data, the appearance of sleep-onset REM periods could be assessed only on the first recording day of each session.

## Multiple Sleep Latency Test Results

The data presented in the accompanying tables list the group mean (and standard deviation) values for each daily sleep latency test and for subjects' overall mean daily scores. Because means were calculated using a value of 20 minutes when no sleep occurred during the test, we have also listed the number of subjects who did *not* fall asleep on any of the tests. The mean values in these cases are therefore spuriously low because of the built-in ceiling created by limiting the tests to 20 minutes. In addition, the occurrence of sleep-onset REM periods is noted in the tables.

Tables 4B 1–6 list the multiple sleep latency test findings in the five Tanner stage groups and in the group of older adolescents given a ten-hour time in bed. Gender comparisons (*t* test) showed no consistent significant effects of gender. Analysis of variance was performed for days and groups. There was no significant days effect on the SLT parameters. Table 4–6 lists the mean values for significant effects attributed to group. These data show a trend for reduced daily mean SLT values reflected in reduced SLT scores at 0930, 1130, 1330, and 1530. Previous analysis of these data across the five Tanner stages *(22)* showed a significant reduction in SLT scores at Tanner stages 3 and 4 and suggested that the scores remained low at Tanner stage 5. The additional data on older adolescents confirm that SLTs remain low after Tanner stage 3.

Table 4–7 lists the SLT findings in older adolescents permitted to sleep only eight hours. Gender analyses (*t* tests) in this group also showed no significant differences, nor were any significant changes attributable to a days effect (analysis of variance). Comparisons of SLT scores between the two groups of older adolescents showed a consistent trend for lower scores in the group with an eight-hour time in bed.

# Assessing Sleep Disorders in Adolescents

## Introduction

Many adolescents who have a sleep complaint do not come to the attention of a sleep disorders center until the disturbance begins to affect school performance or has a disruptive effect on family life. Children who come to a sleep center, therefore, may not be aware of the problems (as in the cases of sleepwalking or night terrors) or may be less concerned about the disorders than their parents or teachers. In the older adolescents, who have begun to take a greater interest in the body and bodily functions, the patients may tend to exaggerate the significance of the complaints. Many of these adolescent patients may, apart from their sleep complaints, be "healthy adolescents."

Initial screening of these patients should make allowances for their ages and take into account the special physical, psychological, and social dynamics of the adolescent. One example of an adolescent-screening paradigm has been presented in a recent symposium on adolescent medicine *(27)*. This symposium also contains very helpful reference materials for normative values in the evaluation of adolescents *(28)*. Relevant sleep and daytime-sleepiness history information can be obtained from parents, teachers, and siblings; but the child should always be consulted as well, because his perception of the problem often differs from that of observers. When sleep diaries are

**Table 4-6** Effects of Groups on Multiple Sleep Latency Tests (Time to Sleep Onset in Minutes)

| Time of Test | Mean Values | | | | | |
|---|---|---|---|---|---|---|
| | Tanner 1 | Tanner 2 | Tanner 3 | Tanner 4 | Tanner 5 | Older Adolescents* | $p <$ |
| 0930 | 19.6 | 18.7 | 15.9 | 16.0 | 17.6 | 15.9 | .002 |
| 1130 | 19.0 | 18.8 | 13.3 | 15.2 | 18.3 | 15.4 | .001 |
| 1330 | 18.6 | 17.1 | 16.1 | 13.7 | 13.6 | 14.3 | .001 |
| 1530 | 18.5 | 17.9 | 16.1 | 14.0 | 12.5 | 11.8 | .001 |
| Daily mean | 19.0 | 18.5 | 16.1 | 15.7 | 16.6 | 15.7 | .001 |

*Older adolescents in the group with a bedtime of 2200 to 0800.

**Table 4–7** Multiple Sleep Latency Tests in Older Adolescents
(Time to Sleep Onset in Minutes, Bedtime = Midnight to 0800, N = 14)

| Time of Test | Day 1 Mean | SD | Day 2 Mean | SD | Day 3 Mean | SD |
|---|---|---|---|---|---|---|
| 0930 | 14.8 | 5.9 | 13.0 | 6.2 | 12.9 | 7.3 |
| 1130 | 12.2* | 6.8 | 11.1 | 7.5 | 13.1 | 6.3 |
| 1330 | 12.2* | 6.7 | 11.8 | 7.4 | 11.7 | 6.8 |
| 1530 | 10.2 | 6.1 | 10.6 | 6.8 | 12.6 | 7.4 |
| 1730 | 16.3* | 4.6 | 15.4 | 6.2 | 15.4 | 6.0 |
| 1930 | 17.1 | 4.8 | 16.0 | 6.5 | 17.8 | 3.8 |
| Daily mean | 13.8 | 3.9 | 12.9 | 5.4 | 13.9 | 4.5 |
| Number with no sleep | 1 | ... | 1 | ... | 1 | ... |

*REM sleep in one female subject at 1130 and in another female subject at 1330 and 1730.

obtained, it may also be helpful to have the patient and parent (or roommate) complete them simultaneously.

An accurate drug- and alcohol-ingestion history is often of particular interest when evaluating sleep complaints. Although parents may be able to provide an adequate description of prescription medications, the adolescent himself must be consulted to obtain information regarding nonprescription-drug use. Given the ready access the modern adolescent has to potent drugs, whether from his parents' medicine cabinet or on the streets, this aspect of the patient's history should be given careful attention.

Because the normative sleep data presented in this chapter emphasize Tanner stages of development, this staging system will be described in sufficient detail so that (along with standard photographs that may be found in a number of sources (9,28)) the clinical polysomnographer will feel comfortable using the system.

## Tanner Staging and Sleep-Related Hormone Secretion

Tanner staging (9) of adolescent development relies on rating genital development and pubic hair growth in boys and breast development and pubic hair growth in girls. These four ratings are made on a scale of 1 to 5; pubic hair growth ratings may be considered comparable between the sexes. The ratings, which are based on visual inspection, acquire greater reliability when performed longitudinally; but according to Tanner (9), a fair degree of accuracy can be achieved with cross-sectional ratings. The pubic hair growth ratings are apparently more reliable than genital or breast development ratings when only a single determination is made.

Table 4–8 paraphrases the descriptions of adolescent development staging given by Tanner (9). The first sign of puberty in boys is generally enlargement of the scrotum and testes; whereas in girls, breast budding tends to be the first sign of puberty (60%

*Sleeping and waking disorders: indications and techniques*

**Table 4–8**  Tanner Stages of Adolescent Development

*I. Genital Development in Boys*
- Stage 1: Preadolescent; testes, scrotum, and penis retain size and proportion of early childhood
- Stage 2: Enlargement of scrotum and testes; reddening and texture change in scrotal skin; little or no enlargement of penis
- Stage 3: Lengthening of penis; further growth of testes and scrotum
- Stage 4: Enlargement of penis, with growth in breadth and development of glans; further growth of testes and scrotum; increased darkening of scrotal skin
- Stage 5: Adult size and shape of genitalia.

*II. Breast Development in Girls*
- Stage 1: Preadolescent; elevation of papilla only
- Stage 2: Breast bud stage; elevation of breast and papilla as a small mound; enlargement of areolar diameter
- Stage 3: Further enlargement and elevation of breast and areola, with no separation of their contours
- Stage 4: Projection of areola and papilla to form secondary mound above level of breast
- Stage 5: Mature stage; projection of papilla only; recession of areola to general breast contour

*III. Pubic Hair Growth in Girls and Boys*
- Stage 1: No pubic hair
- Stage 2: Sparse growth of long, slightly pigmented, downy hair; hair is straight or only slightly curled; hair appears chiefly at the base of the penis or along the labia
- Stage 3: Hair is much darker, coarser, and more curled; hair is spread sparsely over junction of pubes
- Stage 4: Hair resembles adult in type, but is in much smaller area; hair has not spread to the medial surface of the thighs
- Stage 5: Adult in quantity and type; distribution has spread to medial surface of thighs but not up linea alba or above the base of the "inverse triangle"

SOURCE: Tanner JM. Growth at adolescence, 2nd ed. Oxford: Blackwell, 1962.

of cases). There remains some question regarding the accuracy of judging intermediate stages of adolescent development in girls from breast development. According to Tanner (9), the stage 4 occurrence of the areolar mound is not present or is slight in about half of girls, and when it does appear, it may last into adulthood. In about 60% of girls, menarche begins at Tanner stage 4 (28). It should also be kept in mind that girls usually enter puberty at a younger age than boys. On the other hand, there is great variability in the ages at which children attain the various developmental stages (27).

Sleep-related changes in the secretion of the gonadotropins, luteinizing hormone (LH) and follicle-stimulating hormone (FSH), and sex steroids occur in specific relationship to puberty. In older children, before physical changes appear (i.e., Tanner stage 1), there is a sleep-associated rise in gonadotropin secretion *(29)*. This prepubescent sleep-related release of gonadotropins leads to testosterone secretion in boys and estradiol secretion in girls and is thought to be the initiator of puberty *(30)*. During this time, the waking secretory pattern maintains a prepubertal level.

This nocturnal augmentation of gonadotropin secretion is maintained during early (Tanner stage 2) and midpuberty (Tanner stage 3) *(29)*. In midpuberty, the peak nocturnal secretory levels are higher, and waking levels of gonadotropins are also increased *(29)*. One study of sleep reversal in midpubertal boys showed that LH secretion remained high during nocturnal waking and that the LH concentration rose during daytime sleep *(31)*. Thus, the nocturnal gonadotropin secretion during puberty appears to be related to a circadian secretory pattern on which is superimposed a sleep-associated augmentation.

In late puberty (Tanner stage 4), the nocturnal differential in gonadotropin secretion continues, and waking levels are well above prepubertal values *(29)*. In adulthood (Tanner stage 5), the gonadotropin secretion achieves adult levels showing no further sleep-related augmentation *(29)*.

## Sleep Recordings in the Second Decade

Most children and adolescents have an intrinsic fascination with the gadgets used to record sleep. Polysomnographic technologists should schedule plenty of time for a tour of the lab and a thorough, though simple (especially in younger adolescents), explanation of the techniques and apparatus. Younger children may wish to have a parent present during the hookup and explanations. In addition, a great deal of effort should be spent reassuring the young patient that the procedures are entirely harmless and that the machines will not give them electrical shocks, read their minds, or reveal the content of their dreams.

As mentioned previously, a low-frequency filter of 1.0 cps was used to record EEG in the younger adolescent control subjects presented in the chapter. This setting was used to reduce the effects of "sweat artifact" that is sometimes a problem in children (and adults) when air conditioning is not available. This filter setting is rarely a problem in youngsters because slow waves are so predominant in stages 3 and 4 that the faster time constant does not appear to affect scoring.

The amplitude of slow waves in certain youngsters may, however, create problems if the pens block. Occasionally, we have recalibrated the EEG channels at a lower sensitivity (e.g., 100 µV/cm) to avoid this problem. If recalibration is performed, the scorer must be certain to keep it in mind when measuring amplitudes for stage 3 and stage 4 sleep.

Another problem that can arise in scoring the nocturnal sleep stages in these subjects, particularly in the younger adolescents, is missing the first REM period. The chief difficulty that leads to this problem is the brevity of the first REM period when it appears with a relatively short latency. In our control subjects, we have found a significant direct correlation (0.68) between the latency to REM sleep and the length of the first REM period. In approximately 10% of the nights recorded in the control subjects, the duration of the first REM period was two minutes or shorter. It is clear that careless scoring, or even the careful use of a one-minute scoring epoch, could miss these brief REM-sleep episodes.

Multiple sleep latency testing in this age group will also require more time and attention than in adults. Most adolescents tend to be more active than adults and will probably require greater supervision during the breaks between SLTs. If youngsters are physically active between tests, it is a good idea to suspend such activity during the 15 minutes before the start of the test. If activity has been strenuous, electrode impedances should be checked before the tests and electrodes replaced when necessary. Less active and sleepy patients must also be observed between SLTs to make sure they remain awake.

Another very important factor that may affect multiple sleep latency testing is the previous night's sleep. In our older adolescents, we have found that a two-hour reduction in available sleeping time has a marked effect on SLT scores. In younger adolescents, we *(32)* have found that an acute restriction of sleep to four hours for a single night results in a reduction of SLT scores on the following day and even carries over to a subsequent day after 10 hours of sleep. The SLT scores of older adolescents appear to recover much more quickly after a similar experience *(33)*. Nonetheless, sufficient nocturnal sleeping time should be provided on the night before sleep latency testing so that sleep restriction does not affect the SLT scores. The subject's report of his sleeping time from the preceding night may also be useful. Finally, it should be noted that sleep restriction may result in sleep-onset REM periods that are unrelated to narcolepsy on nocturnal or daytime sleep recordings *(33)*.

## Narcolepsy

Retrospective information reported by patients in a number of surveys *(1–3)* has linked the onset of the disorder to the second decade in a large percentage of cases. Daytime sleepiness is usually the first symptom to appear, but most patients do not receive an appropriate diagnosis until long after the onset of the disorder and after auxiliary symptoms have begun *(34)*. A major cause of this delay in diagnosis appears to be the obscurity of the complaint of sleepiness in youngsters. Often the sleepy adolescent is simply dubbed lazy, or the daytime sleepiness may be masked behind behavioral disturbances *(34)*. In addition, other than pupillography *(35)*, no tool has been available for objectively measuring daytime sleepiness until recent use of multiple sleep latency testing.

Thus few cases of narcolepsy have been evaluated during childhood or adolescence. The Mayo group *(36)* has reported 16 children (aged 7 to 15) with narcolepsy, although only 12 of these cases (aged 9 to 15) would probably receive the diagnosis using more recent criteria *(15)*. In eight of these 12 patients, the onset of symptoms occurred in the second decade. Certain common diagnostic errors were reported in these children, including hypothyroidism, emotional disorders, intracranial disease, viral encephalitis, or epilepsy *(36)*.

At the present time, considerable evidence exists to suggest that narcolepsy is a familial disorder *(37–40)*; consequently, many patients with the disorder are concerned about the risk their children face for developing narcolepsy. As our normative data illustrate, children tend to become sleepy during the pubertal years, even if nocturnal sleep time is unchanged from prepubertal levels. We have suggested that youngsters may be more vulnerable to narcolepsy during the middle to late stages of puberty *(22)*. We have followed the children of several narcoleptic patients for a number of years, using the same techniques as in the controls, to determine if such a link can be established *(11)*.

In our group of seven children who have a family history of narcolepsy, one has developed the disorder during the study. This child was first evaluated when she was 12 years old, at Tanner stage 2, and without any signs or symptoms of narcolepsy. She was also evaluated at age 13 (Tanner stage 3) and age 14 (Tanner stage 4). Symptoms of narcolepsy were not reported by the child until the third year, although multiple sleep latency tests showed her to be significantly sleepier than controls, with a daily mean SLT score of 11.8 minutes in the first year and 10.4 minutes in the second year. In the third year, the child reported cataplexy, sleep paralysis, and hypnagogic hallucinations and had a mean daily SLT score of 5.8 minutes. In addition, REM sleep was seen in 13 of 18 sleep latency tests in the third year, including five REM episodes on the first day's SLTs.

None of the other children in this group have developed narcolepsy. Several are somewhat sleepier than controls, and most have not yet reached Tanner stage 5. Thus it is too early to determine the usefulness of these procedures in predicting the development of narcolepsy. Nonetheless, the multiple sleep latency test can be helpful in determining whether a youngster is sleepier than his peers and in determining whether there is an abnormal propensity for REM sleep *(41,42)*. In the case presented above, for example, the abnormal REM latency would have been missed if a single all-night sleep recording had been performed.

The multiple sleep latency test may also be helpful in evaluating therapy. In one case, we have recorded the multiple SLT when a 20-year-old male patient was given eight or ten hours of nocturnal sleep. Mean daily SLT scores improved from 4.8 to 10.4 minutes with the extended nocturnal sleep. In addition, the number of REM episodes declined from an average of 3.7 per day to 1.5. Parenthetically, such a sleep extension program may be a viable therapeutic alternative when there is reluctance to prescribe drugs to adolescents.

---

This research was supported in part by grants from the Spencer Educational Foundation, William and Flora Hewlett Foundation, and NIMH Award MH 31845. I thank William Dement, Thomas Anders, Iris Lift, Helena Kramer, Kim Harvey, and many student technicians for their assistance and support in this project.

*Sleeping and waking disorders: indications and techniques*

**Table 4A–1** Nocturnal Sleep at Tanner Stage 1
(Time in Minutes, N = 15)

|  | Night 1 Mean | Night 1 SD | Night 2 Mean | Night 2 SD | Night 3 Mean | Night 3 SD |
|---|---|---|---|---|---|---|
| Total dark time | 592 | 16 | 593 | 18 | 595 | 17 |
| Total wake time | 67 | 37 | 35 | 22 | 40 | 26 |
| Wake after sleep onset | 34 | 35 | 8 | 11 | 17 | 22 |
| Latency to stage 1 | 29 | 23 | 25 | 22 | 21 | 15 |
| Latency to stage 2 | 37 | 25 | 37 | 28 | 27 | 19 |
| Stage 1 time | 52 | 23 | 42 | 14 | 52 | 13 |
| Stage 2 time | 248 | 42 | 250 | 44 | 245 | 38 |
| Stage 3 time | 32 | 10 | 35 | 20 | 40 | 14 |
| Stage 4 time | 88 | 17 | 99 | 36 | 93 | 21 |
| REM Time | 96 | 22 | 122 | 24 | 114 | 23 |
| Total sleep time | 516 | 40 | 549 | 34 | 545 | 35 |
| Latency to REM | 169 | 76 | 136 | 71 | 143 | 62 |
| Number with spontaneous arousal | 6 | ... | 2 | ... | 2 | ... |

**Table 4A–2** Nocturnal Sleep at Tanner Stage 2
(Time in Minutes, N = 12)

|  | Night 1 Mean | Night 1 SD | Night 2 Mean | Night 2 SD | Night 3 Mean | Night 3 SD |
|---|---|---|---|---|---|---|
| Total dark time | 594 | 17 | 594 | 20 | 595 | 19 |
| Total wake time | 78 | 38 | 34 | 13 | 44 | 21 |
| Wake after sleep onset | 34 | 37 | 8 | 8 | 11 | 16 |
| Latency to stage 1 | 36 | 16 | 21 | 9 | 29 | 17 |
| Latency to stage 2 | 47 | 21 | 25 | 11 | 37 | 21 |
| Stage 1 time | 56 | 20 | 46 | 18 | 49 | 17 |
| Stage 2 time | 244 | 41 | 264 | 24 | 256 | 20 |
| Stage 3 time | 30 | 13 | 36 | 16 | 35 | 12 |
| Stage 4 time | 79 | 20 | 89 | 17 | 84 | 26 |
| REM time | 97 | 13 | 113 | 15 | 118 | 29 |
| Total sleep time | 507 | 31 | 550 | 22 | 541 | 26 |
| Latency to REM | 112 | 42 | 118 | 37 | 105 | 42 |
| Number with spontaneous arousal | 2 | ... | 2 | ... | 1 | ... |

**Table 4A-3** Nocturnal Sleep at Tanner Stage 3
(Time in Minutes, N = 10)

|  | Night 1 Mean | Night 1 SD | Night 2 Mean | Night 2 SD | Night 3 Mean | Night 3 SD |
|---|---|---|---|---|---|---|
| Total dark time | 594 | 10 | 596 | 5 | 599 | 4 |
| Total wake time | 72 | 40 | 36 | 13 | 38 | 22 |
| Wake after sleep onset | 34 | 30 | 9 | 8 | 11 | 14 |
| Latency to stage 1 | 37 | 31 | 25 | 15 | 25 | 13 |
| Latency to stage 2 | 42 | 30 | 32 | 15 | 31 | 12 |
| Stage 1 time | 51 | 25 | 44 | 10 | 40 | 20 |
| Stage 2 time | 250 | 45 | 273 | 29 | 271 | 48 |
| Stage 3 time | 34 | 11 | 32 | 16 | 36 | 11 |
| Stage 4 time | 79 | 24 | 80 | 21 | 76 | 21 |
| REM time | 98 | 16 | 122 | 11 | 118 | 17 |
| Total sleep time | 512 | 42 | 550 | 14 | 549 | 21 |
| Latency to REM | 146 | 79 | 86 | 25 | 74 | 14 |
| Number with spontaneous arousal | 1 | ... | 2 | ... | 3 | ... |

**Table 4A-4** Nocturnal Sleep at Tanner Stage 4
(Time in Minutes, N = 8)

|  | Night 1 Mean | Night 1 SD | Night 2 Mean | Night 2 SD | Night 3 Mean | Night 3 SD |
|---|---|---|---|---|---|---|
| Total dark time | 596 | 5 | 597 | 5 | 599 | 2 |
| Total wake time | 43 | 21 | 40 | 26 | 48 | 37 |
| Wake after sleep onset | 18 | 16 | 14 | 12 | 19 | 28 |
| Latency to stage 1 | 21 | 20 | 24 | 22 | 25 | 11 |
| Latency to stage 2 | 28 | 19 | 30 | 21 | 31 | 10 |
| Stage 1 time | 42 | 20 | 50 | 18 | 51 | 13 |
| Stage 2 time | 287 | 32 | 276 | 45 | 277 | 16 |
| Stage 3 time | 28 | 11 | 24 | 10 | 27 | 7 |
| Stage 4 time | 85 | 26 | 74 | 21 | 68 | 10 |
| REM time | 103 | 16 | 124 | 18 | 121 | 24 |
| Total sleep time | 544 | 28 | 547 | 29 | 541 | 40 |
| Latency to REM | 164 | 56 | 110 | 53 | 96 | 44 |
| Number with spontaneous arousal | 3 | ... | 3 | ... | 0 | ... |

*Sleeping and waking disorders: indications and techniques*

**Table 4A–5** Nocturnal Sleep at Tanner Stage 5 (Time in Minutes, N = 7)

|  | Night 1 Mean | Night 1 SD | Night 2 Mean | Night 2 SD | Night 3 Mean | Night 3 SD |
|---|---|---|---|---|---|---|
| Total dark time | 595 | 3 | 595 | 5 | 599 | 2 |
| Total wake time | 45 | 24 | 47 | 27 | 44 | 31 |
| Wake after sleep onset | 19 | 19 | 19 | 14 | 10 | 9 |
| Latency to stage 1 | 26 | 23 | 26 | 13 | 31 | 21 |
| Latency to stage 2 | 36 | 22 | 37 | 18 | 43 | 32 |
| Stage 1 time | 58 | 31 | 61 | 29 | 67 | 23 |
| Stage 2 time | 303 | 34 | 281 | 39 | 281 | 44 |
| Stage 3 time | 23 | 8 | 19 | 4 | 19 | 6 |
| Stage 4 time | 60 | 13 | 52 | 10 | 65 | 18 |
| REM time | 96 | 14 | 121 | 26 | 111 | 13 |
| Total sleep time | 528 | 39 | 530 | 23 | 542 | 32 |
| Latency to REM | 148 | 58 | 116 | 71 | 108 | 48 |
| Number with spontaneous arousal | 0 | ... | 0 | ... | 1 | ... |

**Table 4A–6** Nocturnal Sleep in Older Adolescents (Time in Minutes, Bedtime = 2200 to 0800, N = 8)

|  | Night 1 Mean | Night 1 SD | Night 2 Mean | Night 2 SD | Night 3 Mean | Night 3 SD |
|---|---|---|---|---|---|---|
| Total dark time | 595 | 1 | 596 | 4 | 598 | 1 |
| Total wake time | 57 | 22 | 44 | 22 | 60 | 41 |
| Wake after sleep onset | 24 | 26 | 16 | 17 | 33 | 43 |
| Latency to stage 1 | 32 | 19 | 26 | 16 | 24 | 19 |
| Latency to stage 2 | 37 | 21 | 31 | 16 | 31 | 21 |
| Stage 1 time | 42 | 16 | 47 | 19 | 52 | 20 |
| Stage 2 time | 294 | 29 | 305 | 16 | 297 | 39 |
| Stage 3 time | 24 | 11 | 27 | 11 | 26 | 10 |
| Stage 4 time | 63 | 17 | 55 | 20 | 68 | 24 |
| REM time | 108 | 10 | 108 | 21 | 105 | 32 |
| Total sleep time | 531 | 19 | 542 | 20 | 530 | 42 |
| Latency to REM | 144 | 39 | 117 | 83 | 108 | 42 |
| Number with spontaneous arousal | 1 | ... | 2 | ... | 2 | ... |

**Table 4B–1** Multiple Sleep Latency Tests at Tanner Stage 1
(Time to Sleep Onset in Minutes, N = 15)

| Time of Test | Day 1 Mean | SD | Day 2 Mean | SD | Day 3 Mean | SD |
|---|---|---|---|---|---|---|
| 0930 | 19.5 | 1.5 | 19.4 | 1.8 | 20.0 | 0 |
| 1130 | 19.2 | 2.1 | 18.9 | 3.3 | 18.8 | 3.1 |
| 1330 | 18.6 | 4.4 | 18.5 | 2.6 | 18.9 | 3.4 |
| 1530 | 18.4 | 4.1 | 17.8 | 4.7 | 19.3 | 1.7 |
| 1730 | 19.5 | 1.9 | 17.9 | 4.5 | 19.3 | 2.6 |
| 1930 | 17.7 | 4.9 | 20.0 | 0 | 20.0 | 0 |
| Daily mean | 18.8 | 1.8 | 18.7 | 2.0 | 19.4 | 1.1 |
| Number with no sleep | 9 | ... | 6 | ... | 9 | ... |

**Table 4B–2** Multiple Sleep Latency Tests at Tanner Stage 2
(Time to Sleep Onset in Minutes, N = 12)

| Time of Test | Day 1 Mean | SD | Day 2 Mean | SD | Day 3 Mean | SD |
|---|---|---|---|---|---|---|
| 0930 | 19.8 | 0.9 | 18.5 | 3.4 | 17.9 | 4.0 |
| 1130 | 18.5 | 2.9 | 18.8 | 3.2 | 19.0 | 2.4 |
| 1330 | 15.7* | 5.4 | 18.3 | 3.1 | 17.4 | 4.7 |
| 1530 | 17.4 | 5.2 | 16.6 | 5.1 | 19.5 | 1.6 |
| 1730 | 19.2 | 2.0 | 18.0 | 3.9 | 19.3 | 1.8 |
| 1930 | 19.3 | 1.7 | 20.0 | 0 | 20.0 | 0 |
| Daily mean | 18.3 | 2.1 | 18.4 | 2.2 | 18.8 | 1.5 |
| Number with no sleep | 5 | ... | 4 | ... | 5 | ... |

*REM sleep in one male subject.

**Table 4B–3** Multiple Sleep Latency Tests at Tanner Stage 3
(Time to Sleep Onset in Minutes, N = 10)

| Time of Test | Day 1 Mean | SD | Day 2 Mean | SD | Day 3 Mean | SD |
|---|---|---|---|---|---|---|
| 0930 | 17.8 | 4.4 | 14.1 | 4.9 | 15.8 | 5.9 |
| 1130 | 14.2 | 6.5 | 11.5 | 6.1 | 14.0 | 7.3 |
| 1330 | 16.0 | 4.6 | 16.5 | 4.7 | 15.8 | 6.1 |
| 1530 | 15.3* | 5.7 | 16.7 | 4.8 | 16.3 | 5.6 |
| 1730 | 16.8 | 5.5 | 16.5 | 5.7 | 17.1 | 6.0 |
| 1930 | 19.2 | 2.5 | 18.8 | 3.8 | 16.9 | 6.6 |
| Daily mean | 16.5 | 2.8 | 15.7 | 3.4 | 16.0 | 5.2 |
| Number with no sleep | 1 | ... | 0 | ... | 4 | ... |

*REM sleep in one female subject.

**Table 4B–4** Multiple Sleep Latency Tests at Tanner Stage 4
(Time to Sleep Onset in Minutes, N = 8)

| Time of Test | Day 1 Mean | SD | Day 2 Mean | SD | Day 3 Mean | SD |
|---|---|---|---|---|---|---|
| 0930 | 14.0* | 6.7 | 17.8 | 2.7 | 16.2 | 5.0 |
| 1130 | 14.4 | 7.6 | 14.1 | 5.2 | 17.2 | 3.6 |
| 1330 | 13.0 | 6.0 | 14.2 | 7.6 | 14.0 | 5.1 |
| 1530 | 15.2 | 5.1 | 12.9 | 6.9 | 13.9 | 6.7 |
| 1730 | 16.8 | 4.7 | 17.1 | 4.1 | 17.5 | 4.4 |
| 1930 | 19.5 | 1.4 | 19.3 | 1.3 | 17.8 | 3.8 |
| Daily mean | 15.5 | 3.3 | 15.7 | 3.4 | 16.1 | 3.5 |
| Number with no sleep | 1 | ... | 1 | ... | 0 | ... |

*REM sleep in two female subjects.

**Table 4B–5** Multiple Sleep Latency Tests at Tanner Stage 5
(Time to Sleep Onset in Minutes, N = 7)

| Time of Test | Day 1 Mean | SD | Day 2 Mean | SD | Day 3 Mean | SD |
|---|---|---|---|---|---|---|
| 0930 | 17.0 | 5.7 | 18.1 | 3.5 | 17.8 | 5.4 |
| 1130 | 16.5 | 3.5 | 19.5 | 1.3 | 18.8 | 3.2 |
| 1330 | 13.8 | 4.5 | 12.9 | 5.8 | 14.1 | 6.5 |
| 1530 | 11.9 | 6.1 | 13.6 | 6.5 | 12.1 | 6.3 |
| 1730 | 19.4 | 1.1 | 16.6 | 4.7 | 20.0 | 0 |
| 1930 | 18.0 | 5.1 | 19.4 | 1.1 | 18.8 | 3.2 |
| Daily mean | 16.2 | 1.5 | 16.7 | 2.8 | 16.9 | 2.1 |
| Number with no sleep | 0 | ... | 1 | ... | 1 | ... |

**Table 4B–6** Multiple Sleep Latency Tests in Older Adolescents
(Time to Sleep Onset in Minutes, Bedtime = 2200 to 0800, N = 8)

| Time of Test | Day 1 Mean | SD | Day 2 Mean | SD | Day 3 Mean | SD |
|---|---|---|---|---|---|---|
| 0930 | 15.3 | 6.7 | 17.6 | 5.2 | 14.9 | 5.6 |
| 1130 | 15.8 | 4.4 | 15.1 | 6.9 | 15.4 | 5.8 |
| 1330 | 15.7 | 4.5 | 11.7 | 5.4 | 15.4 | 5.4 |
| 1530 | 12.2 | 6.6 | 10.8 | 6.0 | 12.6 | 6.1 |
| 1730 | 17.2 | 4.0 | 18.6 | 3.0 | 20.0 | 0 |
| 1930 | 18.2 | 4.2 | 18.1 | 5.3 | 18.2 | 3.9 |
| Daily mean | 15.8 | 3.5 | 15.3 | 3.6 | 16.1 | 3.2 |
| Number with no sleep | 0 | ... | 1 | ... | 1 | ... |

# REFERENCES

1. Daniels L. Narcolepsy. Medicine 1934; 34:1–122.
2. Sours J. Narcolepsy and other disturbances of the sleep-waking rhythm: a study of 115 cases with a review of the literature. J Nerv Ment Dis 1963; 137:525–42.
3. Kessler S, Guilleminault C, Dement WC. A family study of 50 REM narcoleptics. Acta Neurol Scand 1974; 50:503–12.
4. Frank Y, Braham J, Cohen BE. The Kleine-Levin syndrome. Am J Dis Child 1974; 127:412–3.
5. Chiles JA, Wilkus RJ. Behavioral manifestations of the Kleine-Levin syndrome. Dis Nerv Syst 1976; 37:646–8.
6. Billiard M, Guilleminault C, Dement WC. A menstruation-linked periodic hypersomnia: Kleine-Levin syndrome or new clinical entity? Neurology 1975; 25:436–43.
7. Price VA, Coates TJ, Thoresen CE, Grinstead OA. Prevalence and correlates of poor sleep among adolescents. Am J Dis Child 1978; 132:583–6.
8. White L, Hahn PM, Mitler MM. Sleep questionnaire in adolescents. Abstract presented at the 20th annual meeting of the Association for the Psychophysiological Study of Sleep, Mexico City, 1980.
9. Tanner JM. Growth at adolescence. 2nd ed. Oxford: Blackwell, 1962.
10. Anders TF, Carskadon MA, Dement WC, Harvey K. Sleep habits of children and the identification of pathologically sleepy children. Child Psychiatry Hum Dev 1978; 9:56–63.
11. Carskadon MA. Determinants of daytime sleepiness: adolescent development, extended and restricted nocturnal sleep. Dissertation submitted to Stanford University in partial fulfillment of requirements for the degree of doctor of philosophy, 1979.
12. Webb WB, Agnew HW. Sleep and dreams. Dubuque, Iowa: Wm C Brown Company, 1973.
13. Williams RL, Karacan I, Hursch CJ. EEG of human sleep: clinical applications. New York: John Wiley and Sons, 1974.
14. Webb WB, Agnew HW. Are we chronically sleep deprived? Bull Psychon Soc 1975; 6:47–8.
15. Association of Sleep Disorders Centers. Diagnostic classification of sleep and arousal disorders. 1st ed. Prepared by the Sleep Disorders Classification Committee, HP Roffwarg, chairman. Sleep 1979; 2:1–137.
16. Salzarulo P, Pelloni G, Lairy GC. Semeiologie electrophysiologique du sommeil du jour chez l'enfant de 7 à 9 ans. Electroencephalogr Clin Neurophysiol 1975; 38:473–94.

17. Ross JJ, Agnew HW, Williams RL, Webb WB. Sleep patterns in pre-adolescent children: an EEG-EOG study. Pediatrics 1968; 42:324–35.
18. Williams RL, Karacan I, Hursch C, Davis GE. Sleep patterns of pubertal males. Pediatr Res 1972; 6:643.
19. Karacan I, Anch M, Thornby JK, Okawa M, Williams RL. Longitudinal sleep patterns during pubertal growth: four-year follow-up. Pediatr Res 1975; 9:842–6.
20. Marshall WA, Tanner JM. Variations in patterns of pubertal changes in girls. Arch Dis Child 1969; 44:291.
21. Boyar R, Finkelstein J, Roffwarg H, Kapen S, Weitzman E, Hellman L. Synchronization of augmented luteinizing hormone with sleep during puberty. N Engl J Med 1972; 287:582–6.
22. Carskadon MA, Dement WC. Pubertal changes in daytime sleepiness. Sleep 1980; 2:453–60.
23. Barnes HV. Physical growth and development during puberty. Med Clin North Am 1975; 59:1305–17.
24. Rechtschaffen A, Kales A, eds. A manual of standardized terminology, techniques and scoring system for sleep stages of human subjects. Los Angeles: UCLA Brain Information Service/Brain Research Institute, 1968.
25. Agnew HW, Webb WB, Williams RL. The first night effect: an EEG study of sleep. Psychophysiology 1966; 2:263–6.
26. Carskadon MA, Dement WC. Effects of total sleep loss on sleep tendency. Percept Mot Skills 1979; 48:495–506.
27. Marks A. Aspects of biosocial screening and health maintenance in adolescents. Pediatr Clin North Am 1980; 27:153–61.
28. Friedman IM, Goldberg E. Reference materials for the practice of adolescent medicine. Pediatr Clin North Am 1980; 27:193–209.
29. Finkelstein JW. The endocrinology of adolescence. Pediatr Clin North Am 1980; 27:53–69.
30. Boyar RM. Control of the onset of puberty. Annu Rev Med 1978; 29:509–20.
31. Kapen S, Boyar RM, Finkelstein JW, Hellman L, Weitzman ED. Effect of sleep-wake cycle reversal on luteinizing hormone secretory pattern in puberty. J Clin Endocrinol Metab 1974; 39:293–9.
32. Carskadon MA, Harvey K, Dement WC, Anders TF. Acute partial sleep deprivation in children. Sleep Res 1977; 6:92.
33. Carskadon MA, Dement WC. Cumulative effects of sleep restriction on daytime sleepiness. Psychophysiology, 1981; 18:107–13.
34. Navelet Y, Anders TF, Guilleminault C. Narcolepsy in children. In: Guilleminault C, Dement WC, Passouant P, eds. Narcolepsy. New York: Spectrum, 1976:171–7.
35. Yoss RE, Moyer NJ, Ogle KN. The pupillogram and narcolepsy: a method to measure decreased levels of wakefulness. Neurology 1969; 19:921–8.
36. Yoss RE, Daly DD. Narcolepsy in children. Pediatrics 1960; 25:1025–33.

37. Daly D, Yoss R. A family with narcolepsy. Proc Staff Mtg Mayo Clin 1959; 34:313–20.
38. Yoss R, Daly D. Hereditary aspects of narcolepsy. Trans Am Neurol Assoc 1960; 85:239–40.
39. Bruhova S, Roth B. Heredofamilial aspects of narcolepsy and hypersomnia. Arch Suisse Neurol Neurochir Psychiatr 1972; 110:45–54.
40. Baraitser M, Parkes JD. Genetic study of narcoleptic syndrome. J Med Genet 1978; 15:254–9.
41. Richardson G, Carskadon M, Flagg W, van den Hoed J, Dement W, Mitler M. Excessive daytime sleepiness in man: multiple sleep latency measurement in narcoleptic and control subjects. Electroencephalogr Clin Neurophysiol 1978; 45:621–7.
42. Mitler M, van den Hoed J, Carskadon M, Richardson G, Park R, Guilleminault C, Dement W. REM sleep episodes during the multiple sleep latency test in narcoleptic patients. Electroencephalogr Clin Neurophysiol 1979; 46:479–81.

# FIVE
# ELECTRONIC PUPILLOGRAPHY IN DISORDERS OF AROUSAL
HELMUT S. SCHMIDT,
LINDA D. FORTIN

## Introduction

The eye is unique among the sense organs in being intimately associated with sleep-wake rhythms and the cycling of dream periods within sleep (1). The pupil serves as a unique window into the central nervous system and is the most directly observable indicator of autonomic nervous system activity. Autonomic nervous system balance has long been thought to reflect fatigue and wakefulness (2); high adrenergic tone and mydriasis correlate well with cortical arousal and a hyperalert state, whereas parasympathetic predominance and miosis correlate with cortical underarousal and sleep. Clinical examination of the pupil, however, reveals only a small fraction of pupillary behavior and cannot appreciate the subtle but important alterations in autonomic imbalance. The purpose of this brief chapter is to review the development of pupillography, its techniques, and clinical applications as they pertain to sleep-related disorders.

Electronic pupillography (EPG) is a precise technique of continuous infrared scanning (60 times per second) and recording of the maximum diameter of the pupil either at rest or during response to stimuli, most often light (3). Depending on available instrumentation, either eye can be scanned, or both simultaneously. The latter capacity can be helpful in localizing organic lesions (4) but is not essential for purposes of differentiating levels of wakefulness.

Peripheral autonomic manifestations have long been associated with states of arousal/excitation as well as sleep on the continuum of sleep-wakefulness, and the behavior of the pupil is recognized as a classical index for such autonomic activity (5). Over two hundred years ago, pupillary constriction was observed to be associated with sleep (6), and a parasympathetic state during sleep was postulated as early as 1932 (7). Pupillary constriction during sleep was confirmed by Berlucchi and his associates (8), and they also described slow tonic variations as well as rapid pupillary dilations synchronous with REM bursts that they concluded were due to phasic parasympathetic inhibitions.

Spontaneous pupillary movement in darkness in the normal awake individual has been described as reflecting "tiredness," "fatigue," and "sleepiness" *(2,5)*. Unfortunately, these descriptors have been used very loosely and interchangeably, with emphasis on Webster's Dictionary definition of fatigue *(2)*. Lowenstein's concept of the phenomenon of psychosensory restitution *(9)*, emphasized in his most recent paper as well *(5)*, has been appropriately replaced by the concept of arousal phenomenon as evidenced in the new sleep-disorders nosology. Alterations in the sleep-arousal continuum obviously occur that have little or no relationship to being tired or fatigued; for example, the fatigued but hyperalert insomniac, or the very sleepy but nontired narcoleptic. A parsimonious interpretation of pupillary behavior in individuals without an organic lesion suggests that it does indeed reflect autonomic nervous system balance and that it is consequently an indirect but accurate indicator of sleepiness or arousal level. EPG provides, therefore, a simple, objective, reproducible, and accurate assessment of moment-to-moment sleepiness-arousal level.

# Normal Pupillary Stability and Reflex Curves

The integrity of normal spontaneous and reflexive pupillary movements, i.e., normal autonomic nervous system integration, is dependent on four complex and interacting mechanisms: (*a*) intact light reflex neural pathways (the parasympathetic reflex arc-afferent retinal impulses transmitted through the optic nerve for relay in the brainstem pertectal area of the Edinger-Westphal nucleus, with efferent fibers returning via the ciliary ganglion to innervate the iris sphincter); (*b*) several inhibitory mechanisms modulating the parasympathetic tone of the Edinger-Westphal nucleus (supranuclear inhibitory influences—cortical and diencephalic, and reticular formation afferent sensory input); (*c*) the iris dilator muscle innervated by impulses originating in the cortex and traveling via the thalamus, posterior hypothalamus, cervical cord, and peripheral sympathetic chain; and (*d*) humoral adrenergic stimulation, more important in slow tonic pupillary behavior *(4,5)*.

In most of the EPG studies by Lowenstein and Loewenfeld *(2,5,10)*, light stimuli were of high intensity (15 footcandles or more) and long duration (one second), with short intervals between stimuli (three seconds). Extent of pupillary constriction under these conditions ranged from 2–3 mm in normal subjects at various levels of alertness, and a "fatiguing" of the pupillary reflex resulted. Emphasis was placed on intersubject variation in the shape and the "fatiguability" of the stimulus-response curve. It is our opinion that low-intensity reactions are more sensitive indicators of arousal level, as shown by Lee and Knopp *(11)*. Using a 15-footcandle light stimulus "of 1/10 second duration" and attenuated by a 4.0-log neutral-density filter, they found that the mean extent of contraction (EC) for 25 healthy third-year medical students (18 male, 7 female) was 0.81 mm (SD 0.37). This is illustrated in Figure 5–1, an actual recording of a stimulus-response curve in a normal medical student whose polysomnogram for two

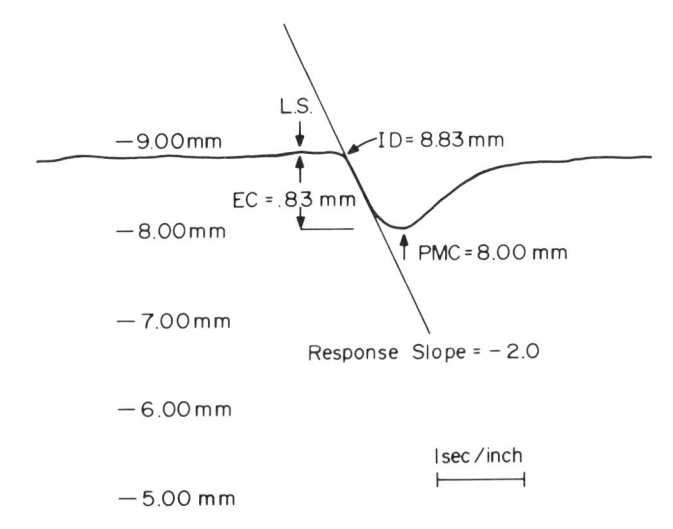

**Figure 5–1.** A normal pupil reflex recording in a 24-year-old medical student. The light stimulus (LS) is given for one-tenth of a second and is of 15-footcandle intensity attenuated by a 4.0-log neutral-density filter. Maximum pupillary constriction (PMC) is reached at the indicated arrow. The extent of contraction (EC) is calculated by substracting the PMC from the initial diameter (ID), i.e., EC = ID − PMC. The response slope for the initial (primary) contraction phase is shown. The pupillary diameter is indicated in millimeters by the vertical scale on the left.

consecutive nights was entirely normal. The initial diameter (ID) of the pupil at light stimulus (LS) impact is 8.83 mm. A latency period of almost 0.5 second transpires before the initial (primary) contraction phase occurs. The slope of this contraction phase in normal young adults at this laboratory using the above criteria for light stimulation of the dark-adapted pupil ranges from −1.0 to −2.0. The response slope is determined by parasympathetic reflex activity and antagonistic sympathetic tone *(10)*, i.e., the level of supranuclear inhibition (SNI) of parasympathetic reflex activity. A slower secondary contraction phase follows until the point of maximum contraction (PMC) is reached and redilation begins. Increasing sympathetic antagonism is thought to be the primary influence in shaping this secondary contraction phase. The initial phase of redilation is for the most part a result of parasympathetic relaxation and is followed by a slower redilation phase thought to be due to cortical sympathetic stimulation *(10)*. Increasing the intensity and duration of the light stimulus shortens the response latency, increases the EC, delays the point of maximum contraction, and is likely to obscure subtle alterations in autonomic nervous system activity, specifically the state of supranuclear inhibition. The EC to a light stimulus is thus determined by five variables: (*a*) stimulus intensity, (*b*) stimulus duration, (*c*) stimulus frequency, (*d*) state of retinal (dark) adaptation, and (*e*) intensity level of supranuclear inhibition at stimulus impact. During standard EPG procedures, the first four variables are held constant and a measurement of the EC is then obtained that is thought to reflect in an inverse relationship the state of supranuclear inhibition and of arousal *(12)*. As will be seen later, however, a number of puzzling and paradoxical observations have been made, suggesting that a more complex interpretation is probable.

# Pupillary Instability and Reflex Curves in Pathologic Arousal States

A normal alert individual sitting quietly in total darkness can maintain a stable pupil diameter, usually well above 7 mm, for at least ten minutes without subjective difficulty or pupillary oscillations *(5)*. A sample recording of the ninth minute of the test, in total darkness, during the first hour awake following normal all-night sleep is shown in the left half of Figure 5–2. A stable pupil is recorded throughout the ten-minute test at about 8.7 mm, and the light reflex is normal, suggesting optimum autonomic balance

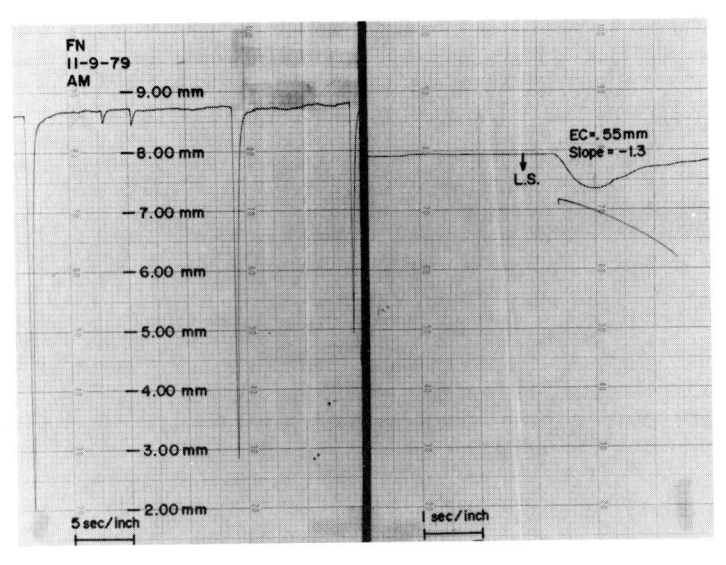

**Figure 5–2.** A segment of dark-adapted stable pupil diameter recording with three large eye blinks is illustrated on the left. On the right an essentially normal (highly alert) pupillary reflex response to attenuated light stimulation is shown. The recording was obtained following normal all-night sleep. LS = light stimulus (time of stimulus impact).

and arousal level. A similar sample at bedtime the night before in the same individual is shown in Figure 5–3. Occasional, small pupillary oscillations of less than 0.5 mm were recorded, suggesting an arousal level that is somewhat less than optimum, and the subject may experience a mild sensation of sleepiness. This is further emphasized by the increased EC of 1.32 mm and a steeper initial contraction phase, suggesting a slight shifting towards parasympathetic dominance (Lowenstein's "Type 2" individual?).

With increased sleepiness in a normal subject, the reflex curve takes on more prominent V- and/or W-shapes. An example of V-shaping is seen in Figure 5–4, a recording of a 37-year-old male with chronic insomnia (REM sleep interruption insomnia) following a night in the sleep laboratory with 375 minutes of sleep. The dark-adapted pupil diameter remains well above 7 mm, but there is increased pupillary instability with occasional oscillations over 0.5 mm. The reflex-response slope is very steep and the EC is as excessive as on the previous evening. It is similar in extent to responses seen in normal subjects who are given a high-intensity light stimulus. More than six hours of sleep in this patient have apparently not resulted in optimization of autonomic nervous balance, and this agrees with the patient's subjective complaint of not feeling refreshed or normally alert. It is premature to state categorically that EPG is a useful procedure in the assessment and treatment of insomnic conditions, but our

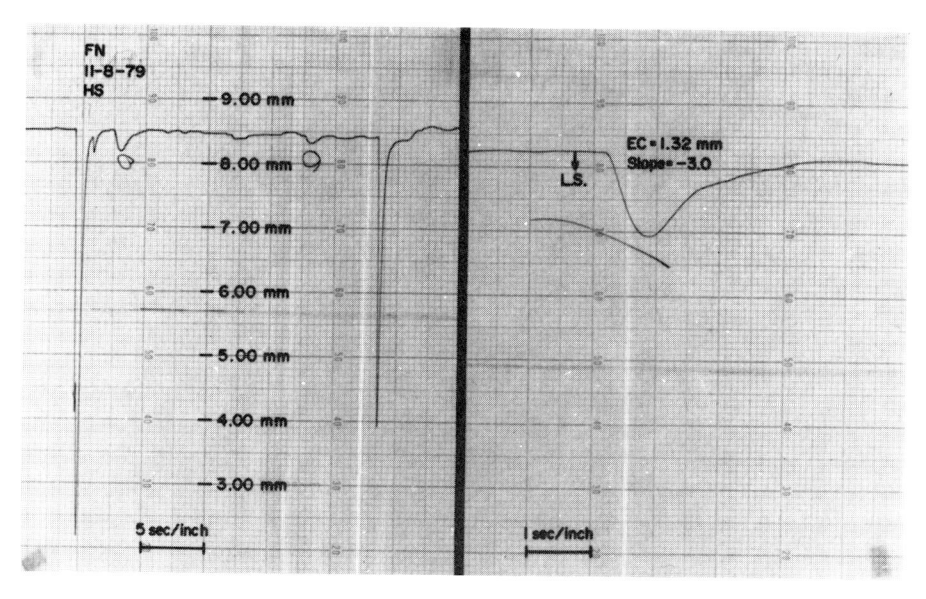

**Figure 5–3.** A bedtime recording of a normal male medical student. Mild underarousal is indicated by small pupillary oscillations, an increased extent of contraction (EC), and a steeper primary contraction slope.

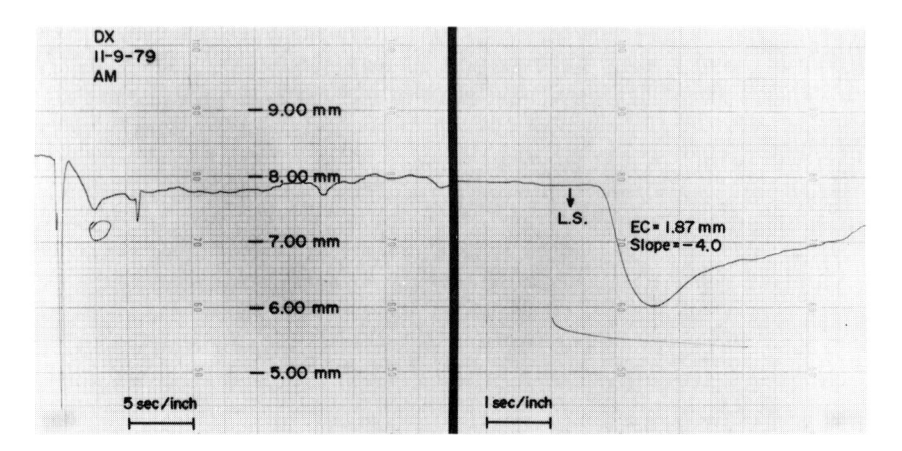

*Sleeping and waking disorders: indications and techniques*

**Figure 5–4.** Moderate oscillations of the dark-adapted pupil (left half) of a 37-year-old male with REM sleep interruption insomnia. The pupillary reflex to attenuated light stimulation shows a steep primary contraction phase and a large extent of contraction (EC), despite preceding 375 minutes of sleep. The very slow secondary redilation (following the initial rapid redilation due to parasympathetic relaxation) reflects weakened cortical sympathetic stimulation.

early observations suggest that EPG procedures may have some promise in differentiating and managing some of the disorders of initiating and maintaining sleep.

Marked changes in pupillary stability and extent of oscillations have been consistently shown to occur in normal "tired" subjects *(2,5,10)* as well as in individuals with pathologic somnolence diagnosed as narcoleptics *(13)*. However, differences in pupil reflex response to light stimuli have not been observed. In fact, Yoss et al. categorically state that "in patients with narcolepsy, the pupillary response to light and convergence is normal" *(13)*. It is noteworthy, however, that Lowenstein and Loewenfeld describe pupillary responses to low-intensity stimuli (0.2 footcandles) but attach much greater importance to high-intensity reactions and indications of "fatiguability" *(10)*. They also assert that the slope of the primary contraction phase "depends primarily on the intensity of the stimulus, and secondarily on the sympathetic-parasympathetic balance of the subject at the time the stimulus is applied" *(10)*. Although this may have validity in normal individuals, it is not likely to be applicable in patients with insomnia or excessive somnolence, where the balance and stability of sympathetic-parasympathetic tone would assume primary importance. Figure 5–4, for example, illustrates a very steep contraction slope to a low-intensity stimulus in a case of insomnia; in contrast, a very shallow slope is apparent in Figure 5–5 with a very small EC to the same standard low-intensity stimulus in a narcoleptic patient.

The EPG procedure used at our center includes an initial ten minutes of dark-adaptation recording followed by a series of light stimuli of 15-footcandles intensity

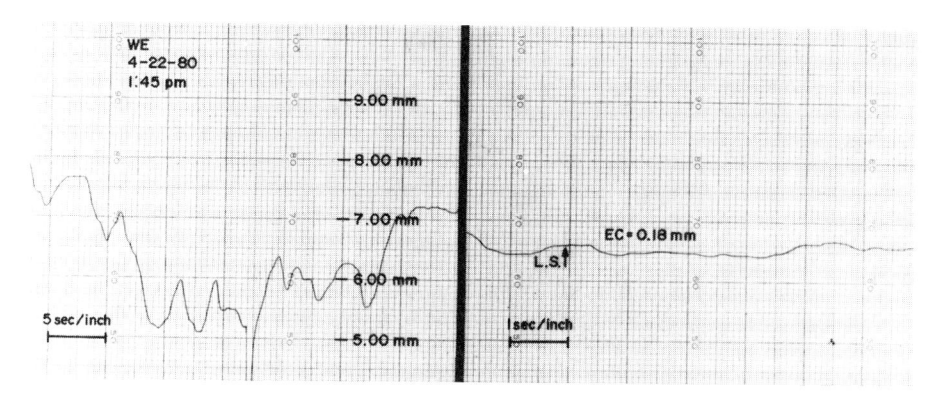

*Electronic pupillography in disorders of arousal*

**Figure 5–5.** The dark-adapted pupil and light reflex in a narcoleptic patient. Frequent large pupillary oscillations are evident. The extent of contraction (EC) in response to a 4.0-log neutral-density filter-attenuated 15-footcandle light stimulus (LS = time of stimulus impact) is very, very small.

attenuated by a 4.0-log neutral-density filter, and of 1/10 sec duration given every 9.9 seconds. Under these conditions, we have confirmed the work of Yoss et al. *(13)* and found that narcoleptics show a very unstable pupillary diameter in the dark-adapted period, with oscillations frequently over 1 mm. This is illustrated in the left half of Figure 5–5, a segment in the second minute of recording in a 32-year-old female narcoleptic subject. She had the classic symptoms of narcolepsy, including cataplexy, and a REM period was recorded within one minute of sleep onset in a routine all-night polysomnogram. However, responses of narcoleptics to a low-intensity light stimulus are paradoxical, as can be seen for this patient in Figure 5–5. Her response is in the opposite direction of the "sleepy normal" (Figure 5–3) or the "tired" insomniac (Figure 5–4). This pattern is consistently observed in the majority of narcoleptic patients recorded by us and contradicts earlier assertions of normal pupillary responses to light stimuli. It suggests the paradoxical state of heightened supranuclear inhibition in the presence of parasympathetic predominance, i.e., large pupillary constrictions during darkness and lower ID but small EC to light stimulus. An analogous observation was made in schizophrenic subjects who were given the same low-intensity light stimulus and who had the same ID as normal subjects but who responded with a small EC *(12)*. During dark adaptation, retinal (parasympathetic) influences on the Edinger-Westphal nucleus are eliminated; so the pupillary diameter recorded under this condition reflects the sum total of supranuclear inhibition. An uncoupling of two modulating systems was postulated to explain the paradoxical finding in schizophrenic subjects *(12)*: the noradrenergic-serotonergic hypothalamic modulation of the ID, and the predominantly dopaminergic mesencephalic modulation of the Edinger-Westphal nucleus. To explain the paradoxical findings in our narcoleptic patients, we need to take into account the third supranuclear modulating system already described by Lowenstein and Loewen-

*Sleeping and waking disorders: indications and techniques*

feld, i.e., sympathetic stimulation of cortical origin primarily modulating pupillary diameter and responsible for the pupillary oscillations in subjects with excessive daytime sleepiness. The paradoxical pupillographic findings in our narcoleptic patients would therefore suggest an uncoupling of cortical (sympathetic) stimulating influences as well as an uncoupling, or out-of-phase activity, of the two subcortical supranuclear inhibitory modulators suggested by Knopp and Hakerem *(12)*. The apparent paradox of excessive sleepiness and associated signs of peripheral adrenergic excess in narcoleptic patients *(14)* is, therefore, congruous with our pupillographic findings suggesting a sleepy cortex and a hyperaroused brainstem.

In patients where the diagnosis of narcolepsy is firmly established by the presence of the ancillary symptoms, particularly cataplexy, and the documentation of sleep-onset REM periods, the above pattern appears to be consistent (personal preliminary observations). Where the ancillary symptoms of narcolepsy are not at all prominent or are absent and REM latency in all-night polysomnograms is normal, a diagnosis of idiopathic CNS hypersomnolence is suggested. These individuals show a similar pattern of pupillary instability during the dark-adaptation period, but their pupil reflex responses to low-intensity light stimulation are normal. Figure 5–6 is a sample EPG recording of a 52-year-old woman diagnosed with idiopathic CNS hypersomnolence. Ancillary symptoms of narcolepsy were absent and the polysomnogram showed a sleep latency of one minute, a REM latency of 72 minutes, and, aside from minimal slow wave sleep, an entirely normal polysomnogram. During dark adaptation, the overall pupillary diameter is under 5 mm and frequent oscillations are present. However, the pupillary response curve is entirely normal. This would suggest an uncoupling of cortical mod-

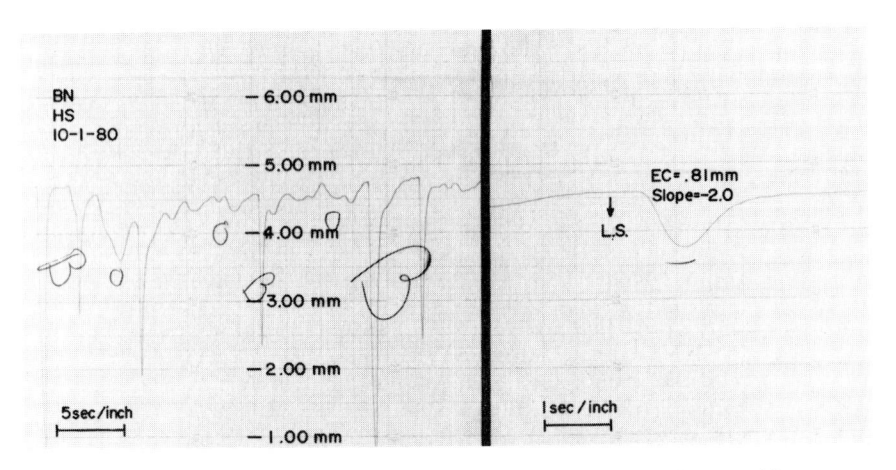

**Figure 5–6.** Large oscillations of the dark-adapted pupil in a 52-year-old woman with idiopathic CNS hypersomnolence. The notations of "O" (oscillation) and "B" (blinks) were made by the technician at time of recording. Note the normal pupil reflex to attenuated light stimulation (LS), in contrast to the greatly reduced or absent reflex response in patients with classic narcolepsy.

*Electronic pupillography in disorders of arousal*

ulation, as in the narcoleptic patient, but an optimum balance between the two subcortical modulating systems. Work is currently in progress to further document these observations and to assess any correlation with the results of multiple sleep latency testing.

## EPG Instrumentation

The essential physical requirements consist of a small dark room with a comfortable chair, preferably with armrests and elevation capability, and a sturdy, secure table for the mounting of a TV pupillometer camera (Figure 5–7). The base under the movable platform (Item 5 in Figure 5–7) is firmly secured on the table, and minor adjustments

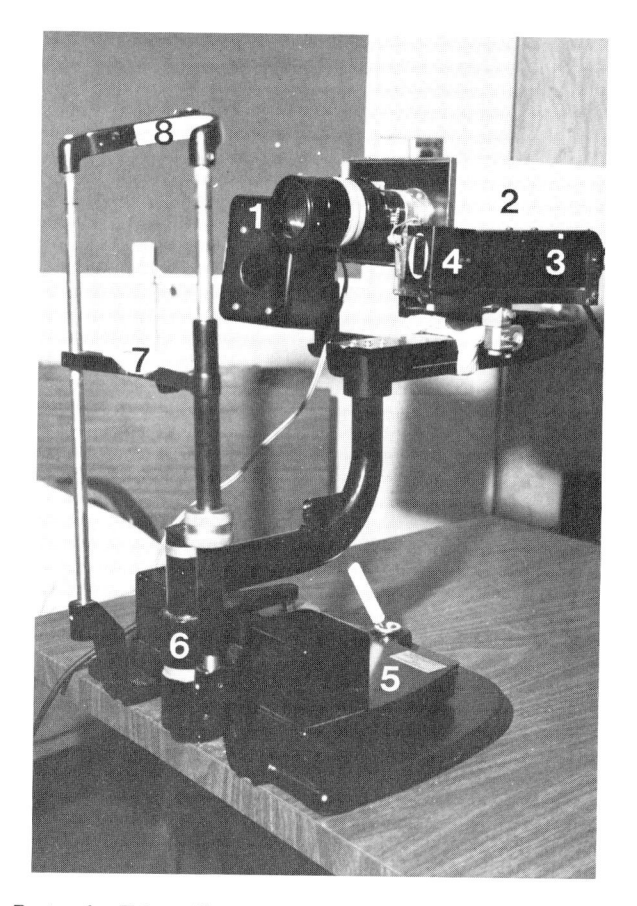

**Figure 5–7.** Parts of a TV pupillometer system located in the dark-adaptation room. 1 = infrared illuminator, 2 = TVP camera, 3 = light stimulator, 4 = light filter (4.0-log neutral-density filter in place), 5 = movable base with joystick, 6 = angular indicator for camera, 7 = chin rest, 8 = head (forehead) rest.

135

*Sleeping and waking disorders: indications and techniques*

can then be made using the joystick of the movable platform and the angular indicator for the camera (Item 6 in Figure 5–7). The light source (Item 1 in Figure 5–7) is provided by invisible near-infrared filtered incandescent lamp illumination centered at 8500 angstroms. The TV camera (Item 2 in Figure 5–7) is equipped with a silicon-matrix vidicon tube and is focused in this particular setup on the subject's left eye. It is connected by coaxial cable to the TV pupillometer control unit (Figure 5–8) located immediately outside of the dark room and in direct view of, and control by, the technician. The light stimulator (Item 3 in Figure 5–7) is mounted next to the camera and aligned so that, when light flashes are given, the light stimulus centers on the subject's left eye. The direct pupillary reflexes of the left eye are therefore monitored by the TV camera and control unit. The light stimuli are brief square wave pulses with rapid rise and decay produced by a Sylvania glow modulator tube (R 1131 C). The intensity of the stimulus can be altered by the placement of a filter (Item 4 in Figure 5–7), in this particular case a 4.0-log neutral-density filter. The light-stimulus control unit (Item 1 in Figure 5–9) is located with the TV control unit (Figure 5–8) and the strip chart recorder (Item 2 in Figure 5–9) within easy range and visibility of the technician outside the dark room. The stimulator control unit should allow adjustment of the duration, frequency, and number of light stimuli given for each testing procedure.

The chart recorder can be a single-channel system (dual-channel if binocular

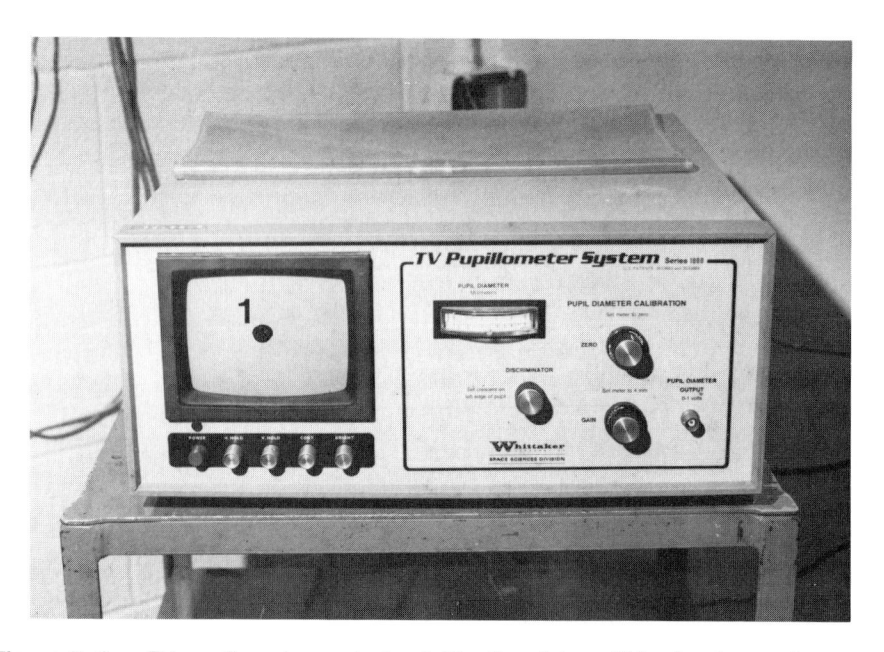

**Figure 5–8.** TV pupillometer control unit. The "model pupil" is showing on the screen.

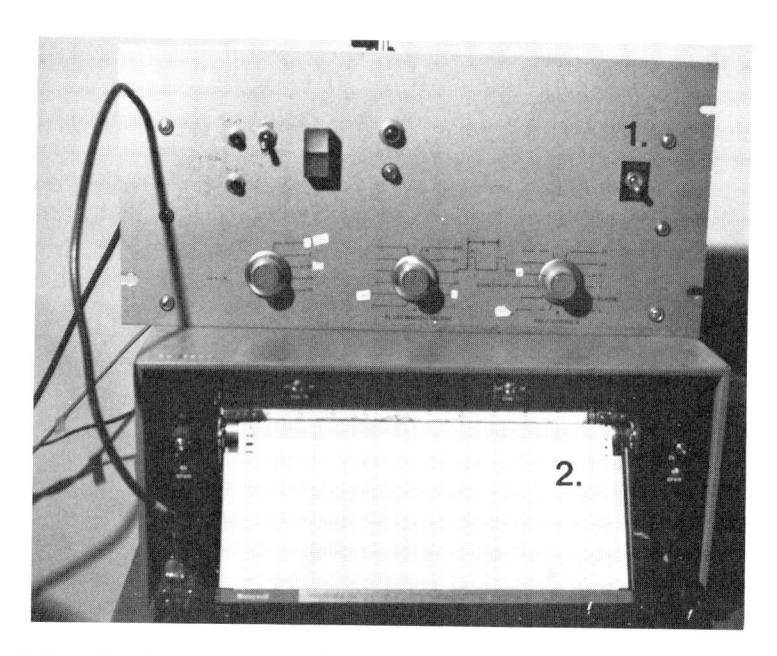

*Electronic pupillography in disorders of arousal*

**Figure 5-9.** The light stimulator (1) and strip chart recorder (2) are located with the TVP control unit outside the dark room and in control of the operator (technician).

monitoring and recording capabilities are desired) and must have variable-speed control and a stimulus time (event) marker. It should have a high-frequency response to record pupil dynamics with high fidelity and be able to record blinks with sufficient precision so that these various components can be readily distinguished. Most pen recorders with sufficient bandwidth will prove satisfactory. The Whitaker TV Pupillometer used at the OSU Sleep Disorders Evaluation Center, and portrayed in Figures 5-7 and 5-8, has an output of 0 to 1 volt, corresponding to 0 to 10 mm of pupil diameter. This output signal may saturate the preamplifier of most chart recorders designed to handle small bioelectrical signals. It is therefore necessary to set the chart-recorder attenuator to (for example) 10 $\mu$V/mm, and to set the zero-suppression feature on the recorder to allow the recording of the desired pupil-diameter segment, for example 3 to 9 mm. The chart recorder illustrated in Figure 5-9 is a Honeywell Electronik 196 two-pen recorder with disposable ink cartridge. A variety of other equally satisfactory recording systems are available.

The range of pupil diameters measurable with standard TV pupillometer equipment is 2.3 mm to 10.0 mm, but can be extended with minor equipment modification (not essential for most purposes). For accurate recording of pupil diameter, the allowable range of eye movement in the horizontal plane is 30° and in the vertical plane, 25°. Accuracy is increasingly reduced beyond these ranges.

## EPG Techniques

The pupillographic procedure should be performed by an experienced technician who is able to readily establish rapport with patients to avoid extraneous anxiety-inducing factors that can affect pupillary diameter and responsiveness to light stimulation (15). The procedures outlined below are routinely employed at this center and may have to be altered if instrumentation is markedly different.

1. The TV pupillometer system must be turned on for a warm-up period of approximately five minutes.
2. The pupillometer must then be calibrated using the "model pupil" of 4.0 mm diameter, which is attached on the chin rest in front of the TV camera. To focus the model pupil on the TV screen, the base of the camera may be moved from side to side or the chin rest may be moved vertically. Calibration is then checked for zero position. Next, the discriminator knob (Figure 5–8) is turned clockwise to set off delimiters and produce a white crescent around the model pupil. The alignment of the illuminator (Item 1 in Figure 5–7) is then checked by turning the discriminator knob to within one turn of full scale. If this cannot be accomplished without losing the delimiters or the white crescent at the edge of the model, then the illuminator is out of alignment and must be realigned. Once the illuminator is realigned, the system must be recalibrated at 0 mm and 4.0 mm. The technician is then ready to calibrate the chart recorder to the 0-mm and 4.0-mm settings of the pupillometer.
3. The patient is then seated in a comfortable chair or stool in front of the TV camera and is prepared for the test in the following ways:
   a. The patient is asked to remove glasses or contact lenses because the reflection from them may cause artifacts in the recording.
   b. The patient is informed that the test will take place in darkness and will last about 15 minutes.
   c. The patient is positioned comfortably in the chair with his chin placed on the chin rest (Item 7 in Figure 5–7) and forehead rested against the head restraint (Item 8 in Figure 5–7). The patient is then instructed to focus on a small light six feet away while alignment and focusing of the pupil are performed.
   d. The patient should sit still with arms on the armrests, away from the equipment, and fixate on a target of a small red light (about six feet from the eyes at optical infinity to keep the direction of gaze and accommodation constant). The fixation light is approximately 15° above eye level so that the subject has to look slightly up and thereby help keep the eyelids above the pupil. The patient should be instructed to blink as little as possible during the dark-adaptation period.
   e. The patient is instructed that at the end of the dark-adaptation recording (ten minutes at this center) he will receive a series of light flashes during which he must try not to blink. The patient is reassured that the light flashes will not be very bright or disturbing.

4. The discriminator knob is then turned clockwise to set off the delimiters and produce a white crescent at the edge of the pupil on the TV screen.
5. The patient is once again instructed to sit as still as possible and to blink as little as possible.
6. All lights in the patient's room are then turned off and the door is closed to provide total darkness.
7. The technician initiates the recording in the next room for the specified period of dark adaptation. Because it is important to assess the patient's spontaneous pupillary diameter and stability, and therefore his arousal level, it is important to avoid noise and other stimulation during the dark-adaptation period, if at all possible. If a patient is restless, moves his head, or is not able to keep the eyelids elevated, additional instructions through an intercom system may be necessary to obtain a readable recording. A relatively slow paper speed of 5 mm/sec is used for this procedure.
8. The patient is again instructed to remain still and to avoid blinking if at all possible, and is told that a series of light stimulations will begin. The routine procedure includes ten light stimuli, each one-tenth of a second in duration, given every ten seconds. This series may need to be repeated if excessive blinking has produced too much artifact in the recording of light reflex response. This procedure is performed with the 4.0-log neutral-density filter in place (Item 4 in Figure 5–7).
9. If high-intensity stimulation is desired, the technician must reenter the patient's room (after dimming light in the immediate area to the lowest necessary level) and remove the filter. A soft, persistent glow produced by the stimulator makes it possible to align the point of stimulus impact directly onto the right pupil, and this should be checked before light stimulation is initiated.
10. An appropriately fast paper speed of one inch per second must be used during the light-stimulation procedure to allow an accurate recording and differentiation of the contraction phases of the light reflex-response curve.

The entire procedure as outlined above may take from 20–30 minutes and is very well tolerated by the vast majority of patients. The dark-adaptation recording is reviewed for overall stability and extent of pupillary diameter and number of oscillations in the categories of small (less than 0.5 mm), moderate (0.5 to 1.0 mm), and large (over 1.0 mm). Marked pupillary constrictions with lid drooping and closure are noted as indicators of severe underarousal and probable sleep onset.

The light reflex responses are measured for initial diameter (ID), commonly taken at point of light-stimulus impact, the extent of contraction (EC) as shown in Figure 5–1, and the slope of the initial contraction phase. These data are analyzed for each artifact-free light stimulus and the mean ID, EC, and initial contraction slope are calculated. The same calculations can be made for reflex responses to high-intensity stimuli for longer durations and in rapid succession to assess the pupil's "fatiguability." To ensure accurate differentiation of artifact from genuine pupillary activity, the tech-

*Sleeping and waking disorders: indications and techniques*

nician must carefully monitor pupillary activity on the TV screen while at the same time observing the recording produced on the chart recorder and providing appropriate notations as much as possible, as can be seen, for example, in Figure 5–5. This becomes particularly important when artifacts are created by instrument noise, such as discriminator problems, or by movement of the patient's head or eye. Useful information and appropriate interpretation can thus be maximized.

# Problems and Limitations of EPG

*Physical and medical limitations* include extreme obesity, which often produces excessive somnolence and respiratory impairment in sleep. The obese individual often cannot be appropriately seated in an EPG chair. Very tall individuals, or those with large heads, encounter difficulties with appropriate positioning and camera alignment. Patients with ocular problems and lesions (e.g., blindness, cataracts, iridectomy), or with autonomic and CNS lesions (e.g., Argyll-Robertson pupil and Horner's syndrome), must be identified and excluded.

*Ability and willingness to cooperate* are essential. Hyperactive patients who are unable to sit still for several minutes, or anxious subjects whose anxiety and autonomic nervous system imbalance may be further aggravated by an unskilled or insensitive operator, are poor candidates for this procedure. When recording is attempted in such patients, useful information is obscured by movement artifacts or incessant blinking, as seen in Figure 5–10A. If eye or head movement disrupts alignment of the pupil, it is best to enter the patient's room and make necessary adjustments rather than attempt to give instructions to the patient from outside the room.

*Avoiding lid drooping or closure* may be difficult or impossible for some patients with disorders of excessive somnolence, and it may be difficult to record a long enough segment of pupillary diameter measurement for appropriate interpretation. In order to compensate at least partially for this problem, the TV camera should be mounted so that the pupil is scanned horizontally rather than vertically and the maximum pupil diameter can still be recorded as long as drooping of the eyelid does not extend beyond the pupil's midpoint. In severe cases of somnolence, a lid crutch has been recommended *(13),* although simply taping the eyelid open for several minutes may be adequate. Again, a skilled technician is necessary for this procedure and caution must be observed to avoid damage to the cornea. The maximum time the eyelid may be kept open with this modified procedure should not exceed five minutes to avoid corneal damage due to drying.

Patients with *small initial pupil diameters* may require the capability to record below the 2.3-mm limit set with the TV pupillometer. An adjustment can be made by the manufacturer to extend this lower limit to within the mechanical limits of the iris sphincter muscle.

Patients with very *dark irises* may be difficult to record. Adjustments may be

*Electronic pupillography in disorders of arousal*

necessary in the f-stop of the camera to differentiate more clearly between the iris and the pupil.

*Excessive eye makeup* and long eyelashes may pose similar problems, and again an adjustment of the f-stop will usually resolve the recording difficulty.

Finally, *interpretation* of the data obtained may be difficult, particularly if the recording conditions are not well-standardized and the recording quality is mediocre. In the sleepy individual, spontaneous pupillary oscillations may obscure or alter pupillary reflex responses. Figure 5–10*B* suggests a very low extent of contraction if the time of stimulus impact is taken as the initial diameter, whereas the opposite would occur in Figure 5–10*C*, where the extent of contraction would appear unduly exaggerated. The initial diameter might be taken approximately 0.5 seconds after the beginning

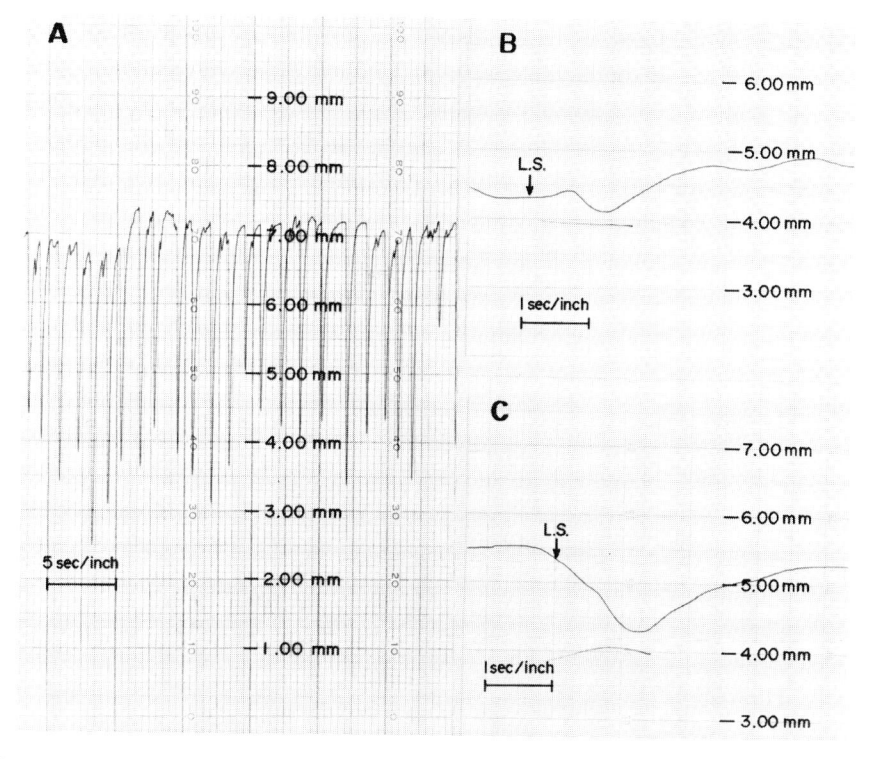

**Figure 5–10.** Examples of frequently encountered recording problems. Excessive blinking in Section A, frequently observed in anxious individuals, makes identification of background pupillary diameter very difficult. Spontaneous pupillary oscillations during the light stimulus testing procedure can minimize (Section B) or exaggerate (Section C) apparent extent of contraction if the initial diameter is taken at time of stimulus impact.

141

of stimulus impact (the usual response latency in normal subjects with this type of stimulus), but it is not clear to what extent the spontaneous dilation or contraction phase of the pupil may influence the extent of contraction. Calculations are therefore best made when reflex responses are free from artifact or indications of spontaneous pupillary changes. It is also recognized that EPG is a relatively new procedure, highly sensitive to external as well as internal stimuli of all kinds, and very little is as yet known about pupillographic parameters in relationship to sleep disorders diagnosed according to the new nosological system. The dark-adapted pupil diameter reflects the underarousal or sleepiness present in all of the "primary" disorders of excessive somnolence but does not differentiate between them. Pupillary reflex responses to light stimuli of different intensity, duration, and frequency may eventually assist us in differentiating between specific sleep disorders, or help to identify specific subcategories of patient populations. In the meantime, cautious optimism for the usefulness of EPG in the diagnosis and management of sleep disorders is certainly warranted.

---

We wish to thank Debbie Starr for assembling, and Mitzi Prosser for preparing, the illustrations. Equipment described in this paper was purchased in part by funds from the Office of Program Program Evaluation and Research, Ohio Department of Mental Health, Contract No. 411-416-95-01.

# REFERENCES

1. Aserinsky E, Kleitman N. Regularly occurring periods of eye motility and concomitant phenomena during sleep. Science 1953; 118:273–4.
2. Lowenstein O, Loewenfeld I. Pupillary movements during acute and chronic fatigue: a new test for the objective evaluation of tiredness. Invest Ophthalmol Vis Sci 1963; 2:138–57.
3. Lowenstein O, Loewenfeld I. Electronic pupillography—a new instrument and some clinical applications. Arch Ophthalmol 1958; 59:352–63.
4. Lowenstein O. Pupillary reflex shapes and topical clinical diagnosis. Neurology 1955; 5:631–44.
5. Lowenstein O, Loewenfeld I. The sleep-wake cycle and pupillary activity. Ann NY Acad Sci 1964; 17:142–256.
6. Fontana F. Dei moti dell' iride. Lucca: Stanyseria Jacopo Guisti, 1765.
7. Hess WR. The autonomic nervous system. Lancet 1932; 223:1259.
8. Berlucchi G, Moruzzi G, Salvi G, Strata P. Pupil behavior and ocular movements during synchronized and desynchronized sleep. Arch Ital Biol 1964; 102:230.

9. Lowenstein O. Der psychische Restitutionseffekt: das Prinzip der psychischen bedingten Wiederherstellung der ermüdeten, der erschöpften, und der erkrankten Funktion. Basel: Benno Schwabe and Company, 1937.
10. Lowenstein O, Loewenfeld I. Types of central autonomic innervation and fatigue: pupillographic studies. Arch Neurol Psychiatry 1951; 66:580–99.
11. Lee SH, Knopp W. Pupillary reactivity in medical students, schizophrenia without phenothiazines and schizophrenia treated with trifluoperazine. Eye Ear Nose Throat Mon 1968; 47:426–33.
12. Knopp W, Hakerem G. Pupillographie, Bioamine und Verhaltenspathologie. In: Dodt E, Schrader KE, eds. Die normale und die gestörte Pupillenbewegung. Munich: JF Bergmann Verlag, 1973.
13. Yoss RE, Moyer NJ, Ogle KN. The pupillogram and narcolepsy. Neurology 1969; 19:921–8.
14. Clark RW, Boudoulas H, Schaal SF, Schmidt HS. Adrenergic hypersensitivity and cardiac abnormality in primary disorders of sleep. Neurology 1980; 30:113–9.
15. Janisse MP. Pupillometry. The psychology of the pupillary response. New York: John Wiley and Sons, 1977.

# SIX

# THE MULTIPLE SLEEP LATENCY TEST AS AN EVALUATION FOR EXCESSIVE SOMNOLENCE

MERRILL M. MITLER

## Introduction

Excessive daytime somnolence is a complaint associated with many disorders of the wakefulness-sleep cycle. Increasingly, physicians require objective evaluation of patients who have the complaint of excessive somnolence.

There are several approaches to the objective quantification of somnolence. Such measures as performance testing and pupillography have been described elsewhere *(1,2)* and also in this volume.

The present chapter discusses the technique of polysomnographically measuring sleep latency at various times throughout the wakefulness-sleep cycle. Increasingly, workers have found this objective measure of tendency to fall asleep scientifically and clinically useful *(3,4,5)*.

The multiple-nap approach to the evaluation of sleepiness has two important theoretical advantages. First, the approach has face validity: someone who is sleepy should fall asleep more quickly than someone who is not sleepy. Furthermore, polygraphically measured sleep latency has been shown to correlate highly with the subjective feeling of sleepiness as measured by the Stanford Sleepiness Scale *(6)*. Second, polygraphic evaluation of daytime napping can precisely measure the onset of sleep and evaluate ensuing sleep structure to check for abnormalities such as sleep-onset REM periods, which might indicate the presence of narcolepsy *(7)*.

Several workers have published important studies involving electrographic sleep monitoring during several opportunities to sleep ("naps") offered throughout one or more 24-hour intervals. Weitzman et al. *(8)* studied the effects on sleep structure of permitting sleep for one hour out of every three hours for ten days. Carskadon and Dement *(9)* studied sleep during successive 30-minute sleep opportunities separated by

60 minutes of enforced wakefulness for five days. Moses et al. *(10)* described the sleep structure of one-hour naps offered every 220 minutes throughout a 40-hour period. Some consistent findings have emerged from this type of work: most important is that sleep tendency, measured in terms of time required to fall asleep or total sleep time per sleep opportunity, has a marked 24-hour periodicity. Sleep tendency is greatest during that interval of the 24-hour clock when the subject normally sleeps, regardless of how much or how little sleep occurred during the preceding days. Another key finding is that sleep structure is time-dependent, with a marked predisposition for REM sleep during the hours that, prior to the experimental sleep schedule, marked the end of the subject's sleep phase. A logical step after these data were available was to study the effect on sleep tendency of such variables as age and sleep loss. Using a protocol designed to (*a*) assess sleep tendency and (*b*) minimize the effects of sleep during the testing, Carskadon *(11)* has gone far in this direction. In an elegant series of studies, five or six sleep opportunities were offered at two-hour intervals throughout most of the waking hours. Each opportunity was terminated after a 30-second epoch of sleep occurred. Children were longitudinally and cross-sectionally studied at points in development ranging from prepubescence to sexual maturity. The effects of reduced nocturnal sleep and total sleep deprivation were also evaluated. For the purposes of this chapter, it is sufficient to mention two of her findings. In a situation where opportunities to sleep are offered at two-hour intervals during waking hours, age and prior sleep are crucial variables. The tendency to fall asleep increases (i.e., sleep latency decreases) with age and with sleep loss.

The remainder of this chapter deals with a clinical version of the multiple sleep latency test. The clinical procedure differs from that used by Carskadon and her associates in several ways. Most importantly, up to ten minutes of continuous sleep is permitted during each opportunity to sleep. Secondly, only five nap times are used, the first at 1000 hours and the others at two-hour intervals. The reader is referred to the methodology section of this chapter for a detailed protocol. Results obtained with this clinical protocol have been published elsewhere *(4,5)*. Table 6–1 summarizes these earlier data combined with more recent data using the identical protocol on narcoleptic patients, patients complaining of excessive daytime somnolence who do not have narcolepsy or sleep apnea, and control subjects who do not complain of excessive somnolence or insomnia.

It is clear from the data presented in Table 6–1 that the multiple sleep latency test distinguishes narcoleptic patients from noncomplaining control individuals. There is no overlap in the distributions of the mean sleep latencies for these two groups.

The narcoleptics also appear to differ from the nonnarcoleptic patients. But the nonnarcoleptic patients are diagnostically heterogeneous, so statistical tests between narcoleptics and this group are not informative. Some patients in this group have sleep latencies well below the five-minute criterion for pathology, whereas others do not sleep at all during multiple sleep latency testing. The important advantage in obtaining sleep latency data for nonnarcoleptic patients with the complaint of excessive somnolence is that patients who are candidates for treatment with stimulant medication can be objectively distinguished from those who are not pathologically sleepy.

**Table 6–1** Mean Scores on MSLT for Various Groups (Time to Sleep Onset in Minutes)

|  | Time of Nap |  |  |  |  |  |
|---|---|---|---|---|---|---|
|  | 1000 | 1200 | 1400 | 1600 | 1800 | Mean |
| Narcoleptics (N = 49) 21 females, 28 males Mean age: 43.8 ± 11.7 | 3.05 (2.4) | 2.74 (3.5) | 2.42 (3.2) | 2.26 (2.6) | 4.07 (5.4) | 2.91 (2.7) |
| Nonnarcoleptics with EDS (N = 63) 33 females, 30 males Mean age: 38.6 ± 13.0 | 8.93 (6.2) | 7.55 (5.9) | 7.81 (6.1) | 8.16 (6.6) | 11.23 (6.9) | 8.74 (4.9) |
| Controls (N = 13)* 9 females, 4 males Mean age: 35.5 ± 10.3 | 14.33 (6.1) | 13.71 (6.7) | 13.17 (5.9) | 11.95 (5.5) | 13.75 (6.4) | 13.38 (4.3) |

NOTE: The standard deviation for each mean is given in parentheses below each entry.

*Two male offspring (ages 19 and 17) of a narcoleptic male patient and the same mother volunteered to be control subjects. Neither presented with excessive somnolence or other clinically significant complaints concerning their wakefulness-sleep cycles. They were not habitual users of alcohol or "street drugs," and they were not taking medications at the time of testing. The protocol consisted of nocturnal polysomnography followed by MSLT. For the 19-year-old, nocturnal sleep was unremarkable. On the MSLT, sleep latencies were 6.5, 7.5, 5.5, 9.5, and 20.0 minutes for the five naps beginning at 1000 (mean = 9.8), and there was one REM-sleep episode 9.5 minutes after sleep onset during the 1000 nap. For the 17-year-old, nocturnal sleep was also unremarkable. Sleep latencies on the MSLT were 3.5, 6.5, 5.0, 8.0, and 20.0 (mean = 8.6), and there were three REM-sleep episodes. These occurred 3.0, 6.5, and 10.0 minutes after sleep onset on the first three naps. These data were not included in any other group because they can be interpreted in several ways.

Abnormal latencies to REM-sleep are reflected in the number of REM-sleep episodes recorded throughout the five naps, with the restriction that only one REM-sleep episode can be counted per nap. Table 6–2 summarizes the number of REM-sleep episodes recorded in each group.

To date (October 1980), no control has shown a sleep-onset REM-sleep period on this protocol. However, Webb et al. *(12)* have shown that normal volunteers can have sleep-onset REM periods during early morning opportunities to sleep. Therefore, one must always be alert to the possibility of clinically nonsignificant REM-sleep episodes during the 1000 and 1200 naps. Recently Czeisler et al. *(13)* have reported data and reanalyzed other data on the temporal distribution of REM sleep, concluding that the predisposition to have REM sleep is coupled to the rising phase of the body-temperature rhythm. Since the trough of body temperature in the nominal wakefulness-sleep cycle is around 0400 or 0500 hours, our data can be considered consistent with their proposition.

Because of the tendency for much REM sleep to occur during the end of the sleep phase and (if permitted) during the beginning of the wake phase, it is also important to consider such normal REM sleep when interpreting clinical electroencephalographic reports of REM-sleep onsets. The time when such EEG procedures are done is of crucial importance.

In terms of the temporal distribution of REM-sleep episodes during the multiple sleep latency test, the 49 narcoleptics showed a trend, although statistically nonsignificant (chi-square $< 1.0$, $df = 4$), to have more REM sleep in the early naps of the day. Table 6–3 shows the number of REM-sleep episodes recorded by the 49 narcoleptics over the five nap times.

The data summarized in Table 6–3 indicate that narcoleptics readily show REM sleep throughout the multiple sleep latency test. It further implies that, like the normal subjects recorded by Webb et al. *(12),* narcoleptics have an increased likelihood for REM sleep in the morning.

## General Discussion

Available data indicate that the multiple sleep latency test, when properly administered and interpreted, can be a useful diagnostic tool. It (*a*) effectively identifies patients with pathologic sleepiness and (*b*) effectively distinguishes narcoleptics from other patients with pathologic sleepiness.

In a clinical setting, it is extremely difficult to evaluate the crucial measures of false-positive and false-negative scores of the multiple sleep latency test. For pathologic sleepiness, there is a diagnostic category in the Association of Sleep Disorders Centers' diagnostic system entitled "Subjective DOES Complaint without Objective Findings" (B.10.b.) *(14)*. This category could contain people who actually are pathologically sleepy although they show no pathologic sleepiness on the multiple sleep latency test

**Table 6–2** Number of REM-Sleep Episodes Recorded versus Percent of Group

|  | \multicolumn{6}{c}{Number of Rem-Sleep Episodes Recorded} |
| --- | --- | --- | --- | --- | --- | --- |
|  | 0 | 1 | 2 | 3 | 4 | 5 |
| Narcoleptics (N = 49) | 2% | 2% | 25% | 12% | 25% | 34% |
| Nonnarcoleptics with EDS (N = 63) | 92 | 8 | 0 | 0 | 0 | 0 |
| Controls (N = 13) | 100 | 0 | 0 | 0 | 0 | 0 |

(average sleep latencies are about five minutes). The data of Carskadon and her colleagues (3,11) on sleep-deprivation studies and multiple sleep latency testing would argue that such a possibility is extremely remote. Their data show that sleep latencies as measured on the multiple sleep latency test are extremely sensitive to increased sleepiness operationally defined by sleep deprivation. Conversely, it is possible that someone who is not pathologically sleepy may fall asleep readily under testing conditions and produce an average sleep latency below five minutes. This possibility can be minimized by not testing individuals who are sleep-deprived. One way to assure standardized sleep prior to testing is to precede multiple sleep latency testing by nocturnal polysomnography. This provides an adequate idea of preceding nocturnal sleep and helps in interpreting multiple sleep latency test results. Nocturnal polysomnography that involves ear oximetry or other exceptionally disruptive monitoring procedures should be categorically avoided on nights prior to multiple sleep latency testing.

False-positives and false-negatives for abnormal tendencies to REM sleep can be operationally minimized by running tests only on drug-free patients. It is certain that some narcoleptics will produce false-negative result on a single multiple sleep latency test. For example, one of the 49 narcoleptic patients had five naps without REM sleep

**Table 6–3** Occurrence of REM-Sleep Episodes and Their Latencies for 49 Narcoleptics
(As a Function of Nap Time)

|  | \multicolumn{5}{c}{Time of Nap} |
| --- | --- | --- | --- | --- | --- |
|  | 1000 | 1200 | 1400 | 1600 | 1800 |
| Number of REM-sleep episodes recorded | 39 | 33 | 37 | 34 | 33 |
| Mean REM-sleep latency after sleep onset | 3.14 | 2.89 | 2.95 | 3.35 | 3.76 |
|  | (3.2) | (2.5) | (2.4) | (2.6) | (2.1) |

NOTE: The standard deviation for each mean is given in parentheses below each entry.

in the present protocol and six naps without REM sleep in a two-day research study before showing four episodes of REM sleep in a row on the second day of the research protocol.

Nevertheless, the multiple sleep latency test seems to be a useful tool in the clinical evaluation and diagnosis of patients presenting the complaint of excessive somnolence.

# Methodology

## Protocol

This polysomnographic procedure is designed to evaluate (*a*) the complaint of excessive daytime somnolence by quantifying the time required to fall asleep and (*b*) the possibility of narcolepsy by checking for abnormally short latencies to REM sleep. Polygraphic variables include central and occipital electroencephalogram (EEG), electromyogram (EMG) for muscles on and beneath the chin, electro-oculogram (EOG), and electrocardiogram (ECG). Patients are monitored throughout five 20-minute opportunities to sleep. Monitoring is usually begun after nocturnal polysomnography (done to rule out patients with sleep disorders that might artifactually produce short sleep latencies on this test).

The first nap is scheduled at 1000 and remaining naps are at two-hour intervals. For each nap, the patient is allowed 20 minutes to fall asleep. Sleep onset is defined as any of the following:

1. The first three consecutive epochs of stage 1 NREM sleep.
2. Any single epoch of stage 2, 3, or 4 NREM sleep; or REM sleep.

Sleep offset is defined as two consecutive epochs of wakefulness after sleep onset. Sleep scoring is done while the data are coming off the polygraph by the criteria of Rechtschaffen and Kales *(15)*.

A nap is terminated after any of the following conditions:

1. At minute #20 if no sleep has occurred.
2. After ten minutes of continuous sleep as long as sleep-onset criteria are met before minute #20. Note that this criterion might lead to a bedtime per nap of up to 30 minutes if sleep first occurs in minute #20.
3. At minute #20, or any point thereafter if the patient is awake, even though some sleep may have occurred earlier in the nap. Note that this criterion permits a maximum of 19 minutes of sleep on each nap. For example, a patient could fall asleep before minute #10 of any nap, sleep for nine minutes, awaken, and then fall asleep again on minute #20 of the same nap. In such an event, the nap is terminated when the patient awakens or after ten minutes of sleep during the second sleep bout, even though he slept for nine minutes prior to that bout in the same nap.

**Table 6-4** Parametric Analysis

|  | Time of Nap |  |  |  |  |
|---|---|---|---|---|---|
|  | 1000 | 1200 | 1400 | 1600 | 1800 |
| Sleep latency (minutes to sleep onset) | | | | | |
| Latency to REM sleep (after sleep onset) | | | | | |
| Patient's estimated sleep latency | | | | | |
| Did patient have a dream-like experience? | | | | | |

*Mean sleep latency.* Naps during which no sleep occurred contribute to the mean with a value of 20 minutes, thus producing some skewing of the latency distribution across subjects. A value less than five is considered abnormal.

*Number of REM sleep episodes.* There can be no more than one episode per nap. A value greater than one is consistent with a diagnosis of narcolepsy.

*Patients should be drug-free for multiple sleep latency testing.* Failing this, the patient should be free of drugs known to alter the latency and/or amount of REM sleep (particularly amphetamine and antidepressant compounds). It should be emphasized that results on the multiple sleep latency test for subjects not free of these compounds are extremely difficult to interpret.

It is imperative that the technician observe the patient throughout testing. Between naps, the patient is to be kept as alert as possible. It should also be noted that this protocol does not minimize daytime sleep in the laboratory. The sleep allowed in each nap optimizes the likelihood of capturing abnormally short latencies to REM sleep on polygraphic records.

---

Dr. Mitler is supported by the Long Island Research Institute, New York State Department of Mental Hygiene. Thanks are due to Mr. Pierre Hahn for his valuable assistance in computerized reduction of the data.

# REFERENCES

1. Wilkinson R. Sleep deprivation: performance tests for partial and selective sleep deprivation. In: Abt L, Riess B, eds. Progress in clinical psychology, vol. 8. New York: Grune and Stratton, 1968:28–43.
2. Yoss R, Moyer N, Ogle K. The pupillogram and narcolepsy: a method to measure decreased levels of wakefulness. Neurology (Minneap) 1969; 19:921–8.
3. Carskadon M, Dement W. Sleep tendency: an objective measure of sleep loss. Sleep Res 1977; 6:200.
4. Richardson G, Carskadon M, Flagg W, van den Hoed J, Dement W, Mitler M. Excessive daytime sleepiness in man: multiple sleep latency measurement in narcoleptic and control subjects. Electroencephalogr Clin Neurophysiol 1978; 45:621–7.
5. Mitler M, van den Hoed J, Carskadon M, Richardson G, Park R, Guilleminault C, Dement W. REM sleep episodes during the multiple sleep latency test in narcoleptic patients. Electroencephalogr Clin Neurophysiol 1979; 46:479–81.
6. Dement W. Daytime sleepiness and sleep "attacks." In: Guilleminault C, Dement W, Passouant P, eds. Narcolepsy. New York: Spectrum, 1976:17–42.
7. Wilson R, Raynal D, Guilleminault C, Zarcone V, Dement W. REM sleep latencies in daytime sleep recordings of narcoleptics. Sleep Res 1973; 2:166.
8. Weitzman E, Nogeire C, Perlo M, et al. Effects of a prolonged 3-hour sleep-wakefulness cycle on sleep stages, plasma cortisol, growth hormone and body temperature in man. J Clin Endocrinol Metab 1974; 38:1018–30.
9. Carskadon M, Dement W. Sleep studies on a 90-minute day. Electroencephalogr Clin Neurophysiol 1975; 39:145–55.
10. Moses J, Hord D, Lubin A, Johnson L, Naitoh P. Dynamics of nap sleep during a 40 hour period. Electroencephalogr Clin Neurophysiol 1975; 39:627–33.
11. Carskadon MA. Determinants of daytime sleepiness: adolescent development, extended and restricted nocturnal sleep. Dissertation submitted to Stanford University in partial fulfillment of requirements for the degree of doctor of philosophy, 1979.
12. Webb W, Agnew H, Sternthall H. Sleep during the early morning. Psychonomic Science 1966; 6:277–8.
13. Czeisler C, Zimmerman J, Ronda J, Moore-Ede M, Weitzman E. Timing of REM sleep is coupled to the circadian rhythm of body temperature in man. Sleep 1980; 2:329–46.

14. Association of Sleep Disorders Centers. Diagnostic classification of sleep and arousal disorders. 1st ed. Prepared by the Sleep Disorders Classification Committee, HP Roffwarg, chairman. Sleep 1979; 2:1–137.
15. Rechtschaffen A, Kales A, eds. A manual of standardized terminology, techniques and scoring system for sleep stages of human subjects. Los Angeles: UCLA Brain Information Service/Brain Research Institute, 1968.

# SEVEN
# SLEEP AND BREATHING

CHRISTIAN GUILLEMINAULT

## Introduction

Sleep and breathing are two basic, vital biologic functions that often are not considered in association. Breathing and its control undoubtedly are affected by sleep and sleep states, and sleep abnormalities affect breathing. Unfortunately, for many years the physiology of the control of breathing has been studied only on anesthetized animals, completely eliminating consideration of one regulatory system.

The control of breathing during non-rapid eye movement (NREM) and rapid eye movement (REM) sleep has been studied recently in dogs, cats, and infants. These investigations were initiated when sleep apnea syndromes in adults and sudden infant death syndrome (SIDS) in infants finally received the attention of the medical community. We are still deciphering the multiple mechanisms responsible for the control of breathing during the sleep/wake cycle (see Orem for review [1]) and the interactions between breathing and sleep. In this chapter, we shall limit discussion to known interactions between breathing and sleep disorders.

Respiratory physiology and respiratory diseases are included in medical school curricula; however, sleep physiology and sleep disorders are not. This oversight no doubt is responsible for some erroneous physiopathogenic explanations of clinical presentations and for ineffective therapeutic recommendations. Perhaps because sleep physiology is not taught in medical schools, many physicians believe it is of little or no "medical" (by which is often meant "organic") impact. Very little, if any, attention is given to a patient's sleep complaint, whereas a report of sleep disturbance should lead to inquiries similar to those provoked by reports of weight loss or mild but continuously elevated core temperature. Although most physicians would consider it to be malpractice to prescribe analgesics without first undertaking a complete clinical investigation of a patient presenting recurring headaches, many fail to recognize a similar responsibility to investigate patient complaints such as "chronic insomnia," "frequent awakenings during sleep," or "falling asleep inappropriately during the day" before prescribing nonspecific medications such as hypnotics or stimulants.

In addition, investigation of a patient's sleep-disorder complaint must include a detailed study of respiration. Periodic hypersomnia, for example, is noted in patients with severe respiratory allergy (e.g., allergic rhinitis, hay fever): the combination of sudden nasal or airway load, coupled with antihistaminic medication intake (central nervous system depressant drugs), leads to nocturnal sleep disturbance, sleep fragmentation, and progressive feelings of tiredness, fatigue, and daytime somnolence. Cases of periodic hypersomnia thus are more likely to occur during seasons that heighten allergic reactions.

Zwillich, in Colorado, has demonstrated experimentally the role of nasal occlusion in the appearance of sleep complaints. He monitored volunteers who wore nose clips while awake and asleep, and found that all subjects presented nocturnal sleep disturbances and complained of "bad sleep," despite the fact that the nose clip was well tolerated while the subject was awake (Zwillich, personal communication).

These examples illustrate the importance of systematic studies of breathing during sleep in cases of chronic sleep complaints. Daytime somnolence and insomnia may be associated with numerous breathing changes during sleep. Sleep-related respiratory problems may cause, for example, alveolar hypoventilation, hypoxemia, and increased respiratory load; these in turn often lead to a sleep complaint.

## Sleep and Breathing Interaction

Sleep and sleep states affect breathing, and *a patient who has a breathing problem while awake will experience a systematic worsening of this complaint during sleep*. Several factors contribute to "sleep-related worsening":

1. The *recumbent position* tends to intensify breathing disorders. Most human physiologic studies have been performed on patients who are awake and are standing or seated. Comparative studies should be performed with both normal subjects and those with breathing problems lying on their backs, sides, and abdomen. We conducted studies on five female patients, all of whom weighed at least 100% above ideal body weight (corrected for height and age). None of these women presented a sleep apnea syndrome or any significant lung pathology, yet all displayed nocturnal sleep disruptions with at least four complete awakenings per night (mean = 5.5 awakenings). None complained of a sleep disorder; all acknowledged taking short naps during the day. We monitored each patient for 30 minutes before she fell asleep, having her lie flat on her back. All presented tachypnea and expressed feelings of discomfort related to their position and to respiration. Unfortunately, since the study was performed in 1971 (Guilleminault, unpublished data), no appropriate evaluation of oxygen saturation during sleep was obtained.

Results of daytime blood gas and pulmonary function were within normal range (corrected for age).
2. *Age* is another factor. Sorbini et al. *(2)* demonstrated that arterial oxygen pressure ($PaO_2$) decreases with age during wakefulness. Further, when a subject assumes a supine posture, $PaO_2$ decreases at a rate of 0.42 mm/Hg per year after the age of 14. (The change in $PaO_2$ is greater when the subject is supine rather than upright.)
3. Physiologic changes related to *sleep states* must be emphasized. During REM sleep, a continuous antigravity muscle atonia is present. This muscle atonia involves the accessory respiratory muscles and, as demonstrated by Duron *(3,4)*, the intercostal muscles. The Toronto school has studied the sudden abnormal laxity of the rib cage, induced by intercostal muscle atonia during REM sleep, in infants. There is no doubt that muscle atonia plays an important role in REM sleep-related hypoxia noted in subjects who have borderline ventilation while awake. Hypoxia is likely to occur in patients with muscle disorders involving the thorax *(5,6,7)*, thoracic deformities, lung diseases, and neurologic disorders or motor-component complaints involving the thorax *(8,9,10,11,12)*.
4. The ability to adjust to *environmental factors* during sleep also should be considered. For example, the decrease of oxygen at higher altitudes requires compensation in breathing. Interestingly, genetic factors influence the potential adaptation of a subject to high altitudes. We note that the Incas always planned mass migrations to locations at the same altitude. High altitude, genetic inability to adapt, and consequential sleep disturbance have been shown to be responsible for "chronic mountain sickness syndrome" *(13)*. Factors influencing adaptability include the ability to switch from nose breathing to mouth breathing during sleep and the sharpness of hypercapnic and hypoxemic responses during different sleep states.
5. *Iatrogenic decreases in central respiratory adaptive responses,* which may be induced by alcohol, most drugs, sleep deprivation, or sleep fragmentation, also may contribute to sleep-related worsening of breathing problems leading to sleep disruption.

## Arousal: A Defense Mechanism

Arousal is perhaps the most important defense mechanism in cases of breathing abnormalities during sleep. Arousal is responsible for sleep disturbances that often lead to a clinical complaint. We would suggest the following operational definition.

Webster's Dictionary defines "arousal" as "excitation." "Arousal" does *not* mean "systematic awakening with full consciousness." Physiologically, "arousal" is a stimulation ("excitation") of a nonspecific system, the reticular activating system (RAS). Stimulation varies in intensity and may produce complete awakening from sleep, or it may simply produce a change in the level of operation of the autonomic nervous system through stimulation of the RAS. Sympathetic and parasympathetic discharges, which affect many organs and interact as forces of opposite signs (i.e., + and −), are affected abruptly by sudden stimulations of the RAS. In humans, the arousal response during sleep will lead to EEG, cardiac, and respiratory changes. The EEG changes are not necessarily equivalent to those of "awakening"; in fact, the EEG changes may be limited to a shift from high-amplitude slow waves to the appearance of a fast theta rhythm, appearance of K complexes, or bursts of slow alpha recorded in the central leads ($C_3$ or $C_4$ of the 10/20 International Placement System), all indicative of a change from stage 3–4 NREM sleep to stage 2–1 NREM sleep. In children (i.e., subjects who have not reached puberty), sleep disturbances or cortical arousal produce a sudden burst of high-amplitude waves—very hypersynchronic fast delta or slow theta.

In addition, *persistence of a sleep EEG does not negate the existence of "arousal response."* This is noted frequently in obstructive sleep apneic patients at the end of an apneic event. The arousal response is associated with many autonomic nervous system changes, of which cardiovascular and respiratory changes are easiest to identify polygraphically. Tachycardia, change in amplitude of finger pulse, tachypnea, and changes in electrodermal reaction—all have been used as indexes of arousal by sleep researchers. For example, finger pulse monitoring was used as the single criterion for arousal during human studies performed at Stanford between 1968 and 1973.

To reiterate, arousal as a defense mechanism is a nonspecific response to many breathing problems during sleep; of course, episodes of arousal change an individual's sleep profile. If repetitive, arousals will lead to numerous sleep problems, such as complete awakenings, sleep fragmentation, sleep deprivation, secondary daytime tiredness, fatigue, and somnolence. While asleep, humans are unaware of the primum movens of their sleep disturbances, but the secondary problems of insomnia or daytime somnolence will be very obvious to them and thus often will be the reported symptom. Any treatment of the symptom, which of necessity must be nonspecific, risks potential impairment of this major defense mechanism against the underlying breathing disorder.

In the context of sleep, *arousal may be a valid and significant respiratory response*. It may be detected by various sleep-stage changes during polygraphic monitoring and also may cause short awakenings. It may be associated with the feeling of air hunger, with free-floating anxiety, or with tachycardia. Because airway obstruction and hypoxemia may cause similar complaints, a patient may associate awakening from sleep with fear and anxiety. The autonomic nervous system reactions may be so pronounced that the subject may not be able to fall asleep again immediately and may, in turn, be upset by this condition.

In most cases, *if the causes of arousal are not investigated and ameliorated, the sleep disturbance will become more severe*. Arousal patterns disrupt a patient's normal biologic status. To counteract this, a series of reactions may occur. For example, the receptors may "reset" their sensitivity level so that arousal does not occur as frequently. This, of course, may be dangerous because arousal is a necessary defense. Unfortunately, the interaction between the physiologic mechanisms of breathing and sleep is such that when one is disturbed, the other reacts immediately; vicious circles can develop progressively and place the patient in jeopardy. Phillipson et al. have demonstrated how interaction between sleep fragmentation and control of breathing in dogs leads to alteration of the chemical control of ventilation *(14)*. We have shown, using sleep apneics as models, how vicious circles can be initiated *(15)*.

# The Sleep Apnea Syndromes

The sleep apnea syndromes have been much publicized during the past ten years, perhaps because they are easy to diagnose when investigated. One must remember, however, that sleep apnea syndromes are only one kind of breathing abnormality that may be present during sleep.

Apnea is a cessation of airflow at the level of the nostrils and mouth lasting at least ten seconds. There are three types of sleep apnea: *obstructive, central,* and *mixed.* Sleep-related apnea may occur secondary to a sleep-induced airway obstruction (obstructive or upper-airway apnea). Apnea may be related to decreased diaphragmatic activity during sleep (central or diaphragmatic apnea). Finally, apnea may result from the combination of both factors (mixed apnea).

Apnea may be seen in individuals of all ages during sleep. Normative data exist for infants *(16,17,18)*, children *(19)*, and adults *(20,21,22)*, but the data from adults are of limited value because age was not taken into consideration. It appears that gender, and endocrine status in women, also influences normal values for apneic events. It is difficult to measure the impact of apneic events on an individual, because factors such as "daytime somnolence" are subjective. Carskadon has performed the only study using objective criteria such as reaction time to measure apneic event impact *(23)*.

To measure the severity of a sleep apnea syndrome, we developed an *Apnea Index (AI)*: the total number of apneic episodes during sleep divided by the sleep time in minutes and then multiplied by 60. This allowed us to take into account variation in total sleep time (whereas the number of apneas per night did not) and to obviate confusion resulting from the equation of "sleep time" to "total time in bed" or "time with light out."

We performed a study in 1977 that indicated that an AI of up to 5.0 was within normal limits. We monitored normal subjects between the ages of 32 and 47 years during one summer, using individual rooms normally assigned to students in one of the Stanford campus sorority buildings. Each subject was monitored on four successive nights. Each followed his daily schedule and a minimum of 6.5 hours of sleep was recorded for each night.

In another study designed to collect normative data *(20)*, we found that men have a higher AI than premenopausal women. This finding was confirmed in a study by Block et al. *(21)*. We also noted the interesting fact that AI did not vary with sex in children (age 9 to 13 years) *(19)*.

Our studies also have suggested that some types of apnea are related more to physiologic events occurring during sleep than to overt pathology *(24)*. For example, abrupt independent central apnea seen in association with bursts of rapid eye movements during REM sleep is related to sleep mechanisms and to the existence of bursts of pontine-geniculo-occipital (PGO) waves *(25)*. The interaction between bursts of PGO waves and sudden diaphragmatic inhibition was also clearly demonstrated by Orem in the cat *(26)*. This normal phenomenon, however, can be associated with an abnormality of chemosensitivity during REM sleep and can, on rare occasions, lead to an overt sleep disturbance. Similarly, central apnea normally is seen at sleep onset; this seems to result from the "deactivation" of the RAS that occurs during the transition from wakefulness to sleep.

Some patients demonstrate sleep-related hypopnea: a reduction—but not a complete cessation—of air exchange. Three types of hypopnea, like apnea, can be distinguished: central, obstructive, and mixed. Diagnosis of each of these breathing patterns during sleep has been obtained from polygraphic monitoring of respiration using strain gauges, thermistors, esophageal pressure balloons, or transducers; by monitoring of intercostal electromyographic (EMG) activity; and by measurement of blood oxygen saturation. In selected cases, fiber-optic studies and filming have confirmed data obtained by polysomnography.

Both apnea and hypopnea syndromes may lead to decreased arterial blood oxygen saturation, to complex cardiovascular changes, and to progressive development of daytime complaints. The impact of abnormal sleep-related breathing patterns on oxygen saturation varies with the duration of the event, the type, the oxygen-saturation level prior to the event, and (probably) the sleep states. We studied adult patients with chronic obstructive airflow disease and sleep apnea syndrome to assess the impact of each type of abnormal breathing pattern on oxygen saturation *(27)*. Obstructive apnea during REM sleep caused the most marked desaturation; central hypopnea during NREM sleep had the least impact. We performed a similar study on infants considered near-miss for SIDS and obtained analogous results—i.e., obstructive apnea resulted in a lower oxygen saturation than did central apnea of similar duration *(28)*.

Apnea and hypopnea during sleep, with resulting impaired oxygenation, are associated with different known pathologies. However, they can also appear as independent, isolated syndromes. In every patient, all three apneic patterns are seen, but usually one is predominant. Two basic sleep apnea syndromes have been differentiated by the predominant type of breathing abnormality—the predominantly obstructive sleep apnea syndrome and the predominantly central sleep apnea syndrome. These two syndromes can be associated with a complaint of disorder of maintaining sleep (insomnia) or a disorder of excessive sleepiness.

A recent survey performed by the Association of Sleep Disorders Centers (ASDC), encompassing ten sleep-disorders centers with different orientations, tabulated the different diagnoses of patients seen in the centers during the first six months of 1980. All patients had been given complete evaluations, including polygraphic monitoring. A total of 4192 patients were studied: 29% complained of a disorder of initiating or maintaining sleep (DIMS); 2% were diagnosed as having sleep apnea insomnia (6% of the total DIMS); 51% complained of a disorder of excessive sleepiness (DOES); and 20% suffered from sleep apnea hypersomnia (42% of the total DOES).

The following review of the two syndromes—obstructive and central sleep apnea—is based primarily on our experience with over 500 sleep apneic patients.

## The Predominantly Obstructive Sleep Apnea Syndrome

*Clinical Symptoms.* Persistent sleepiness, tiredness, and fatigue are the leitmotiv of the predominantly obstructive sleep apnea syndrome. In addition, the patient often complains of deterioration of memory and judgment (particularly occurring in the morning), early morning confusion (which may be so pronounced that toxic status or brain tumor has been suspected in some cases), automatic behavior, and personality changes involving sudden episodes of irrelevant behavior, jealousy, suspicion, anxiety, and/or general depressive outlook. Recurrent morning headaches and morning nausea also are common and may increase the suspicion of an intracranial expansive process or other neurological insult. The degree of incapacity ranges from drastic impairment of daytime activities because of irresistible urges to sleep (often leading to occupational and/or driving accidents) to only moderate daytime sleepiness resulting in drowsiness or falling asleep during quiet situations, such as watching television or reading.

Family members report that these patients snore loudly at night. Their noisy pharyngeal snoring is associated with snorting and is interrupted by periodic silences (apneic episodes). Apneic patients also move about abnormally during sleep; this may involve gross movements of the entire body or, at other times, only simple movements of the extremities. Episodes of sleepwalking or falling out of bed have been reported. Nocturnal enuresis is mentioned infrequently; the most common complaint is of significant nocturia.

At examination, patients with obstructive sleep apnea syndrome often are overweight and/or have a short, fat neck. However, severe obstructive sleep apnea syndromes have been documented in individuals of normal weight who have normal neck features. Hypertension, in varying degrees, is observed often. In the idiopathic type, waking pulmonary-function tests are normal (or show slight impairment related to body conformation in the case of obese patients). In normal-weight patients, we have found no evidence of abnormal responses to hypercapnic and hypoxemic challenges.

In rare cases, patients report frequent arousals during sleep, occasionally associated with sensations of choking or shortness of breath. But the chief complaints are of excessive daytime sleepiness and feelings of tiredness and fatigue during the daytime.

*Polygraphic Monitoring.* The key tests that enable diagnosis of this syndrome are performed during sleep. Various techniques are available to document the number and predominant type of apneic episodes, the level of oxygen saturation, and the severity of the syndrome. Screening techniques may disclose the presence of a sleep apnea–related syndrome and, in severe cases, may indicate the appropriate therapy. For other patients, more sophisticated invasive techniques are indicated.

We caution the reader that *it is important to monitor physiological nocturnal sleep when investigating a sleep apnea syndome problem.* Some researchers advocate monitoring short daytime naps (with or without prior sleep deprivation). We would like to point out the drawbacks of this technique in obtaining a correct diagnosis: (a) The patient may not present any REM sleep during daytime naps and the severity of the sleep-related breathing problem may be masked by this because REM sleep causes lower $O_2$ saturation and has its own impact on the autonomic nervous system. (b) It has been demonstrated recently that apnea syndromes follow a circadian rhythm in infants, with peak in AI occurring between 0300 and 0600 hours (29). Failure to monitor nocturnal sleep will result in the possibility of an investigator missing the period during which the apnea syndrome is most severe. (c) Sleep deprivation or sleep-inducing medications may lead to diagnosis "in excess." Sleep deprivation has been shown to lead to increased severity in patients with moderate sleep apnea syndrome (15). Explanations for the exacerbation of sleep apnea syndromes by sleep deprivation are several—there is a change in arousal threshold with delayed response to arousal, and sleep deprivation affects polysynaptic reflexes. Similarly, central nervous system depressant drugs will increase the severity of a moderate sleep apnea syndrome.

In view of the above, it would seem unwise to use daytime nap monitoring for diagnosis, least of all as a basis for recommending specific therapeutic approaches. We observed an unfortunate case in which a patient underwent only daytime nap monitoring (following sleep deprivation) when sleep apnea syndrome was suspected. On the basis of data obtained during the nap monitoring, a trachcostomy was performed. Six weeks later, the trachcostomy was closed. An all-night study had demonstrated that such a therapeutic approach was unwarranted for this patient (Guilleminault, unpublished data).

We have already introduced the concept of the AI (Apnea Index). In addition, we have developed a similar index that includes the occurrence of hypopnea (H); the $(A + H)I$. To obtain the $(A + H)I$, the total number of abnormal respiratory events during sleep is divided by the total sleep time in minutes, and this result is multiplied by 60. Thus, the $(A + H)I$ gives the number of abnormal respiratory events per sleep hour. The $(A + H)I$ may indicate the severity of the syndrome but may not be sufficient to describe the entire disorder.

Because the $(A + H)I$ represents an average, it may be misleading. For example, some patients breathe normally in specific sleep states; we have reported patients with severe apnea syndrome during NREM sleep and normal respiration during REM sleep (30). (It is more common for apneic events to increase during REM sleep.) An additional consideration is that the longest periods of REM sleep occur during the second half of the night; it is then that oxygen blood levels are lowest and the most severe cardiovascular impact is seen in association with bursts of rapid eye movements. Finally, the distribution of apneic events throughout sleep may be an important factor, particularly if the investigator wishes to examine the hemodynamic effects of the syndrome.

Like the AI, an $(A + H)I$ of up to 5.0 is within normal limits in adults. The investigator also must examine the impact of apneic events during sleep on oxygen saturation and on the cardiovascular system to draw a complete picture of the patient's disorder.

*Cardiac Arrhythmias in the Obstructive Sleep Apnea Syndrome.* Since our first report of the impact of sleep apnea syndromes on cardiac rhythms *(31)*, a number of authors have confirmed the life-threatening risk to these patients during sleep *(32,33)*.

As a rule, normal sinus rhythm is present during wakefulness in these patients, but a cyclic pattern of marked sinus arrhythmia appears during sleep in association with apnea. This rhythm is characterized by progressive sinus bradycardia during apnea (less than 30 beats per minute is not uncommon), with abrupt reversal and sinus acceleration at the onset of ventilation. This rhythm pattern is so characteristic of the sleep apnea syndromes that we have used a 24-hour ambulatory ECG (Holter monitor) as a screening technique in populations at risk for obstructive syndromes (Figures 7–1*a* and *b*).

Second-degree atrioventricular block, prolonged sinus pauses, limited runs of ventricular tachycardia, and paroxysmal tachycardia also may occur in association with apneic events. In some cases, atrial fibrillation (unresponsive to medication and treated by cardioversion) has appeared at the end of long apneic events (Figure 7–2).

Atropine sulfate and oxygen blunt the marked sinus rhythm variations, although the cyclical sinus arrhythmia pattern is still noticeable. Edrophonium hydrochloride enhances the cyclical pattern. Propranolol was given to four patients but had no obvious effect on the cyclical pattern during the following five hours of nocturnal sleep *(31)*.

*Hemodynamic Changes in the Obstructive Sleep Apnea Syndrome.* Systemic and pulmonary arterial pressures rise in association with episodes of sleep apnea. Pressures rise with each episode and return toward control levels when ventilation is resumed. When apneic episodes occur in rapid succession, pressures do not return to control values and show a stepwise increase. Upon awakening (with unobstructed respiration), both systemic and pulmonary arterial pressures return to control levels. Similarly, in a recent study, we documented that pulmonary wedge pressure may rise with repetitive obstructive sleep apnea—in some cases the monitored pulmonary wedge pressure values occurring during apneic events approached those producing pulmonary edema *(34)*. Thus, variations in left ventricular function, and secondary pulmonary congestion, may play a role in the hypoxemia frequently noted in sleep apnea patients.

The hemodynamic impact of obstructive apnea varies with the frequency of apneic events during nocturnal sleep. If apneic events occur repetitively throughout the night, during both REM and NREM sleep, then the longer the sleep period, the greater the pressure increase. We recorded pressures in patients who, in the awake supine control measurement, had pressures of 130/80 and 160/94 (systemic) and 30/20 and 34/20 (pulmonary), and who showed pressure increases to 200/100 and 280/170 (systemic) and 80/54 and 68/40 (pulmonary) respectively, after five hours of repetitive sleep apneic events. Patients in whom apneic events are intermittent (with periods of normal respiration during sleep) will not demonstrate the high pressure values noted in patients with continuous, repetitive apneic events.

Undoubtedly, the Müller maneuver that occurs during obstruction plays a significant role in the rise in systemic and pulmonary arterial pressures. This is obvious when the impact on hemodynamic variables of a single apneic event is compared with

*Sleeping and waking disorders: indications and techniques*

## SLEEP APNEA

**A** BEFORE TRACHEOSTOMY      **B** TRACHEOSTOMY

OBSTRUCTED AIRWAY    OPEN    CLOSED

RR INTERVAL (msec): 1,500 — 1,000 — 500

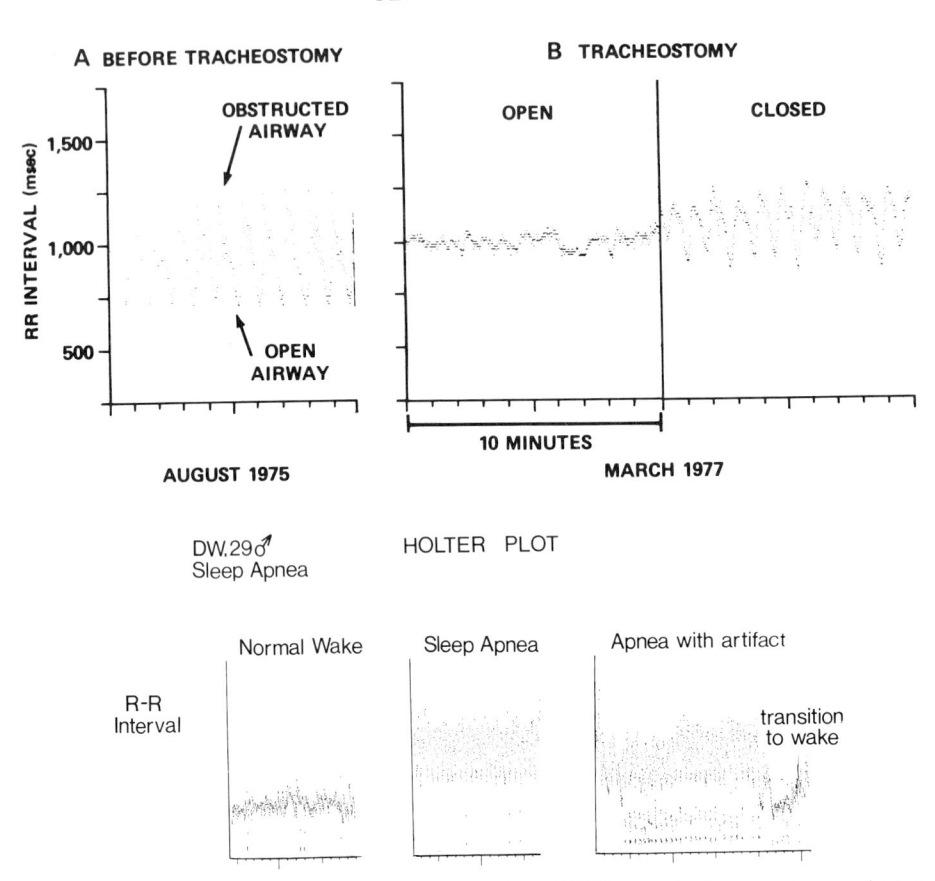

OPEN AIRWAY

10 MINUTES

AUGUST 1975     MARCH 1977

DW.29♂
Sleep Apnea     HOLTER PLOT

R-R Interval: Normal Wake | Sleep Apnea | Apnea with artifact (transition to wake)

**Figures 7–1a & 7–1b.** Holter (24-hour ambulatory) ECG monitoring can be used as a screening technique for abnormal breathing patterns during sleep, providing computer analysis of the R-R interval is available. In association with abnormal breathing patterns, stimulations of the autonomic nervous system occur; the stimulations involve the sympathetic and parasympathetic systems, depending on factors such as respiratory load, hypoxemia, etc. Progressive bradycardia will develop in association with the onset of an episode of apnea or hypopnea. When breathing is resumed, with a concomitant rise in the patient's alertness, important sympathetic responses will be observed. Plotting of the R-R interval will display a very characteristic pattern, similar to saw-tooth waves. The peak-to-peak distance between each saw-tooth wave indicates the duration of the abnormal breathing event. One must remember, however, that this zigzag pattern is not indicative of apnea per se, but rather is only a sign of abnormal breathing. Respiratory-load and state-of-alertness changes (such as from stages 3–4 to stages 1–2 NREM sleep) also will induce parasympathetic/sympathetic tone-balance changes. (This phenomenon is seen in children with enlarged tonsils and adenoids who snore but have no apnea and no significant changes in oxygen saturation.)

*Sleep and breathing*

**CENTRAL SLEEP APNEA IN STAGE 3 NREM SLEEP**

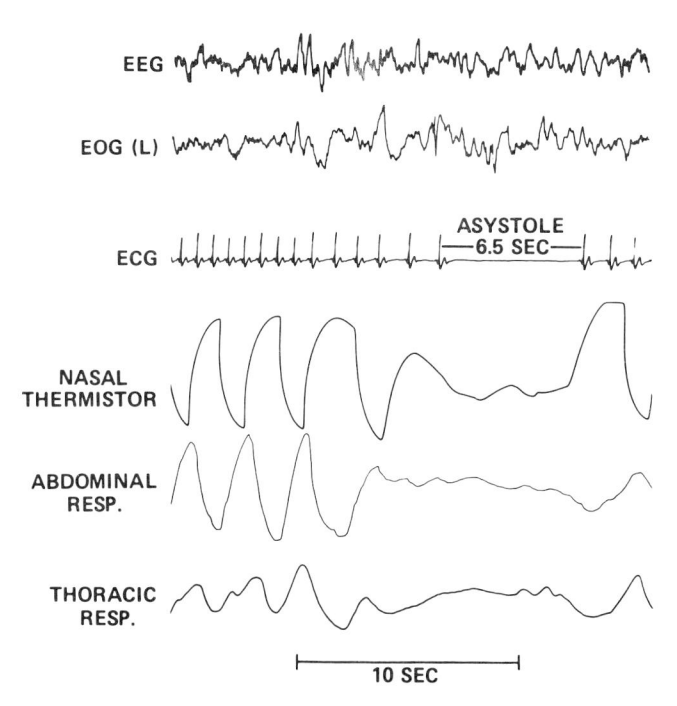

**Figure 7–2.** Example of cardiac arrhythmia associated with central apnea during NREM sleep. Channel I = EEG $C_3/A_2$. Channel II = EOG. Channel III = ECG (lead II). Channel IV = monitoring of airflow (labeled "nasal thermistor"; three thermistors—two nasal and one oral—are used and airflow monitored by them is recorded on this channel. This technique does not allow differentiation of oral versus nasal respiration, but does permit measurement of the presence or absence of airflow with the ambient air). Channel V = abdominal movement (measured with a mercury strain gauge). Channel VI = thoracic movement (measured with a mercury strain gauge). Paper speed is 10 mm/sec.

---

Because the peak-to-peak interval of the saw-tooth wave may provide a clue about apnea and hypopnea, continuous Holter ECG monitoring, or monitoring with a low-cost portable, digital device that records only R-R intervals, allows screening for abnormal breathing patterns during sleep. Figures 7–1a & 7–1b present R-R interval plots. The former was recorded with a classic Holter ECG with analog monitoring, and the latter was recorded with a digital device being developed by Vitalog Company. The difference between the R-R intervals during normal and abnormal sleep can be seen clearly.

that of a single obstructive event, or when the effect of a train of central apneic episodes is compared to the effect of a train of obstructive apneic episodes of similar duration. Rises in systemic, pulmonary, and wedge pressure are much more pronounced in association with obstructive apnea than they are with central apnea.

Thus, as noted above, hemodynamic changes should be investigated in addition to ascertaining the (A + H)I, if prognosis and therapeutic recommendations are to be determined. Hemodynamic considerations emphasize the importance of evaluating patients during several hours of continuous nocturnal sleep. Temporal distribution of apnea, and the impact of apneic events on blood oxygen levels, should be determined (Figure 7-3).

*The Obstruction: Location and Mechanisms.* In 1967, Schwartz and Escande reported a fiber-optic study during sleep in an obese, Pickwickian-type patient in whom they located the site of the obstruction in the oropharynx *(35)*. Since then, other studies—particularly those of Weitzman and his colleagues *(36)* and our group at Stanford *(37)*—have confirmed that *the oropharynx is the site of the obstruction.* Remmers et al. studied supraglottic pressures and confirmed this location *(38)*. To date, the only dissenting report has come from Krieger et al., who located the obstruction at the vocal-cord level after fiber-optic study of one obese, Pickwickian-type patient *(39)*.

Our studies have indicated that the posterolateral pharyngeal walls are first to invaginate and, at times, are the only anatomic structure involved in the obstruction. Various other anatomic structures, including the tongue, may participate in inspiratory obstructive phenomena, but obstructive sleep apnea may occur without involvement of the genioglossus.

At this time, the consensus is that sleep-related obstruction occurs in most patients at the level of the oropharynx without lower-structure involvement.

*The mechanisms of obstruction are not yet fully understood.* On the basis of fiber-optic studies, Weitzman et al. have suggested that an active contraction of the constrictors of the pharynx is responsible for obstruction *(36)*. Previously, Sauerland and Harper monitored the activity of the genioglossus muscle and reported decreased tone in association with obstructive apnea *(40)*.

We performed a study on three control and 19 obstructive sleep apneic patients in which we recorded muscle activity surrounding the pharynx during sleep in combination with fiber-optic scope studies *(37)*. Recordings of the palatoglosseus, palatopharyngeus, genioglossus, superior and middle constrictors of the pharynx, and stylopharyngeus demonstrated a sudden decrease in muscle tone just prior to the development of an obstructive apnea. Muscle tone returned just prior to resumption of airflow. In obstructive hypopnea, loss of muscle tone was complete in the superior and middle constrictors of the pharynx and in the stylopharyngeus but was only partial in the genioglossus.

Recently, Remmers et al. performed studies with simultaneous recording of the genioglossus and the tensor palatini, and confirmed that oropharyngeal closure may not be related to involvement of the genioglossus *(38)*. This negated the hypothesis that an active contraction of the constrictors of the pharynx was responsible for the obstruction

*Sleep and breathing*

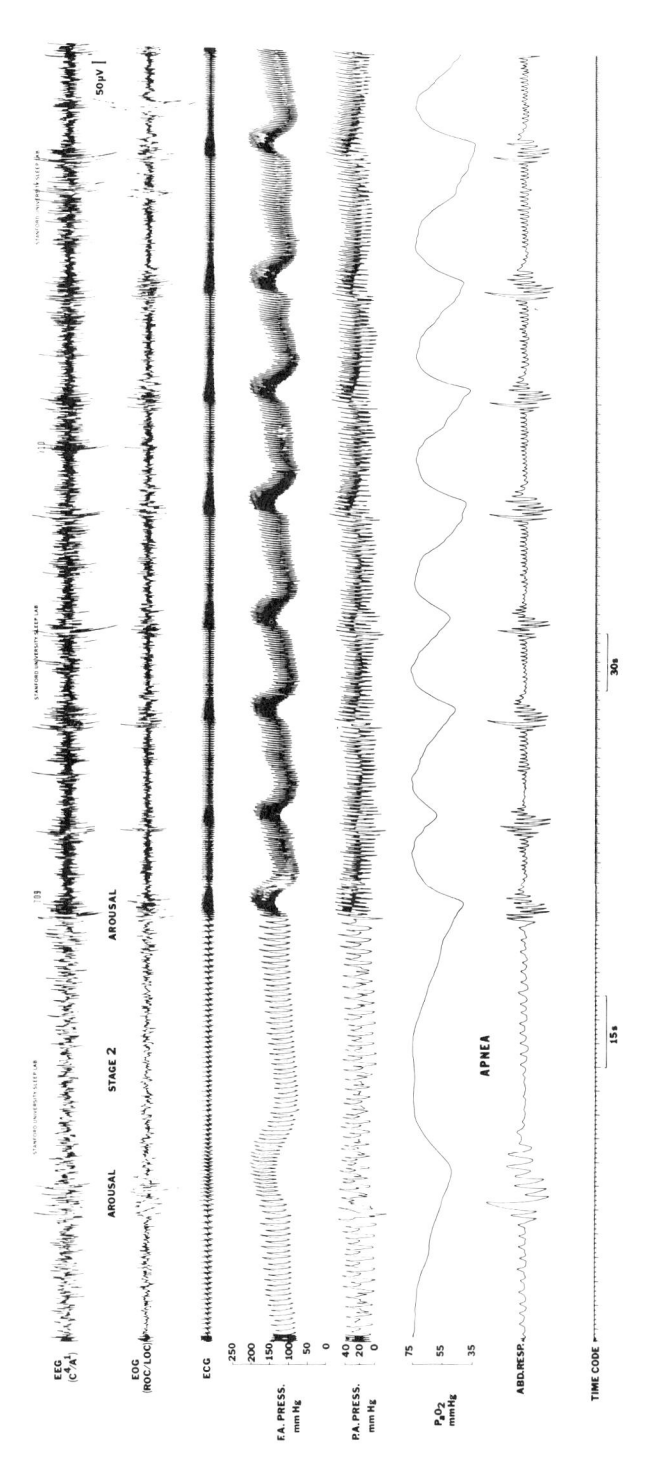

**Figure 7–3.** Polysomnogram performed on an obstructive sleep apneic patient with simultaneous hemodynamic study. Channel I = EEG $C_4/A_1$. Channel II = EOG. Channel III = ECG (lead II). Channel IV = femoral arterial pressure. Channel V = pulmonary arterial pressure. Channel VI = arterial oxygen (continuous monitoring by means of an intra-arterial electrode). Channel VII = abdominal respiration. Channel VIII = time code. (Time code was necessary because two polygraphs were used to make this recording. As is obvious from the figure, airflow and chin EMG were not monitored here. These variables were monitored, with others, on a second polygraph.) Paper speed is 5 mm/sec on the right and 1 mm/sec on the left. This recording emphasizes monitoring of cardiovascular variables. The changes in systemic and pulmonary arterial pressures with oxygen desaturation can be appreciated easily. Similarly, the relationship between EEG changes and hemodynamic changes are displayed.

and allowed them to propose a dynamic explanation. We also monitored central apneic events during sleep and observed inhibition of muscle tone in the oropharyngeal muscle and intercostal muscles simultaneous with diaphragmatic pause; i.e., during central apnea, a general inhibition of muscle tone was observed in the muscles involved in breathing. This is quite different from what we had observed during obstructive apneic events (Figure 7–4).

Recently, Dr. P. Lynne-Davies's technique for diaphragmatic monitoring with an endoesophageal diaphragmatic electrode allowed us to demonstrate that diaphragmatic activity increases, up to a point, with each inspiratory effort until the obstruction is resolved *(15)*. Thus, there is a clear dissociation between diaphragmatic and oropharyngeal muscle tone activity.

*The patency of the upper airway is controlled partially by the central nervous system* and is maintained by adjustment of muscular tone of the pharyngeal muscles. Tactile and proprioceptive messages from the pharyngeal mucosa and musculature supply the sensory input necessary for automatic adjustments. The pharyngeal muscles, particularly those responsible for maintaining the patency of the "pharyngeal tent," must increase their tone to overcome the tendency to collapse during inspiration. The forces that contribute to the tendency toward collapse during inspiration are: (*a*) the surrounding atmospheric pressure (a constant), (*b*) the weight of the soft tissue of the neck (which varies with individuals and usually is high in patients with obstructive sleep apnea syndrome), (*c*) the local compliance of the airway walls (which varies depending on fatty infiltration, edema, etc.), (*d*) the negative pressure inside the lumen of the airway during inspiration.

Normally, airflow varies inversely with the resistance and directly with the pressure developed between the alveoli and the airway opening. If resistance is high, negative inspiratory pressure must increase to counterbalance it and thus maintain normal tidal volume and oxygen saturation.

Sukerman and Healy *(41)* summarized the dynamics of the flow in the airway with the following mathematical formula, where $V_A$ = flow in the airway, $P_O$ = atmospheric pressure, $P_I$ = inspiratory pressure, and $R$ = airway resistance:

$$V_A = \frac{\Delta P (P_O - P_I)}{R}$$

Our studies demonstrated that a decrease in muscle tone, at the level of the "pharyngeal tent," and/or neck fat (neck infiltration and submucosal infiltration) increase resistance. Finally, the Bernoulli effect also contributes to collapse: if the volume of airflow is constant, the velocity of air at the constriction will decrease. Thus, if there is a narrowing of the airway at one point, the tendency to collapse will increase during inspiration.

Apparently, various central and peripheral factors play a role in the development of obstructive sleep apnea syndrome. During heavy snoring, there is a partial obstruction of the airway. Obstructive sleep apnea patients often report a history of heavy

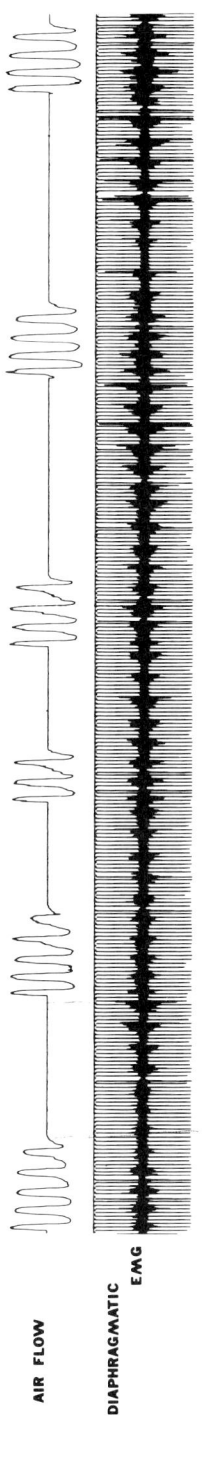

**Figure 7–4.** This figure presents the progressive increase in diaphragmatic EMG discharges, monitored with an endoesophageal electrode, that occur in association with each inspiratory effort during obstructive apnea. Channel I = airflow. Channel II = diaphragmatic EMG.

snoring during childhood, indicating that their airways were compromised early in life with varying degrees of increased airway resistance due to local and neurologic (central) factors. Sleep and its different states are in themselves central factors. The recent report that strychnine may decrease the severity of NREM sleep–related apnea syndrome indicates that we may be able to manipulate some of the central factors *(38)*.

Feedback loops may develop within central control: abnormal sleep due to frequent arousals increases the need to sleep, and sleep pressure affects muscle tone (not only during frank sleep but also during the "twilight" states so often observed in these patients during apparent wakefulness). Sleep deprivation, further, has general impact on the polysynaptic reflexes, increasing their latency period and slowing response progressively. Blood gas changes due to repetitive hypoxemia and hypercapnia also affect neuronal function. Thus a negative-feedback loop may develop that leads to a progressive decrease in the already compromised pharyngeal muscle tone; the local complication of weight increase and fatty infiltration of the oropharyngeal mucosa, combined with gradual exacerbation of central malfunction, may explain the full-blown syndrome that occurs most commonly when the patient reaches his fourth decade.

The vicious circle of this negative feedback loop can be interrupted by tracheostomy. Findings in long-term, post-surgery follow-up studies, such as immediate increase in percent of REM sleep (up to 30% each night in the first few months following surgery), indicate that these patients have been suffering from sleep deprivation. Not surprisingly, central apneas are frequently observed immediately after surgery but disappear gradually over the next three to six months. The chemoreceptors, presumably "reset" to progressively higher thresholds as the syndrome increased in severity, begin to regain sensitivity, sharpness, and rapid response time after surgical intervention.

## Clinical Symptoms of Predominantly Central Sleep Apnea Syndrome

Patients with predominantly central sleep apnea syndrome primarily complain of difficulty maintaining sleep and report several awakenings throughout each night. Some patients seek medical attention only after their partners observe their apneic events during sleep and become concerned. Depression and impaired sexual function also are symptoms frequently reported by this patient population.

At examination, predominantly central sleep apneics usually are within normal weight range or are underweight. They tend to be older than patients with predominantly obstructive syndromes. (In our patient population, the mean age of predominantly central apneics is 63, compared to a mean age of 46 in predominantly obstructive apneics.) Polygraphic monitoring demonstrates less pronounced oxygen desaturation and more moderate hemodynamic impact than is observed in obstructive syndromes. Central apneic events, however, do lead to cardiac arrhythmias and to arousal.

A difficult problem has been the classification of patients who have very long, repetitive central apneic episodes only during REM sleep. REM sleep–related apnea is a normal physiologic phenomenon, particularly in males. Some patients, however, experience repetitive central apneic episodes with each REM period, sometimes associated with cardiac arrhythmias and/or marked oxygen desaturation. This syndrome may lead to typical REM sleep-related insomnia; patients complain of "too many dreams," of continuous awakenings, and of daytime tiredness and exhaustion. We had the opportunity to study ventilatory responses of one patient with REM sleep–related disturbances. This patient had abnormal hypercapnic and hypoxemic values with REM sleep. No changes in ventilation were noted; $CO_2$ increased to 58 torr. Similarly, no change was induced despite a drop of oxygen saturation to 50%; when the patient reached hypoxemic levels equal to or under 40 torr, he would awaken abruptly. His hypercapnic, hypoxemic, and hyperoxic responses were normal when he was awake.

# Conditions Associated with Sleep Apnea Syndromes

Sleep apnea syndromes may occur in the presence of enlarged tonsils, adenoids, acromegaly, myxedema, micrognathia (birdlike face syndrome), basilar invagination, platybasia, neck infiltration secondary to Hodgkin's disease, and lymphoma. Apnea often complicates neurologic disorders such as myotonic dystrophy, multiple sclerosis, bulbar poliomyelitis, and polyneuropathy involving accessory respiratory muscles. It is seen in association with chronic obstructive airflow diseases and with thoracic deformities.

### Problems That Can Lead to Sleep Apnea Syndromes

As noted, patients who experience hypoxemic episodes during REM sleep may develop progressive central hypopnea and reduction in diaphragmatic activity and may further develop mixed apnea with an undeniable obstructive component.

We documented obstructive components in five patients: two had myotonic dystrophy, two were elderly patients with poliomyelitis, and one patient had moderately severe kyphoscoliosis (Guilleminault, unpublished data). All patients were placed under a Curass ventilator at bedtime. Interestingly, once good ventilation during sleep had been established, with parallel improvement of sleep-related oxygen saturation, the obstructive apnea disappeared. All patients experienced a decrease in daytime somnolence. This study provides insight into the development of mixed apnea and, particularly, the appearance of an obstructive component.

Two factors are implicated: (*a*) central apnea-induced sleep fragmentation and (*b*) sleep-induced hypoxemia and mild hypercapnia. Such repetitive chemical changes impact on the neuronal network involved in the multiple reflexes that normally assure the maintenance of a patent airway and avoid inspiratory mismatch. Other unknown factors may be involved. Certainly the rapid resolution of obstructive apnea by the establishment of good ventilation during sleep is striking and deserves further investigation.

## Hypoxemia During Sleep Without Apnea

Patients with rib-cage involvement (e.g., severe kyphoscoliosis, muscle diseases, and neurologic problems involving the thorax), lung involvement (e.g., chronic obstructive lung disease, asthma, cystic fibrosis), or significant obesity may not present any apneic events yet may experience a sudden decrease in oxygen saturation during sleep that is often associated with moderate changes in $CO_2$ (Figure 7–5). Oxygen saturation drops from wakefulness levels during NREM sleep and decreases further during REM sleep. Complaint of a sleep disorder—most frequently daytime somnolence—develops progressively. The severity of oxygen desaturation during sleep correlates with both the subjective sleep complaint and evidence of cardiac disorders (Figure 7–6).

Hypoxemia is observed in some patients only during REM sleep; in such cases it is associated with cardiovascular changes that occur only during this sleep state. As mentioned previously, intercostal and accessory respiratory muscles are inhibited during REM sleep. This tonic motoneural inhibition arises from the caudal brainstem region of Magoun and Rhines and is related to changes of membrane potential in the alpha motoneuron. The membrane potential of the spinal motoneurons (42) has been shown to be tonically hyperpolarized during REM sleep, involving the accessory respiratory and intercostal muscles. In infants, this sudden REM sleep–related muscle inhibition causes paradoxical motion of the rib cage and chest deflation. In children and adults with already compromised ventilation (e.g., secondary to deformed chest, lung abnormality), this sudden muscle inhibition causes an abrupt REM sleep–related reduction in tidal volume and resulting decrease in oxygen saturation. Values for these subjects are close to the "steep portion" of the oxyhemoglobin-hemoglobin saturation curve while the subjects are awake—thus a moderate change in tidal volume leads to noticeable desaturation, whereas a normal individual (with normal waking ventilation and oxygen saturation) will experience little desaturation due to moderate decreases in tidal volume. The difference in impact is due to the "inverse S" shape of the oxyhemoglobin-hemoglobin curve.

# Other Breathing Disorders

## Central (Primary) Alveolar Hypoventilation Syndrome

In 1970, Coccagna et al. reviewed 40 cases of "Ondine's curse" (primary (idiopathic) alveolar hypoventilation syndrome) and added their own cases (43). They emphasized that 16 of 40 cases presented obvious excessive daytime somnolence. Subsequently, "alveolar hypoventilation with normal lung, or the syndrome of primary or central alveolar hypoventilation," has been investigated. The introduction of diaphragmatic pacing led to a better understanding of the syndrome. Central hypoventilation syndrome may occur in adults, children, or infants. It can be "idiopathic" or congenital and can be secondary to brain insult.

*Sleep and breathing*

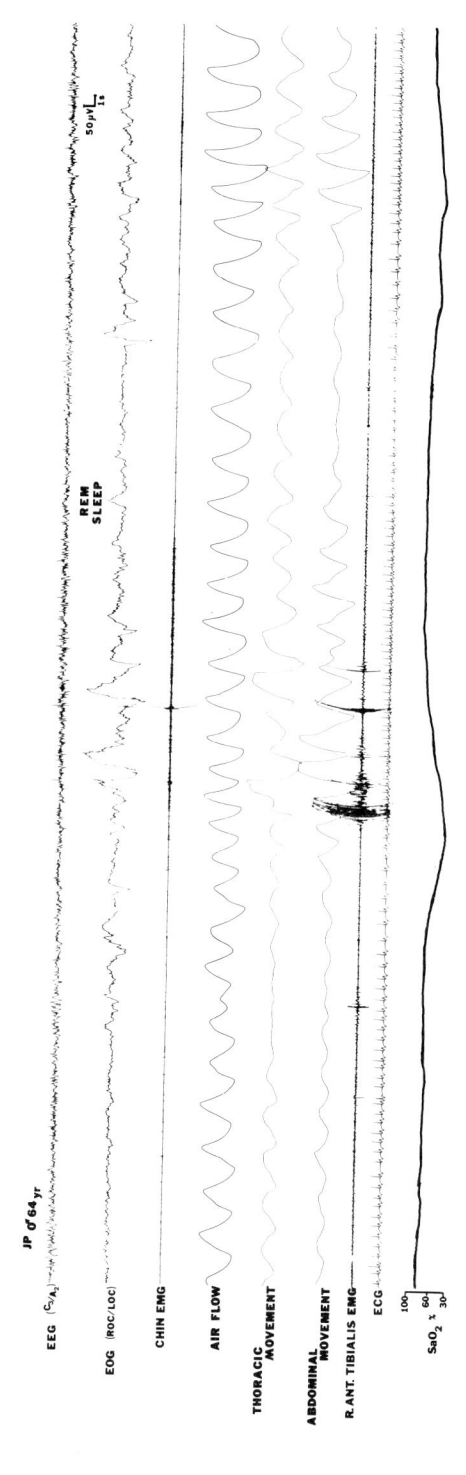

**Figure 7–5.** Monitoring obtained on a 64-year-old white male with severe chronic obstructive pulmonary disease (COPD). During REM sleep, intercostal and respiratory accessory muscles are "turned off" and oxygen desaturation occurs, associated with some bradycardia. Note that when hypoxemia is severe, an arousal response can be observed. During NREM sleep, ventilation is more even, and there are no abrupt hypoxemic "dives" such as those seen during REM sleep.

173

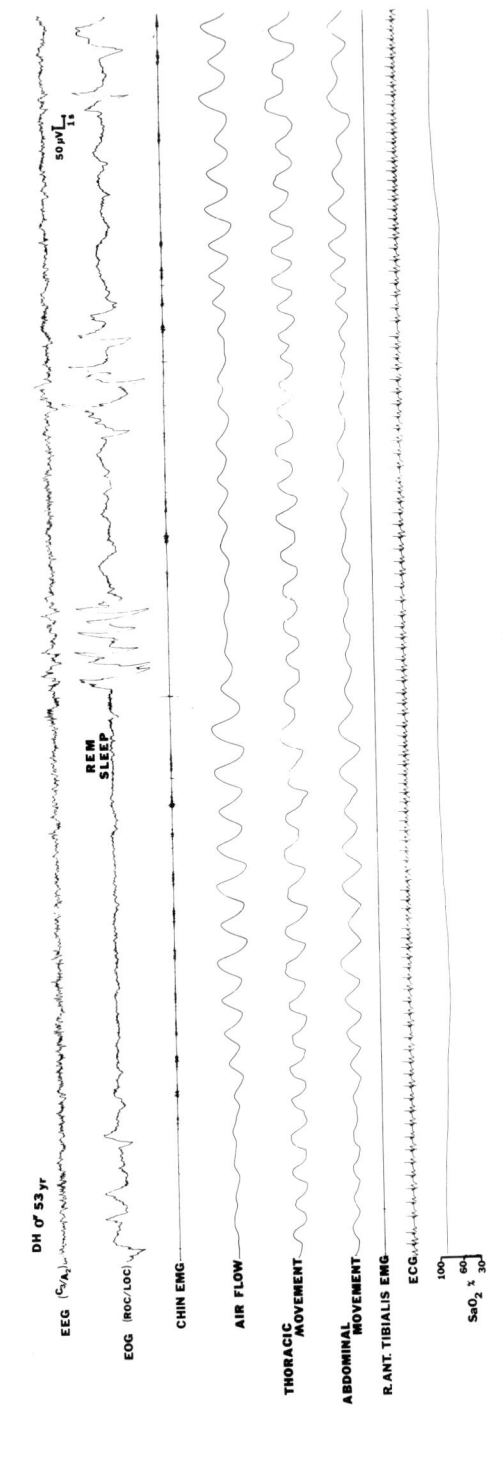

*Sleeping and waking disorders: indications and techniques*

**Figure 7-6.** Monitoring obtained on a 53-year-old black male with active tuberculosis and important lung lesions. As seen in COPD patients (see Figure 7-5), noticeable hypoxemia and mild sinus arrhythmia can be observed during REM sleep in association with the abrupt physiologic inhibition of intercostal and respiratory accessory muscles. During NREM sleep, no significant hypoxemia was noted.

## Congenital Central Hypoventilation Syndrome (CCHS)

CCHS previously was thought to be a rare defect involving central control of ventilation. It is particularly noticeable during sleep. Of late, CCHS has been diagnosed with increasing frequency during the neonatal period in intensive care units. During the past eight years, we have followed five CCHS cases and have consulted on eight others. Researchers did not perform long-term polygraphic monitoring at first; it is only during the past five years that investigation has focused on sleep-related problems.

Cyanosis and apnea were the initial symptoms noted in all reviewed cases; in 30% of the cases, these were associated with seizure activity. One subgroup presented abdominal distension and failure to pass meconium—they were diagnosed as having Hirschsprung's disease in addition to CCHS. All cases demonstrated marked differences in $Paco_2$ values between wakefulness and behavioral sleep, although blood gas studies indicated that $Paco_2$ was abnormal during wakefulness in most cases.

Unfortunately, evaluation of CCHS infants has not been systematic. Some CCHS infants were not diagnosed at first despite noticeable cyanosis and apnea during the perinatal period. Because CCHS infants present daily variability in the degree of clinical and biologic disruption, several reported cases were not transferred to specialized centers when their symptoms were first noted. When sleep monitoring *was* performed, it was discovered that the state of sleep in CCHS infants had a drastic effect on oxygen tension and end-tidal $CO_2$. In our own studies, all CCHS infants demonstrated normal findings of irregular respiration during REM sleep; however, the number of respiratory pauses and the degree of decrease in esophageal pressure readings (i.e., "shallow breathing" indicative of decreased diaphragmatic activity) were greater than we had expected when compared to normative studies performed in the same laboratory. During REM sleep, we noted sudden drops in recorded values of $Po_2$ that were followed sometimes by an awakening $O_2$ or by an arousal response. The most severe disruptions were noted during NREM sleep. Shannon et al. *(44)* and Barnhart et al. *(45)* report that hypoventilation was, in their cases, "directly related to sleep-state NREM sleep."

In most reported cases, moderate hypoventilation occurs during REM sleep with, at times, a sudden progressive increase in severity that frequently can lead to an arousal response. During NREM sleep, the syndrome is always at its peak with, at times, complete respiratory arrest.

Nocturnal polygraphic monitoring of CCHS infants should be associated with ventilatory studies performed during both wakefulness and sleep. Hypoxemic, hypercapnic, and hyperoxic responses can be obtained during wakefulness and REM and NREM sleep using techniques such as the "steady-state method" or the Read rebreathing method.

Hyperoxic responses can be used in evaluating the integrity of peripheral chemoreceptors in CCHS. Increased $Paco_2$ during hyperoxia indicates decreased alveolar ventilation and suggests functioning peripheral chemoreceptors, which generally is the case in CCHS.

The possibility of sleep-related airway obstruction should be considered during monitoring of CCHS infants. Several infants have been noted to present a stridor during sleep. Hunt et al. *(46)* reported a case in which a tracheostomy was required after implantation of a diaphragmatic pacer; persistent vocal-cord closure during all pacemaker-stimulated inspirations had caused the problem. We emphasize this case because it demonstrates that there are reflexes that precede phrenic input and impinge on the airway. If the reflexes are not present, diaphragmatic pacing will be useless without associated tracheostomy. This case also indicates that the "defect" of CCHS, usually attributed to deficient central chemoreceptors (47), may extend to other "control" cells. Heart rate abnormalities have been noted during sleep in CCHS infants (48); this may be due to some abnormality in the autonomic control of the heart.

When CCHS is suspected, infants should receive a careful autonomic nervous system evaluation during both sleep and wakefulness. Recent data indicate that CCHS often is associated with Hirchsprung's disease (which is characterized by aganglionic bowels) and with ganglioneuroblastoma (49) (often involving thoracic sympathetic chains and adrenals); these conditions should be considered and watched for (50).

## Central (Primary) Alveolar Hypoventilation in Children and Adults

Patients who receive the diagnosis of central alveolar hypoventilation exhibit one or more of the following features of the syndrome: (a) hypercapnia and hypoxemia, which may be present during wakefulness but always increase greatly during sleep; (b) sleep apnea, sometimes associated with respiratory arrest; (c) congestive heart failure; (d) pulmonary hypertension; and (e) polycythemia. The diagnosis may be suspected after a sudden crisis, such as respiratory arrest during sleep, nocturnal epileptic seizure due to anoxia, or severe cardiac arrhythmia; or it may be suspected because of unexplained cardiac failure or excessive daytime somnolence. It may be observed following encephalitis (we have seen cases who had Reye's syndrome), or following midpontine accident or head trauma. Sometimes the etiology cannot be discovered. One variant of the syndrome is presented by patients who had poliomyelitis as young adults (particularly with bulbar involvement) and who, having been free of any respiratory complaint for over ten years, developed excessive daytime sleepiness 20 years after having had poliomyelitis. Farmer et al. (51), in one report dealing with the largest number of patients having ventilatory studies, demonstrated that most of their patients exhibited a respiratory defect while awake. They found impairments in respiratory responses to hypercapnia, hypoxemia, and the combination of the two. Glenn et al. (52) have demonstrated clearly that upper-airway obstruction may be associated with central alveolar hyperventilation in both children and adults. They observed all three classical types of apnea associated with central alveolar hyperventilation and reported cases in which tracheostomy and diaphragmatic pacing were required owing to the obstructive component.

## Respiratory Problems During Sleep Associated with Neck and Head Trauma

Hypoxemia and apnea during sleep can be induced by significant, localized neck trauma without fracture. Severe whiplash syndrome was responsible for development of overt respiratory problems during sleep in eight patients referred to us. Often, patients who experience lower brainstem or upper cervical vertebrae trauma, leading to odontoid fracture *(53)*, or cervical hernia, are not seen by pulmonary-medicine specialists but are referred to neurologists and neurosurgeons. Fracture of the odontoid may be associated with forward displacement and mild compression of the inferior part of the medulla and of the upper cervical cord; immediate improvement is observed if the mild compression is released by moving the fractured odontoid forward.

The cause of sleep apnea following neck trauma is not known; spontaneous recovery is not uncommon. The disorder is, for obvious reasons, of legal as well as medical importance. Five of the eight cases referred to us were entangled in court compensation cases.

Excessive daytime somnolence was the referral complaint in all eight cases; in four cases, this was severe enough to cause complete disability eventually, and in the other four it was marked enough to create noticeable disruption.

The long-term prognosis for patients with respiratory problems during sleep secondary to head and neck trauma is variable. Caution should be exercised before final determination of the extent of disability is made. In some cases, trauma results in permanent disability and necessitates tracheostomy.

Because an investigator's findings are likely to influence legal issues such as long-term compensation in these cases, we strongly recommend that daytime sleepiness be evaluated objectively by sleep-latency tests and that the respiratory evaluation include determination of cardiovascular impact.

## Daytime Complaints Secondary to Respiratory Resistive Load During Sleep

Over the years, we have had the opportunity to study 25 children (10 girls, 15 boys), ranging in age from 2 to 14 years (mean age = 7), who were referred to us either by their schools, their parents (after reports of our work on snoring had been published in the local newspapers), or the otolaryngology division. The children were referred for abnormal daytime behavior, including napping at inappropriate times and snoring during sleep. Their clinical symptom complexes were similar, although symptoms varied in intensity from case to case. (Several of the children were first seen in the otolaryngology division for enlarged tonsils and/or adenoids.) The two most commonly reported daytime symptoms were daytime somnolence (this may represent a bias of our sleep clinic) and abnormal daytime behavior. The latter was of two types: (*a*) aggressiveness toward peers, siblings, or pet animals, refusal to accept adult supervision, and hyperactivity, or (*b*) complete withdrawal, pathologic shyness, absence of interaction with peers, etc. In many cases, the possibility of significant emotional problems or organic brain syndrome had been investigated but not resolved. Lack of coordination had been noted in some children, but examination failed to reveal evidence of cerebellum impairment. Thirty-three percent of the children had been placed in or considered for special-education classes. Enuresis was reported in 60% of the cases (age range 2 to 14 years).

At examination, 66% of these children were underweight or underdeveloped (height and weight). The four children whose ages were between 11 and 14 were still at Tanner stage 1 for secondary sexual characteristics (i.e., prepubertal). Four children had received a neurologic consult for significant limb hypotonia, and muscle biopsies had been performed. In one case the biopsy result was reported as "abnormal" but without clear histologic or clinical diagnoses. All others were completely normal. All of the children had presented enlarged tonsils and/or adenoids; some were borderline enlarged, some were obviously enlarged. History of recurrent colds, pharyngo laryngitis, or upper-airway infections were not common (only 14% of the children).

All patients were monitored polygraphically in quiet supine awake states and during nocturnal sleep. Variables monitored included: sleep parameters (EEG, EOG, chin EMG), ECG (lead II), and respiration. Airflow was monitored systematically using nasal and buccal thermistors. Abdominal and thoracic strain gauges were used to measure abdominal and thoracic movement. In 66% of cases, percentage of expired $CO_2$ was measured continuously using an $LB_1$ $CO_2$ or $LB_2$ $CO_2$ Beckman analyzer. Oxygen saturation was measured by ear oximeter. (Different models were used depending on what year the study was performed and what size ear the patient had.) Recent studies utilized a transcutaneous $PO_2$ electrode, despite obvious limitations in older children. An endoesophageal balloon was used to monitor endocsophageal pressure continuously during sleep.

The results of the recordings surprised us. No apneic events were recorded for any patient. However, every child presented abnormal recordings of respiration. All patients snored heavily throughout the night; some continuously, some intermittently. Twenty percent presented observable tachypnea, which was verified by recording. Most were restless sleepers; they tossed and turned frequently and often slept in unusual positions, e.g., with knees under the chest and neck in hyperextension. Significant sweating was noted in 75% of cases.

A significant increase in endoesophageal pressure without concomitant drop in $O_2$ saturation was noted in association with sleep, particularly during NREM stage 1 and REM sleep. (At times, transient drops in $O_2$ levels were noted during REM sleep only.) Holter (24-hour) ECG monitoring and computer analysis of recorded R-R intervals demonstrated that heart rate changes occurred in association with snoring.

In conclusion, some abnormalities of respiratory load during sleep were indicated clearly by recorded increases in endoesophageal pressure. The lack of concomitant hypoxemia is noteworthy.

All reported patients underwent surgery (tonsillectomy and/or adenoidectomy). We clinically followed each subject for a minimum of one year (mean follow-up, four years; range, one to eight). Monitoring was performed three to six months post-surgery in all cases; respiration was normal and reported symptomatology had receded.

We consider these findings particularly important in view of the great controversy concerning the advisability of performing tonsillectomy and/or adenoidectomy in children. Increased respiratory (inspiratory) load during sleep can lead to significant daytime symptoms ranging from free-floating anxiety, hyperactivity, or aggressiveness to complete withdrawal from social interaction. Children who demonstrate such abnormal behavior at school and at home with nocturnal snoring should receive an evaluation of respiratory load during sleep. Absence of apneic events during sleep does not preclude indication for surgery.

## Conclusion

Breathing during sleep is a complex function that may be impaired easily. Understanding the different components of the control of breathing during sleep forms the basis for investigating the impact of respiration and ventilation on sleep and sleep stages and of the secondary effects of sleep on the control of breathing. Adequate evaluation of respiration and ventilation during sleep requires appropriate protocols and technology. Although nocturnal sleep monitoring may not be convenient, it is necessary for accurate diagnosis and treatment of sleep-related respiratory complaints.

# REFERENCES

1. Orem J. Control of the upper airway during sleep and the hypersomnia–sleep apnea syndrome. In Orem J, Barnes CD, eds. Physiology of sleep. New York: Academic Press, 1981:273–313.
2. Sorbini CA, Brassi V, Solinas E, Muieson G. Arterial oxygen tension in relation to age in healthy subjects. Respiration 1968; 25:3–13.
3. Duron B. Postural and ventilatory functions of intercostal muscles. Acta Neurobiol Exp 1973; 33:355–80.
4. Duron B, Marlot D. Intercostal and diaphragmatic electrical activity during wakefulness and sleep in normal unrestrained adult cats. Sleep 1980:3:269–80.
5. Coccagna G, Mantovani M, Parchi C, Mironi F, Lugaresi E. Alveolar hypoventilation and hypersomnia in myotonic dystrophy. J Neurol Neurosurg Psychiatry 1975; 38:977–84.
6. Guilleminault C, Cummiskey J, Motta J, Lynne-Davies P. Respiratory and hemodynamic study during wakefulness and sleep in myotonic dystrophy. Sleep 1978; 1:19–32.
7. Skatrud J, Iber C, McHugh W, Rasmussen H, Nichols D. Determinants of hypoventilation during wakefulness and sleep in diaphragmatic paralysis. Am Rev Respir Dis 1980; 121:587–93.
8. Leitch AG, Clancy LJ, Leggett RJE, Tweeddale P, Dawson P, Evans JI.

Arterial blood gas tension, hydrogen ions, and electroencephalogram during sleep in patients with chronic ventilatory failure. Thorax 1976; 31:730–5.
9. Muller NL, Francis PW, Gurwitz D, Levison H, Bryan CA. Mechanism of hemoglobin desaturation during rapid eye movement sleep in normal subjects and in patients with cystic fibrosis. Am Rev Respir Dis 1980; 121:463–9.
10. Douglas NJ, Leggett RYE, Calverley PMA, Brash HM, Flenley DC, Brezinova V. Transient hypoxemia during sleep in chronic bronchitis and emphysema. Lancet 1979; 1:1–4.
11. Mezon BL, West P, Israels J, Kryger M. Sleep breathing abnormalities in kyphoscoliosis. Am Rev Respir Dis 1980; 122:617–21.
12. Guilleminault C, Kurland G, Winkle R, Miles LE. Severe kyphoscoliosis, breathing and sleep: the "Quasimodo" syndrome during sleep. Chest 1981; 79:626–31.
13. Kryger M, Glas R, Jackson D, et al. Impaired oxygenation during sleep in excessive polycythemia of high altitude: improvement with respiratory stimulation. Sleep 1978; 1:3–18.
14. Phillipson EA, Bowes G, Sullivan CE, Woolf GM. The influence of sleep fragmentation on arousal and ventilatory responses to respiratory stimuli. Sleep 1980; 3:281–8.
15. Guilleminault C. Sleep apnea syndromes: impact of sleep and sleep states. Sleep 1980; 3:227–34.
16. Guilleminault C, Ariagno R, Korobkin R, et al. Mixed and obstructive sleep apnea and near miss for SIDS. II. Near miss and normal control infants: comparison over age. Pediatrics 1979; 64:882–91.
17. Hoppenbrouwers T, Hodgman JE, Harper RM, Hofman E, Sterman MB, McGinty DJ. Polygraphic studies of normal infants during the first six months of life. III. Incidence of apnea and periodic breathing. Pediatrics 1977; 60:418–25.
18. Hoppenbrouwers T, Hodgman JE, Harper RM, Sterman MB. Respiration during the first six months of life in normal infants. IV. Gender differences. Early Hum Dev 1980; 4:167–77.
19. Carskadon MA, Harvey K, Dement WC, Guilleminault C, Simmons FB, Anders TA. Respiration during sleep in children. West J Med 1978; 128:477–81.
20. Guilleminault C, Dement WC. Sleep apnea syndrome and sleep disorders. In: Williams R, Karacan I, eds. Sleep disorders: diagnosis and treatment. New York: John Wiley and Sons, 1978:9–28.
21. Block AG, Boysen PG, Wynne JW, Hunt LA. Sleep apnea, hypopnea and oxygen desaturation in normal subjects: a strong male dominance. N Engl J Med 1979; 300:513–7.
22. Block AG, Wynne JW, Boysen PG. Sleep disordered breathing and nocturnal oxygen desaturation in post menopausal women. Am J Med 1980; 69:75–9.
23. Carskadon MA. Determinants of daytime sleepiness: adolescent develop-

ment, extended and restricted nocturnal sleep. Dissertation submitted to Stanford University in partial fulfillment of requirements for the degree of doctor of philosophy, 1979.
24. Guilleminault C, Tilkian A, Dement WC. The sleep apnea syndromes. Annu Rev Med 1976; 27:465–84.
25. Aserinsky E. Physiological activity associated with segments of the rapid eye movement period. In: Evants E, Kety S, Williams H, eds. Sleep and altered states of consciousness. Baltimore: Williams & Wilkins, 1967:335–50.
26. Orem J. Neuronal mechanisms of respiration in REM sleep. Sleep 1980; 3:251–68.
27. Guilleminault C, Cummiskey J, Motta J. Chronic obstructive airflow disease and sleep studies. Am Rev Respir Dis 1980; 122:397–406.
28. Guilleminault C, Pereita R, Souquet M, Dement WC. Apneas during sleep in infants: possible relationship with SIDS. Science 1975; 190:677–9.
29. Hoppenbrouwers T, Jensen DK, Hodgman JE, Harper RM, Sterman MB. The emergence of a circadian pattern in respiratory rates: comparison between control infants and subsequent siblings of SIDS. Pediatr Res 1980; 14:345–51.
30. Tilkian AG, Guilleminault C, Schroeder JS, Lehrman RL, Simmons FB, Dement WC. Hemodynamics in sleep induced apnea: studies during wakefulness and sleep. Ann Intern Med 1976; 85:714–9.
31. Tilkian AG, Guilleminault C, Schroeder JS, Lehrman KL, Simmons FB, Dement WC. Sleep induced apnea syndrome: prevalence of cardiac arrhythmias and their reversal after tracheostomy. Am J Med 1977; 63:348–58.
32. Bartall HZ, Tye KH, Roper P, Dessert KB, Benchimol A. Atrial flutter associated with obstructive sleep apnea syndrome. Arch Intern Med 1980; 140:121–2.
33. Shaw TRD, Corrall RJM, Craib IA. Cardiac and respiratory standstill during sleep. Br Heart J 1978; 40:1055–8.
34. Buda AG, Schroeder JS, Guilleminault C. Abnormalities of pulmonary artery wedge pressure in sleep induced apnea. Eur J Cardiol, in press.
35. Schwartz B, Escande J. Etude cinématographique de la respiration hypnique pickwickienne. Rev Neurol 1967; 116:667–78.
36. Weitzman ED, Pollak C, Borowiecki B, Burack B, Shprintzen R, Rakoff S. The hypersomnia sleep apnea syndrome (HSA): site and mechanism of upper airway obstruction. Sleep Res 1977; 6:182.
37. Guilleminault C, Hill MW, Simmons FB, Dement WC. Obstructive sleep apnea: electromyographic and fiberoptic studies. Exp Neurol 1978; 62:48–67.
38. Remmers JE, Anch AM, deGroot WJ, Baker JP, Sauerland EK. Oropharyngeal muscle tone in obstructive sleep apnea before and after strychnine. Sleep 1980: 3:447–54.
39. Krieger J, Kurtz D, Roeslin N. Observation fibroscopique directe au cours des apnées hypniques chez un sujet pickwickien. Nouv Presse Med 1976; 5:2890.

40. Sauerland EK, Harper RM. The human tongue during sleep: electromyographic activity of the genioglossus muscle. Exp Neurol 1976; 51:160–70.
41. Sukerman S, Healy GB. Sleep apnea syndrome associated with upper airway obstruction. Laryngoscope 1979; 89:878–84.
42. Glen LL, Foutz AS, Dement WC. Membrane potential of spinal motoneurons during natural sleep in the cat. Sleep 1978; 1:199–204.
43. Coccagna G, Mantovani M, Berti-Ceroni G, Pazzaglia P, Petrella A, Lugaresi E. Sindromi ipersonniche-ipoventilatore. Minerva Med 1970; 61:1073–84.
44. Shannon DC, Marsland DW, Gould JB, Callahan B, Todres ID, Dennis J. Central hypoventilation during quiet sleep in two infants. Pediatrics 1976; 57:342–6.
45. Barnhart BG, Reynolds W, Lees MH. Sleep ventilation correlates in congenital central hypoventilation syndrome (CCHS). Clin Res 1980; 28:120A (abstract).
46. Hunt CE, Matalon SV, Thompson TR, et al. Central hypoventilation syndrome: experience with bilateral phrenic nerve pacing in three neonates. Am Rev Respir Dis 1978; 118:23–8.
47. Severinghaus J, Mitchell P. Ondine's curse—failure of respiratory center automaticity while awake. Clin Res 1962; 10:122.
48. Haddad GG, Mazza NM, Defendini R, et al. Congenital failure of automatic control of ventilation, gastro-intestinal motility and heart rate. Medicine 1978; 57:517–26.
49. Liu HM, Loew YM, Hunt CE. Congenital central hypoventilation syndrome—a pathologic study of the neuromuscular system. Neurology 1978; 28:1013–9.
50. Guilleminault C, Challamel MJ. Congenital central hypoventilation syndrome (CCHS): independent syndrome or generalized impairment of the autonomic nervous system. In: Korobkin R, Guilleminault C, eds. Progress in perinatal neurology. Baltimore: Williams & Wilkins, 1981.
51. Farmer WC, Glenn WWL, Gee JBL. Alveolar hypoventilation syndrome: studies of ventilatory control in patients selected for diaphragmatic pacing. Am J Med 1976; 64:39–49.
52. Glenn WWL, Gee BL, Cole DR, Farmer WC, Shaw RK, Beckman CB. Combined central alveolar hypoventilation and upper airway obstruction: treatment by tracheostomy and diaphragmatic pacing. Am J Med 1978; 64:50–60.
53. Hall CW, Danoff D. Sleep attacks: apparent relationship to antitoxic dislocation. Arch Neurol 1975; 32:58–9.

# EIGHT
# RESPIRATORY MONITORING DURING SLEEP: POLYSOMNOGRAPHY

SHARON KEENAN BORNSTEIN

## Introduction

The presence of sleep apnea syndrome can be confirmed by polygraphic monitoring of respiration during sleep. The recording can also answer questions concerning the severity of the disease and can quantify disruption of sleep secondary to the disorder. Simultaneous recording of all the relevant parameters is necessary to achieve complete evaluation of the patient's condition.

It is convenient to distinguish between polygraphic monitoring performed as a screening procedure to diagnose sleep apnea syndrome and more extensive studies that may be performed once the diagnosis has been confirmed. Once the diagnosis is established, the more extensive studies provide evaluation of the severity of the syndrome and consequently help with the selection of the best therapeutic approach.

To diagnose sleep apnea syndrome accurately, simultaneous recording of electroencephalogram (EEG), electro-oculogram (EOG), electromyogram (EMG) of the mental and submental muscles, respiration, arterial blood oxygen saturation, and electrocardiogram (ECG) must be recorded over a minimum of six hours of nocturnal sleep *(1)*.

As mentioned in the previous chapter, a short daytime nap protocol (with or without prior sleep deprivation) has specific limitations:

1. The patient may not present rapid eye movement (REM) sleep during the daytime nap, which would cause a masking of the severity of the sleep-related breathing problem. This is true for two reasons: *(a)* the most extreme episodes of $O_2$ desaturation are usually seen during REM sleep and *(b)* a non-REM (NREM) nap would not permit evaluation of the impact of REM sleep on the autonomic nervous system *(1,2,3)*.

2. Another consideration is that, at least in children, there exists a circadian rhythm of episodes of apnea during sleep. That is, between 0300 and 0600 there is an increase in the probability of apneas occurring during sleep *(4)*.
3. Sleep deprivation and hypnotics, frequently used as provocative techniques to induce sleep for daytime naps, can bias the results of the tests in favor of positive findings; i.e., sleep deprivation and hypnotics have been shown to increase the severity of the disease in patients with moderate sleep apnea syndrome *(5)*.

Therefore, findings from daytime nap studies of sleep apnea patients can be ambiguous and may lead to an inappropriate therapeutic approach.

In addition to polysomnography, pulmonary function tests, consultation with ear, nose, and throat specialists, and 24-hour Holter monitor recordings are also part of the screening procedure.

Studies designed to document the progression of the disease, its mechanics, or its long-term effects on body function may include determination of endoesophageal pressure, expired $CO_2$, systemic and pulmonary artery pressures, cardiac output, arterial blood gases, and endoesophageal pH *(1,6,7,8)*. These studies are usually performed within a specific protocol after the screening procedure has confirmed a diagnosis of sleep apnea syndrome.

After discussion of the technical aspects of polygraphic monitoring, there will be a description of typical or representative polygraphic findings in the sleep apnea patient as well as a discussion of terms, definitions, and scoring techniques. The information presented is in no way meant to be an exhaustive description of all reliable techniques used to record patients for sleep apnea syndrome, but these techniques have been found to be reliable and have been used with modification and amendment for a number of years at the Stanford Sleep Disorders Clinic and Research Center.

To accurately diagnose sleep apnea syndrome, recordings should include sleep parameters (i.e., EEG, EOG, EMG), respiration, ECG, and $O_2$ saturation, and should be conducted over at least a six-hour period of nocturnal sleep. Wake after sleep onset should be less than 30% of the total sleep time of the recording. It is very important to record at least one REM period because the most severe respiratory irregularities and most extreme episodes of desaturation usually occur during REM.

# The Screening Procedure for Sleep Apnea Syndrome

## Recording Protocol

As stated in the introduction, the screening procedure involves simultaneous recording of the electroencephalogram, electro-oculogram, submental and mental electromyogram, respiration, arterial blood oxygen saturation, and electrocardiogram (Figure

*Respiratory monitoring during sleep: polysomnography*

8–1). Recordings are performed using a Grass model 7D 10-channel polygraph (see Appendices 8–A through 8–C).

*To Record Electroencophalogram (EEG).* Grass gold-cup electrodes with holes are applied using the collodion technique (see Chapter 1). Electrodes are applied to the $C_3$, $C_4$, $A_1$, and $A_2$ positions following the International 10–20 system of electrode placement, and a ground electrode is applied to the forehead. Impedances of less than 5000 ohms are recommended. (Impedances of less than or equal to 10,000 ohms are acceptable.) Sleep is scored from the monopolar derivation $C_3/A_2$. The electrode at $C_4$ is applied as an alternate recording site in the event that artifact develops at the $C_3$ electrode (Figure 8–2).

*To Record Electro-oculogram (EOG).* EOG is recorded using Beckman silver–silver chloride electrodes applied with electrode collars to the outer canthus of each eye. They are offset from the horizontal with the right outer canthus placement 1 cm above the horizontal and the left outer canthus placement 1 cm below the horizontal. EOG is recorded from outer canthus to contralateral ear (left eye/$A_2$, right eye/$A_1$), or from outer canthus to outer canthus derivations (Figure 8–3).

| CHANNEL NUMBER | DERIVATION |
| --- | --- |
| 1. | $C_3/A_2$ |
| 2. | ROC/LOC |
| 3. | EMG |
| 4. | Nasal Thermistor |
| 5. | Thoracic Strain Gauge |
| 6. | Abdominal Strain Gauge |
| 7. | Optional, see legend |
| 8. | ECG |
| 9. | Off, see legend |
| 10. | Hewlett-Packard ear oximeter |

**Figure 8–1.** An example of protocol used for the screening procedure for sleep apnea syndrome. Note channel 7 is available for monitoring other parameters such as endoesophageal pH, endoesophageal pressure, etc. Channel 9 is not used with this montage because the pen excursion for the ear oximeter analog exceeds the limits of channel 10.

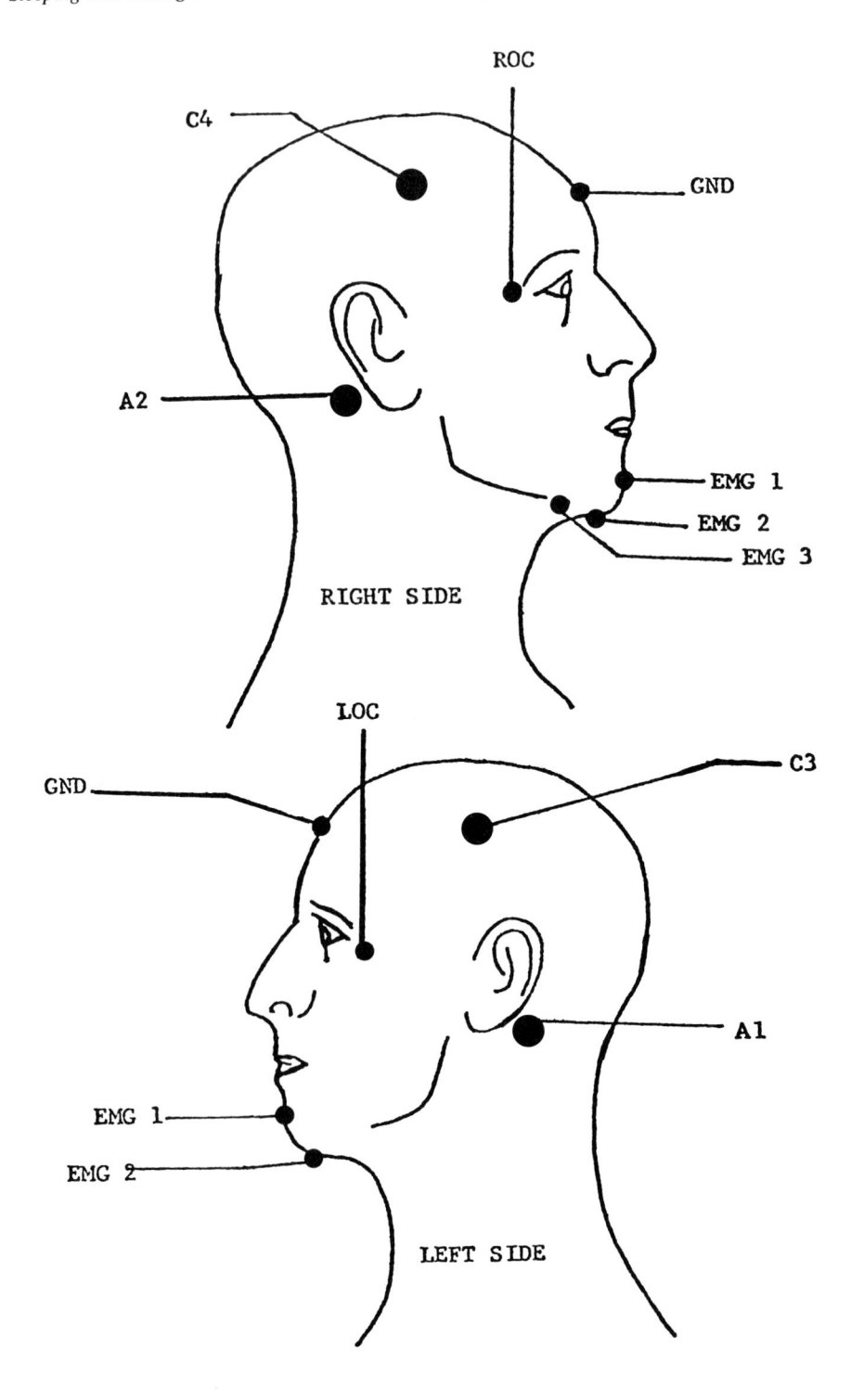

*Sleeping and waking disorders: indications and techniques*

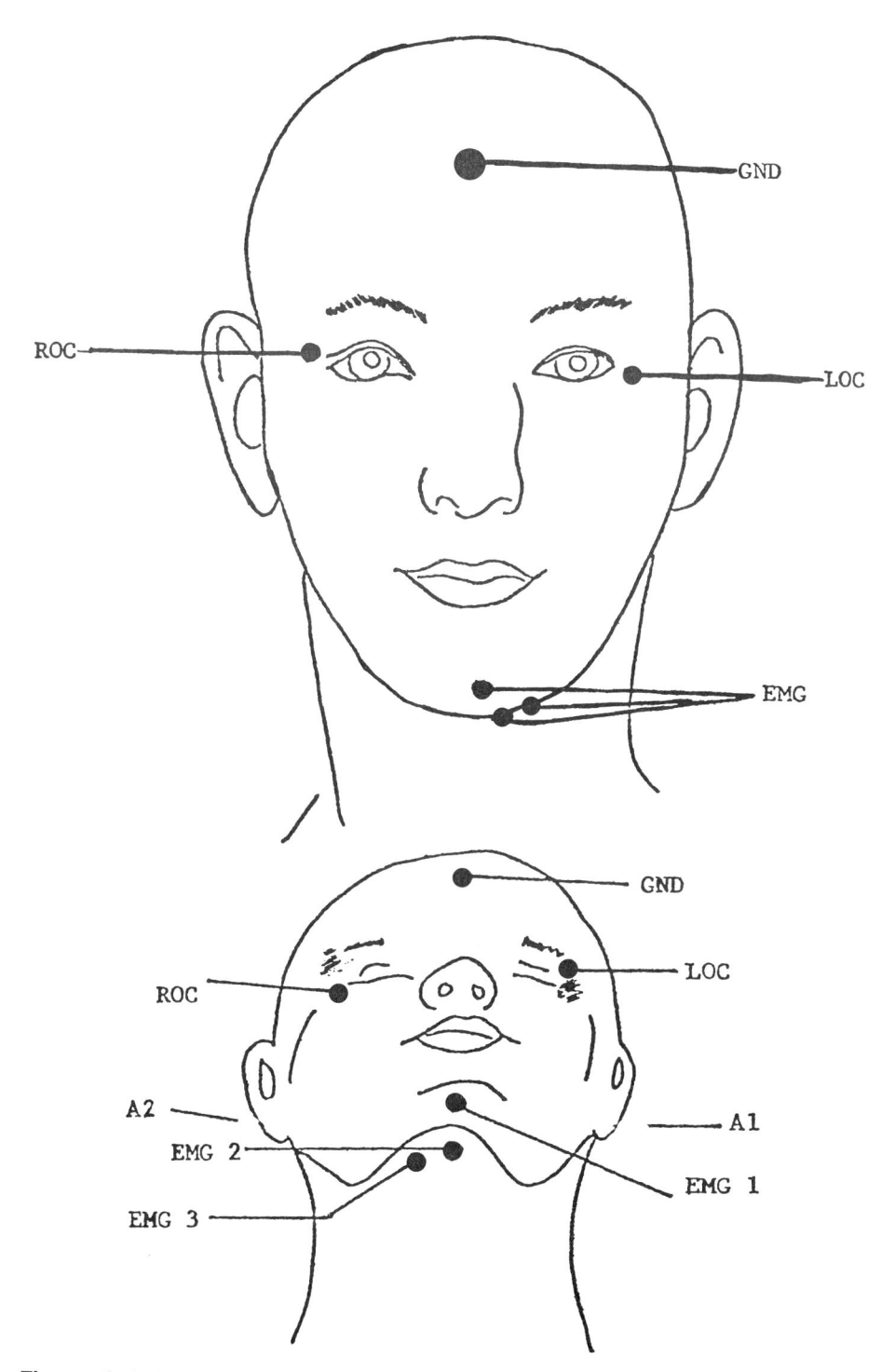

**Figures 8–2, 8–3, & 8–4.** Diagrammatic representation of electrode placement. Placement of reference electrodes $A_1$ and $A_2$ on the mastoid is recommended so as to avoid interference with the oximeter earpiece.

*To Record Electromyogram (EMG).* Mental-submental EMG is recorded using Beckman silver–silver chloride electrodes, identical to the electrodes used for recording EOG (above). One electrode is applied on the center of the chin; two additional electrodes are applied beneath the chin. Application of the third electrode provides an alternate recording site in the event that artifact develops in one electrode (Figure 8–4).

Placement of EOG and EMG electrodes is reinforced by applying surgical tape over the electrodes. Wires from all electrodes (EEG, EOG, EMG) are gathered and taped into a bundle at the crown of the head, forming a "pony tail." This placement is usually more comfortable for the patient. Care must be taken when pulling the electrode wires into the bundle to ensure that the patient has a full range of motion when turning his head. To check this, it is recommended that the technician ask the patient to turn his head from side to side while the wires are held together.

*To Record Respiration.* Respiration can be measured in a variety of ways. One method that is reliable is to measure airflow at the nose and mouth concurrently with measurements of respiratory effort at the abdomen and chest. Such simultaneous recording is necessary to determine the nature of the respiratory problem, i.e., to distinguish between central and obstructive apnea (see definitions later in this chapter).

Airflow is measured with thermistors (see Appendix 8–B) placed at each nostril and at the mouth. Thermistors applied in these positions monitor changes in the temperature of inspired versus expired air.

The nasal thermistors are secured with tape so that the thermistor tips lie firmly in the path of airflow. The oral thermistor is taped securely beside the mouth so that the thermistor tip lies in front of the oral cavity in the airstream that flows into and out of the mouth (Figure 8–5).

There are a few additional considerations to be made when applying thermistors. The technician should check for possible nasal obstruction by asking the patient if he has a deviated septum or other abnormality or if he usually awakens with a dry mouth. (If the patient usually awakens with a dry mouth, it could be an indication that he breathes through his mouth during sleep.) This kind of information will help determine where to place the thermistors for optimal airflow recording.

To amplify the airflow signal, the thermistors are plugged into a battery-powered coupler box, which in turn interfaces with the terminal box of the polygraph (see Appendix 8–B).

Respiratory effort is measured with strain gauges made from mercury-filled capillary tubing (see Appendix 8–B). The strain gauges respond to relative alterations in expansion that occur with efforts to breathe. They are secured with tape over the thorax and abdomen (Figure 8–6a, b, and c). Before applying them, the technician should observe the chest and abdomen to determine the areas of greatest excursion with breathing, then ask the patient which side he prefers to sleep on. If the patient indicates a preference, the gauges should be applied off the midline on the side opposite to the one the patient tends to lie on. After the optimal position for placement has been determined, the area should be cleansed. The skin should be free from surface oils for the best possible adhesion of the tape. If there is much body hair, an area large enough

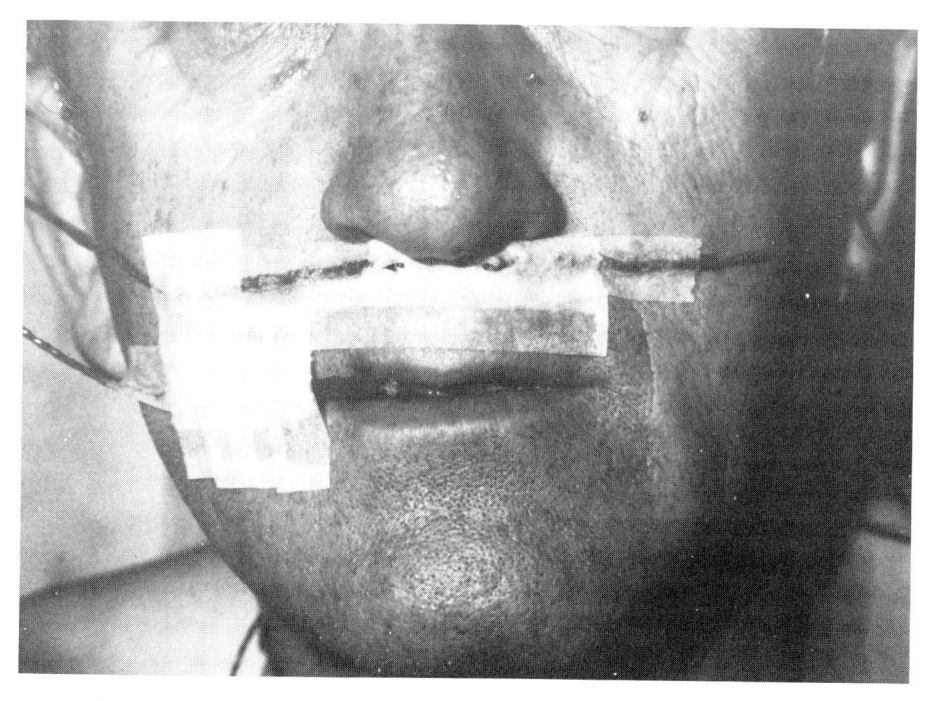

*Respiratory monitoring during sleep: polysomnography*

**Figure 8–5.** Thermistors taped in place to monitor airflow. Note that the glass bead is in the path of airflow at each nostril and in front of the mouth.

for the tape to adhere to the skin should be shaved. Strain gauges are then carefully taped in position. One side of the gauge is secured with surgical tape, the gauge is stretched approximately 2–3 cm, and then the other side of the gauge is secured. If the gauge is too loose, it will not respond to the expansion of the chest and abdomen; if it is too tight, it will be less sensitive and may break. The end wires of the strain gauges are gathered and taped together to minimize discomfort, and the ends are plugged into a coupler box (see Appendix 8–B) that is connected to the terminal box of the polygraph.

This method of measuring airflow and effort to breathe yields qualitative rather than quantitative information. Quantitative analysis can be achieved with a device called Respitrace™ (Respitrace Corporation, Ardsley, New York). A detailed description of this apparatus is presented in Chapter 9.

*To Record Oxygen Saturation.* Measurement of oxygen saturation ($SaO_2$) is accomplished using the Hewlett-Packard ear oximeter (HP 47201A).

$$(SaO_2 = \frac{HbO_2}{HbO_2 + Hb}, HbO_2 = \text{oxyhemoglobin}, Hb = \text{hemoglobin})$$

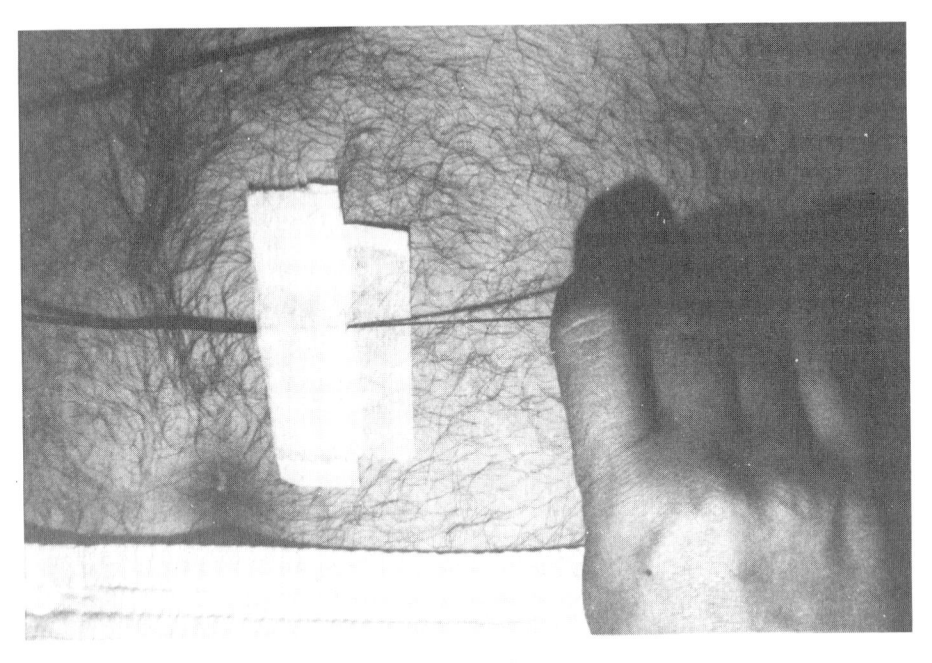

*Sleeping and waking disorders: indications and techniques*

**Figure 8–6a.** One side of the strain gauge is secured with surgical tape, and the gauge is stretched 2–3 cm.

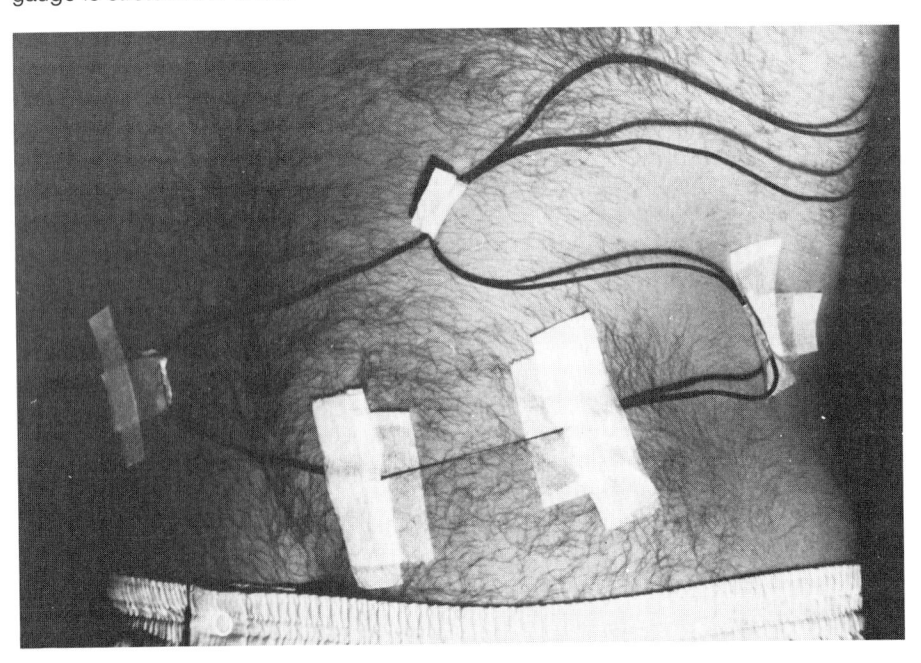

*b.* After the other side of the gauge is secured, stress loops are made on each side of the gauge and then the two wires are taped together.

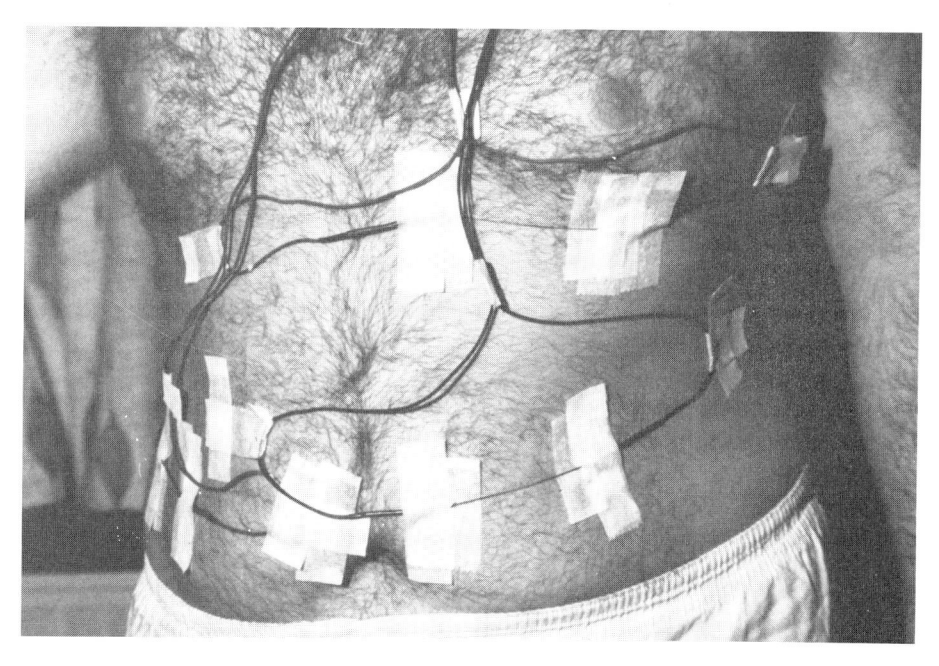

*Respiratory monitoring during sleep: polysomnography*

c.  Three strain gauges in place; two near the umbilicus and one at the level of the seventh rib.

The HP oximeter is an optoelectronic device that computes oxygen saturation and displays it in illuminated figures. The computation is made by analyzing the absorption of certain wavelengths of light passed through the pinna of the patient's ear. An interface (see Appendix 8–C) is placed between the oximeter and polygraph to facilitate graphic display of $Sao_2$, thus enabling the relationship between periods of apnea and subsequent desaturation to be seen clearly (Figures 8–7, 8–8, 8–11).

A complete operating guide for the oximeter is furnished by the Hewlett-Packard Company. The HP ear oximeter technique is noninvasive and is the most reliable instrument for measuring $Sao_2$ to date. One shortcoming of the HP instrument is that the earpiece size is not adjustable and therefore cannot accommodate very small ears.

An alternative to the Hewlett-Packard ear oximeter is the Waters (Waters Instrument Company) ear oximeter. Its design allows for recording on smaller (e.g., children's) ears and gives an indication of relative changes in oxygen saturation, but it is far less accurate for measuring the exact percentage of $Sao_2$ or for representing gradual changes in the patient's blood gases.

Several other devices are being tested now for use in the clinical setting. A device from Corning Company, still in experimental stages, is placed on a finger or toe. The accuracy appears to be within the same range as the HP oximeter, and the main advantage of the Corning oximeter is that it can be used when studying children.

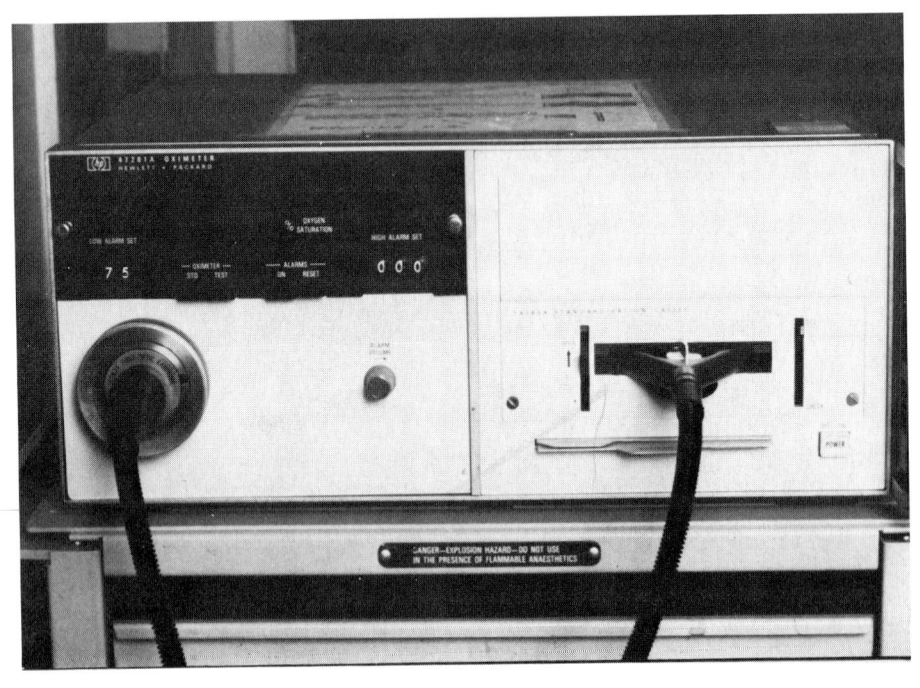

*Sleeping and waking disorders: indications and techniques*

**Figure 8–7.** The Hewlett-Packard ear oximeter. Here the earpiece is shown in place in the earpiece cavity on the right side of the machine. Percent oxygen saturation is a LED display and appears on the left side of the face of the oximeter during calibration and measurement.

*To Record Electrocardiogram (ECG).* ECG is recorded from two Beckman electrodes. One electrode is placed on the right shoulder over the clavicle, the other is placed on the left side in the region of the seventh rib. It is imperative that a visual display of ECG be included on the recording so that cardiac abnormalities may be appreciated. It is important for the technician to be able to see the ECG during the study so he can monitor the cardiac status and call for medical assistance if necessary. The record should accurately document the relationship between incidence of cardiac abnormalities and periods of apnea.

Further appreciation of many of the cardiac abnormalities associated with sleep apnea syndrome may be gained from continuous monitoring of the electrocardiogram during sleep and wakefulness. A 24-hour continuous ECG recording can be made using a Holter monitor (Medilog, Avionics, or Advanced Med), and the data are computer-processed for comparison with the polygraphic record (Figure 8–9).

As mentioned in the preceding chapter, the Holter ECG monitor can be used independently of polysomnography as a screening technique for abnormal breathing during sleep, provided that computer analysis of the R-R interval is available. The use

*Respiratory monitoring during sleep: polysomnography*

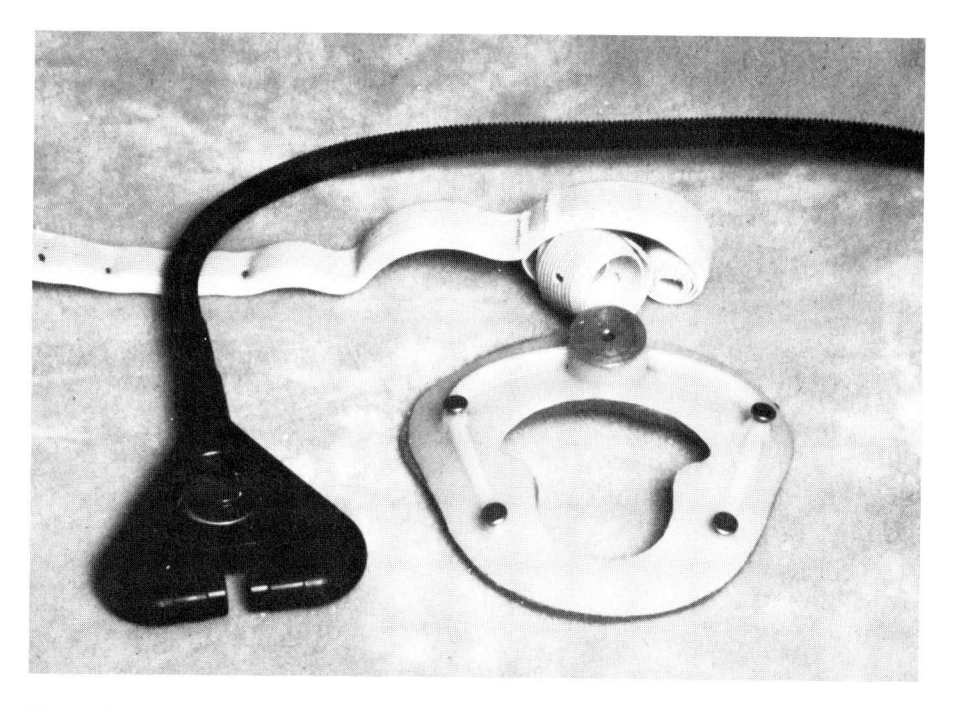

**Figure 8–8.** Shown here are the earpiece (left), head mount (right), and elastic band (above) for the HP oximeter. The head mount is placed over the ear so that the pinna of the ear protrudes through the opening in the center of the mount. The elastic band attaches to the mount and wraps around the circumference of the head to keep the mount in place. The earpiece attaches to the mount via a screw. The threads for the screw can be seen at the top of the mount.

of this technique, however, implies that the user is familiar with the pattern recognition associated with breathing irregularities that occur during sleep, as seen on the Holter plot.

Computer analysis is essential because some of the changes in the R-R interval related to the involvement of the sympathetic and parasympathetic nervous system occur between 500 and 1200 msec (see the legend of Figure 7–1 in the preceding chapter for a theoretical explanation).

The reliability of the technique will vary with the experience of the analyst. An experiment to test the reliability of the technique was performed at Stanford. Dr. R. Winkle of the Cardiology Department and Dr. C. Guilleminault of the Sleep Disorders Clinic reviewed Holter plots from 200 patients. Each subject had a 24-hour Holter monitor, and polysomnography was performed during nocturnal sleep within the same 24-hour period. Each physician was asked to interpret the Holter plot and to determine whether the pattern correlated with abnormal breathing during sleep. Ability to correlate

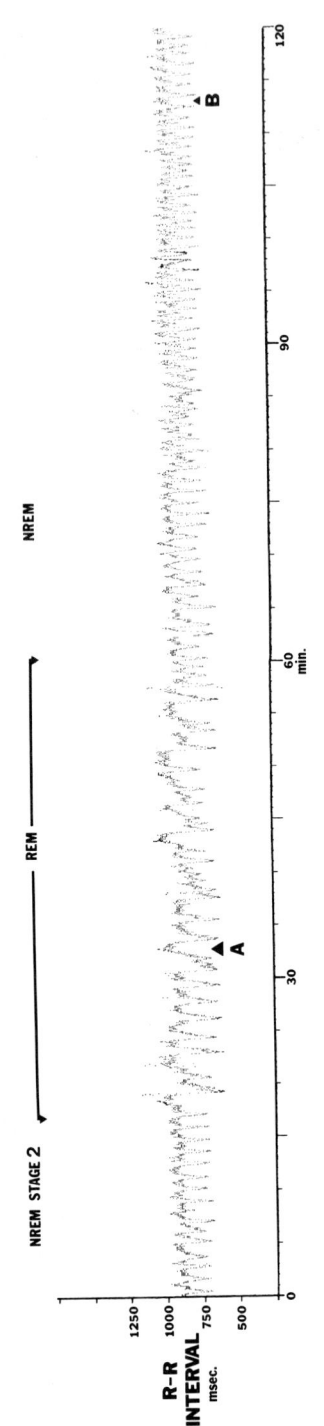

**Figure 8–9.** An example of the computerized plot of the R-R interval of the electrocardiogram of a patient wearing a Holter monitor during sleep. Variations in the R-R interval can be correlated with abnormal respiratory events. Note the difference between point A, found to correlate with REM sleep on the polysomnogram, and point B, which correlates with NREM sleep.

R-R plot and presence of abnormal breathing during sleep ranged between 95% and 99.3%. Errors represented mild cases of sleep apnea syndrome not diagnosed by the Holter plot.

In a second experiment, a random sample of 100 Holter plots was reviewed by Dr. R. Winkle. A total of 11 patients were identified as possibly presenting sleep apnea syndrome by virtue of review of the Holter plot. Polysomnography and 24-hour Holter monitoring was then performed on seven of those 11 patients and all of them presented sleep apnea syndrome.

Therefore, there is potential for ambulatory screening of patients with suspected sleep apnea syndrome as long as the appropriate technology and interpretive experience are available.

## Elaborations on the Screening Procedure Recording Protocol

*Endoesophageal Pressure.* On occasion the standard screening procedure cannot, because of artifact, distinguish between obstructive and central episodes of sleep apnea. Hence a determination of the severity of the disease is difficult, and more refined polygraphic measures may be necessary. A measurement of endoesophageal pressure conclusively determines the type of apnea. This measure is obtained by the insertion of either an endoesophageal balloon (Anode Rubber Plating Company, Houston, Texas) or a catheter-tip pressure transducer (Bio-Tec BT5F, Bio-Tec Instruments, Pasadena, California). A series of increasingly negative endoesophageal pressures, following from and terminated by an interval during which the pressure variation with respiratory effort is consistent with waking values, establishes the presence of airway obstruction. Inspiration may be distinguished from expiration by monitoring percentage of $CO_2$ beneath the nostrils or below the mouth (gas analyzer, Beckman Instruments, Schiller Park, Illinois).

Results obtained from measurement of endoesophageal pressure can illustrate diaphragmatic response to hypoxemia and hypercapnia and may give an indication of diaphragmatic fatigue *(9)*.

*Endoesophageal pH.* In patients with gastroesophageal reflux and/or esophagitis in association with obstructive sleep apnea, it may be helpful to monitor esophageal pH to determine the frequency and duration of reflux episodes during sleep. This is accomplished by placing a pH probe (Microelectrodes, Inc., Londonderry, New Hampshire) in the esophagus 5 cm above the esophagogastric junction for continuous monitoring of esophageal pH (pH meter, Corning, Santa Clara, California). The output of the pH meter is interfaced to the polygraph (J1, J2 input position on the Grass driver amplifier) to enable graphic display. The presence of reflux is documented by a drop in pH below 4.0 lasting approximately ten seconds.

*Hemodynamic Studies.* Evaluation of hemodynamic status during sleep-related respiratory irregularities can be obtained by simultaneous all-night monitoring of aortic and pulmonary arterial pressures, continuous measurement of arterial $Po_2$ by a $Po_2$ electrode (multipurpose differential oxygen analyzer, model 625–001, International Biophysics Corporation, Irvine, California), and intermittent sampling of blood gases.

Standard pressure transducers may be employed (e.g., model MP–15, Micron Instruments, Los Angeles, California) coupled to optically isolated polygraph preamplifiers (model 880 5C pressure amplifier, Hewlett-Packard, Waltham, Massachusetts). The pulmonary arterial pressure tracing significantly aids in evaluating both severity and type of respiratory abnormality. During the course of monitoring, wedge pressures may also be obtained.

Cardiac output, defined as the volume of blood ejected by the heart each minute, can also be measured regularly during sleep using the thermodilution technique. The use of room temperature water rather than ice water is recommended because of the reduced amount of disturbance and chance of subsequent arousal of the patient. Results of the thermodilution method can be confirmed by the Fick method.

## Evaluating the Polygraphic Recording: Terminology, Definition, and Scoring Techniques

*Apnea* has been defined as cessation of airflow at the level of the nostrils and mouth lasting at least ten seconds. Apneic episodes are measured from the end of exhalation to the beginning of the next inhalation. A *sleep apnea syndrome* is diagnosed if, during six hours of nocturnal sleep, at least 30 apneic episodes are observed in both rapid eye movement (REM) and non-rapid eye movement (NREM) sleep, some of which must appear repetitively in NREM sleep. Apneic episodes at sleep onset or accompanying bursts of rapid eye movement during REM periods are not considered pathologic (6).

An *Apnea + Hypopnea Index (A + H)I* is defined as the number of respiratory irregularities per sleep hour and can be calculated as follows:

$$\frac{\text{Total Number of Apneas + Hypopneas}}{\text{Total Sleep Time in Minutes}} \times 60$$

An index of 5 is considered within normal limits.

Three types of apnea can be defined by using the nasal thermistor and strain gauge recording techniques. *Central apnea* is characterized by cessation of both airflow and respiratory movements; i.e., both tracings fall to less than 20% of basal value (Figure 8–10). Arousal need not follow the respiratory irregularity and oxygen desaturation is not an essential characteristic. In *obstructive (or upper airway) apnea*, airflow past nasal and buccal thermistors is absent despite persistent respiratory effort recorded by thoracic and abdominal strain gauges (Figure 8–11). More precisely, obstructive apnea is defined by a fall in amplitude of the thermistor tracing (with or without an associated change in the amplitude of the strain gauge tracings) to less than 50% of the basal value amplitude as judged from the period two minutes before or after the res-

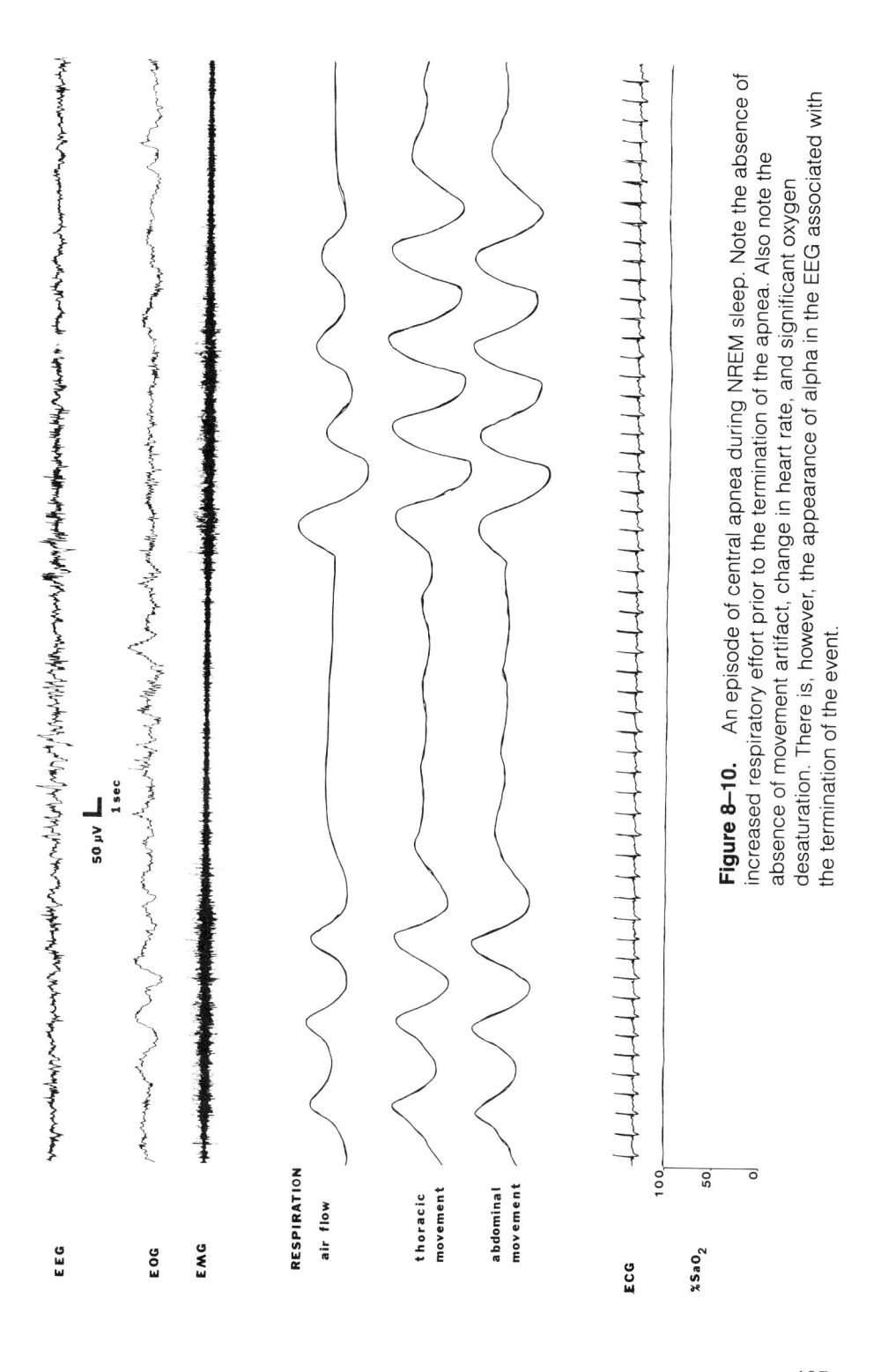

**Figure 8–10.** An episode of central apnea during NREM sleep. Note the absence of increased respiratory effort prior to the termination of the apnea. Also note the absence of movement artifact, change in heart rate, and significant oxygen desaturation. There is, however, the appearance of alpha in the EEG associated with the termination of the event.

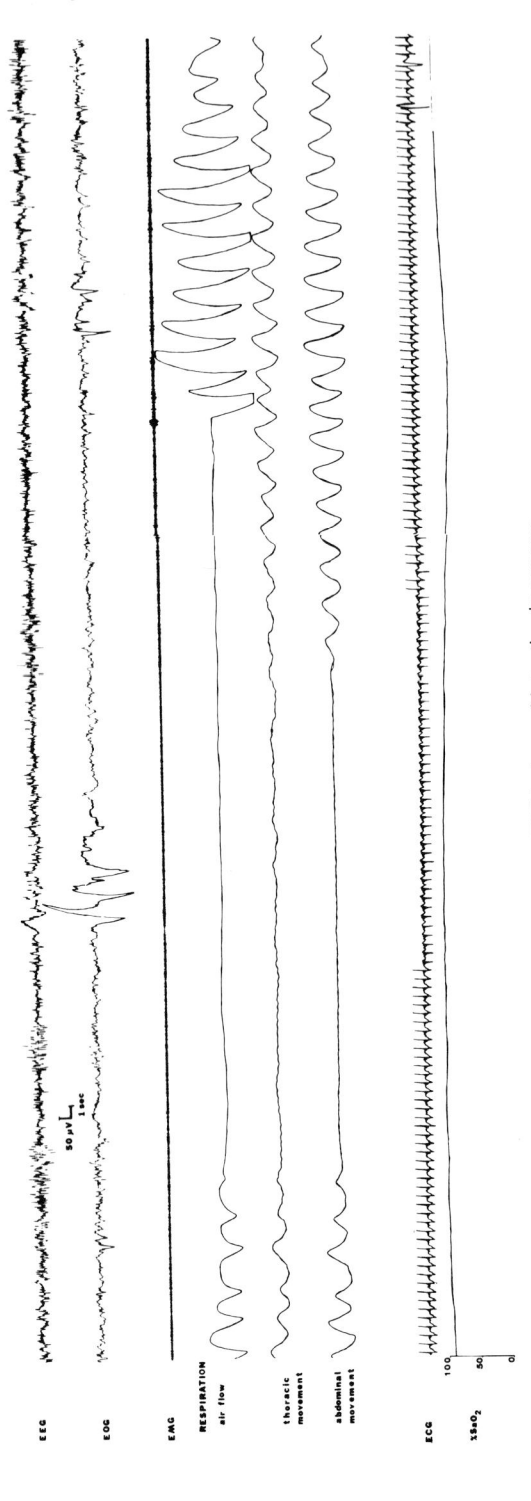

*Sleeping and waking disorders: indications and techniques*

**Figure 8–11.** An episode of obstructive apnea during REM sleep. Note the increase of abdominal and thoracic movement prior to reestablishment of airflow. Also note ECG abnormalities (change in polarity of the "R" wave and PVCs) and oxygen desaturation. This example is somewhat atypical in that there is no movement artifact associated with the termination of the episode.

piratory irregularity in question. To score the episode as obstructive apnea, the strain gauge must continue to fluctuate at the respiration frequency with an amplitude increase of at least 20% when compared with the amplitude of the basal value. This increase in strain gauge trace amplitude occurs in association with the decrease in the amplitude of the thermistor tracing. Obstructive apneas often terminate in significant body movements. Associated with the body movement is an increase in the mental-submental EMG, possible eye movement, and the appearance of movement artifact in the ECG tracing. Frequently, there is muscle artifact in the EEG trace or the appearance of a K complex or a five- to ten-second burst of alpha activity at the end of the apneic episode.

Another feature characteristic of a terminating obstructive apnea is a more than twofold increase in the amplitude of the thermistor tracing with or without a similar change in the strain gauge tracing.

When scoring an obstructive event, if the thermistor tracing decrease in amplitude does not reach or exceed 50% of the basal value amplitude, but there is a persistent increase in the amplitude of the strain gauge trace, the event can be scored obstructive if there is at least a 10% decrease in oxygen saturation as measured by the Hewlett-Packard oximeter or if the oxygen saturation level falls below 90% during or immediately following the apnea.

*Mixed apnea* has both a central and an obstructive component. It is characterized by a cessation of airflow and absence of respiratory effort early in the episode followed by a resumption of respiratory effort in the latter part of the episode that eventually reestablishes airflow. (This sequence of events is true for adults, but a reversal of the sequence—i.e., obstructed breaths, then central apnea—has been seen in studies of infants' respiration on occasion.)

*Hypopnea* (Figure 8–12) is an irregular respiratory event characterized by a decrease in respiratory airflow to one-third of its basal value and a parallel reduction in amplitude of thoracic and abdominal movements associated with a decrease in $O_2$ saturation.

Hypopnea can also be classified as central, obstructive, or mixed. Central hypopnea is associated with a decrease in respiratory muscle activity. Obstructive hypopnea is related to a partial obstruction of the airway, and mixed hypopnea has both central and obstructive components. Recordings performed with strain gauges and thermistors usually will not enable the differentiation of the three types. Hypopnea recorded by the strain gauge–thermistor technique will usually present as a central event. In order to differentiate, it is necessary to record intercostal EMG, diaphragmatic EMG, and endoesophageal pressure. Central hypopnea is indicated by a decrease in intercostal and diaphragmatic EMG and a decrease in endoesophageal pressure changes in association with the decrease in abdominal and thoracic movements, decreased airflow, and $O_2$ desaturation. Obstructive hypopnea can be confirmed by a progressive increase in intercostal and diaphragmatic EMG and a progressive increase in endoesophageal pressure in association with the decrease in airflow and respiratory effort, and $O_2$ desaturation.

Hypopnea, when scored from recordings performed with the strain gauge-thermistor technique, is not differentiated and, as stated above, usually appears as a central

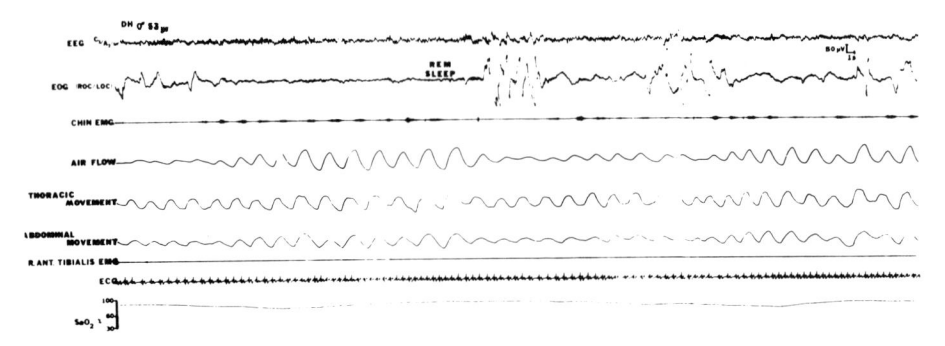

*Sleeping and waking disorders: indications and techniques*

**Figure 8–12.** An episode of hypopnea during REM sleep. Note the simultaneous decrease in amplitude of the airflow and abdominal and thoracic movement channels. Also shown is a decrease in oxygen saturation and the appearance of heart rate changes.

event. Episodes scored as hypopnea are included in the total number of apneas when calculating the apnea index.

## Notes on Sleep Staging

Scoring sleep in the presence of significant respiratory pathology is often difficult. As mentioned above, the EEG often indicates "arousal" (see preceding chapter for definitions of arousal) at the termination of each apneic episode, and the cycle length of the episode may be as short as 20 seconds, in which case no sleep may be scored by the Rechtschaffen-Kales sleep-stage scoring criteria *(10)*. Moreover, there is a significant amount of unscorable artifact, during which the arousal status is unknown.

Therefore, problems arise in the definition of sleep-stage transitions. The following modified rules are suggested to clarify the situation *(11)*. An epoch, following a clear stage wake epoch as judged by the standard rules, shall be scored stage 1 if it contains an interval scorable as stage 1 (by criteria other than duration) of greater duration than cumulative stage wake contained on the same page (epoch). In other words, 50% of the scorable portion of an epoch must meet the conventional criteria for stage 1. Stage 1 is continued through any arousal artifact that is not followed by clear stage wake until the first sleep spindle, K complex, or rapid eye movement. If the sleep spindle or K complex occurs before 50% of the scorable portion of the epoch in which it occurs, that epoch is scored stage 2. Otherwise, it is scored the same as the preceding epoch, and the succeeding epoch is scored stage 2 unless there is an intervening arousal resulting in transition to wake. Stage 2 is continued through any arousals not followed by transition to wake. At the discretion of the scorer, stage 3–4 may or may not be scored, any epochs satisfying the conventional stage 3–4 criteria being regarded as continuations of stage 2. In a central apnea record containing minimal movement artifact, stage 3–4 may be scored according to the standard criteria.

Stage REM following stage 2 is scored from the last sleep spindle or K complex preceding an interval containing a rapid eye movement not associated with an arousal or body movement, irrespective of intervening movement artifact. It continues through an interval of transitional stage wake or stage 2. EMG elevations from snoring or movement artifacts are ignored. A non-stage 2 epoch occurring between stage wake (unambiguous or transitional) and an epoch containing an unambiguous rapid eye movement, when there is no intervening transitional stage wake, is scored stage 1 if the tonic EMG level (excluding snoring and movement-associated increases) is greater than the tonic EMG level of the epoch in which the rapid eye movement occurs; it is scored stage REM if the tonic EMG level is less than or equal to that of the eye movement epoch. Transitional stage wake is an interval of scorable record (i.e., not obscured by artifact) that follows movement artifact or arousal that meets the conventional stage wake criteria other than duration. Movement time is scored by conventional criteria. Body movements are not scored, and movement arousals are only considered when they satisfy the definition of transitional stage wake.

# APPENDIX 8-A

## Standard Sensitivity and Filter Settings

| Derivation | Sensitivity | High-Frequency Filter | Low-Frequency Filter |
|---|---|---|---|
| EEG | 50 μV/cm | 35 Hz | 0.3 Hz |
| EOG | 50 μV/cm | 35 Hz | 0.3 Hz |
| EMG | 20 μV/cm* | 75 Hz | 10.0 Hz |
| ECG | varies† | 15 Hz | 1.0 Hz |
| Respiration | varies‡ | 0.5 Hz | 0.15 Hz |

NOTES: The sensitivity settings of the respiration and EMG channels will vary through the night and must be adjusted when necessary. In particular, the mental-submental EMG might decrease at sleep onset or onset of stage 2. The technician must increase the sensitivity at sleep onset or onset of stage 2 to allow for appreciation of the dramatic decrease in EMG associated with stage REM. Care must be taken, however, not to increase the EMG at the onset of REM.

Sensitivity of respiration channels will need to be adjusted throughout the recording, particularly after a large body movement.
*Mental-submental EMG sensitivity should be adjusted to allow approximately 1 cm pen deflection at patient calibration.
†ECG sensitivity varies with electrode placement. It should be adjusted to allow for a signal of 2 to 2.5 cm in height, showing proper waveform.
‡Sensitivity on respiration channels should allow for a pen swing that is 4 to 6 cm either side of the baseline.

# APPENDIX 8–B

## Strain Gauges, Thermistors, and Their Couplers

The following is a description of the techniques used to manufacture the strain gauges and thermistors that monitor respiratory effort and airflow. Also included is a description of the interface (coupler box) between the thermistor, strain gauge, and polygraph.

### Thermistor

Small glass-bead thermistors available from Victory Engineering Corporation (Springfield, New Jersey) measure relative changes in temperature of air that passes through the nose and mouth with respiration (Figure 8–13).

The thermistor is connected to a 1.5-volt battery. The current flows from the

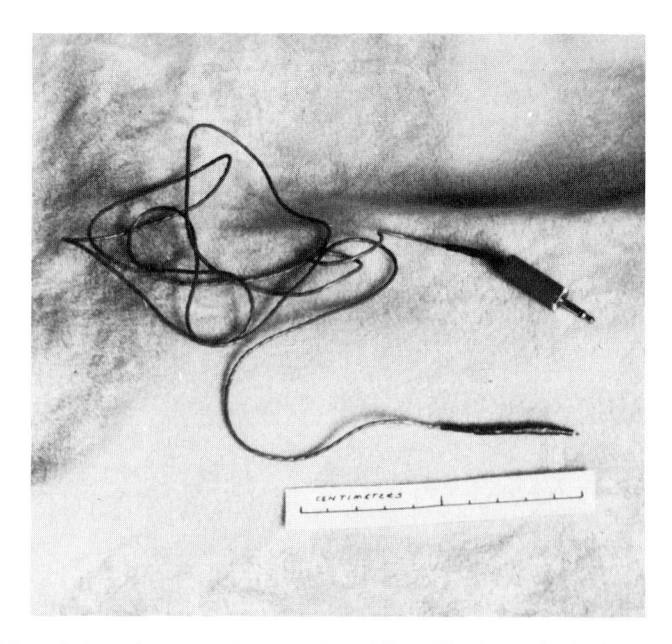

**Figure 8–13.** A thermistor used to monitor airflow. The lower half of the photo shows the glass-bead thermistor. The upper half shows the mini phone jack that plugs into the coupler box.

battery through a resistor, then through the thermistor, and finally back to the battery to complete the circuit (Figure 8–14).

The thermistor responds to changes in temperature by changing its resistance to the current flow. An increase in temperature causes a lower thermistor resistance; a decrease in temperature causes a higher resistance. Consequently, the signal amplified by the polygraph reflects the voltage drop across the variable resistor when it responds to changes in air temperature.

The following equipment is required to make a thermistor to use for monitoring airflow.

1. Thermistor, part no. 32A129 (2000-ohm thermistor) Victory Engineering Corp., Springfield, New Jersey.
2. Mini phone plug
3. Approximately 30 inches of very flexible, lightweight, two-conductor cable.
4. Approximately 1-1/2 inches of appropriate-size shrink tubing (size determined by diameter of cable).
5. Solder and soldering iron (27, 47, or 60 watt).
6. Silicone sealer (optional).

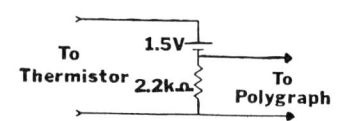

**Figure 8–14.** Circuit diagram for thermistor–coupler box–polygraph interface.

Solder the mini phone plug onto one end of the two-conductor cable, slip an appropriate length of shrink tubing onto the cable, and then solder the thermistor to the other end. It is very important to maintain isolation between the two conducting wires to prevent short-circuiting of the signal. After the soldering is complete, slide the piece of shrink tubing to just beneath the thermistor's tip. It should not cover the glass bead but should be close enough to be supportive. After the shrink tubing is in place, a very small amount of silicone sealer may be applied at the junction of the shrink tubing and the thermistor bead. Avoid covering the bead with sealer. Shrink the tube.

## Strain Gauge

Strain gauges can be used to measure relative alterations in expansion of the chest and abdomen that occur with respiratory efforts *(12)*.

The strain gauge consists of capillary-size silastic tubing filled with mercury and attached by wires to a battery and a resistor in much the same way as the thermistor described above (Figures 8–15 and 8–16).

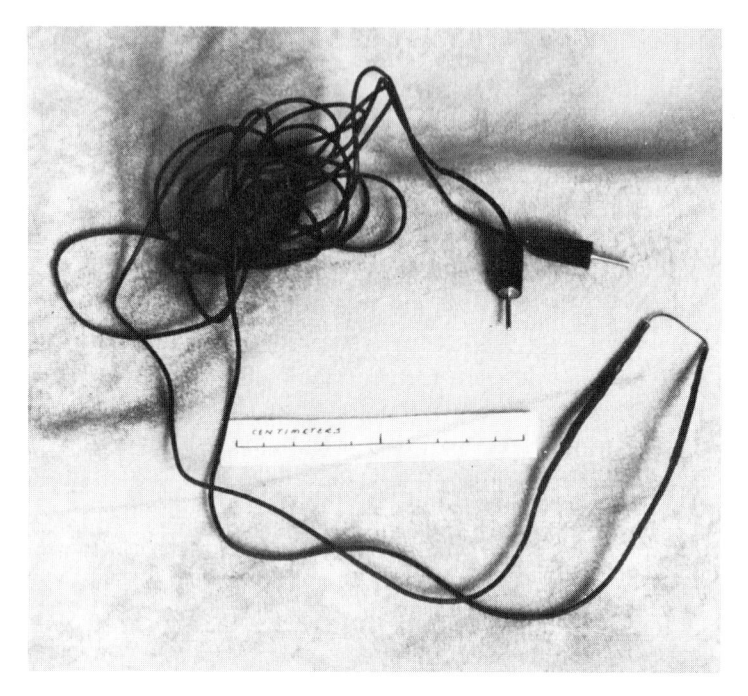

*Sleeping and waking disorders: indications and techniques*

**Figure 8–15.** A strain gauge used to monitor movement of the abdomen and thorax associated with effort to breathe. To the right, the silastic tubing filled with mercury; above that and to the left, the pin plugs that plug into the coupler box.

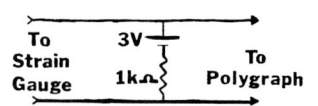

**Figure 8–16.** The circuit diagram for the strain gauge–coupler box–polygraph interface.

As the strain gauge is stretched during inhalation, its diameter is decreased. This results in an increased resistance to current flow through the gauge. With exhalation, resistance drops. The signal amplified by the polygraph reflects the voltage drop across the resistor in response to changes in diameter of the silastic tubing.

The following equipment is required to make a strain gauge to monitor respiratory effort.

1. Approximately 9 cm of silastic tubing, medical grade. (Catalog number 602–135, Dow Corning Corp., Medical Products, 1032 Elwell Court, Palo Alto, California.)
2. Mercury.
3. Two 5- to 6-foot lengths of very flexible, insulated wire (22 awg).

4. Two 1-cm lengths of copper wire (20 awg, solid, enameled).
5. Two pin plugs.
6. Two 3-cm lengths of appropriate-size (1/16-inch) shrink tubing.
7. Some clear silicone glue and seal (RTV or the like).
8. Solder and soldering iron.
9. Some emery cloth or an emery board.
10. One blunt cannula (Luer stub adaptor, 18 gauge).
11. One small syringe (2 cc or 5 cc).

The following procedures are required to make a strain gauge to monitor respiratory effort.

1. Solder one end of each 5- to 6-foot length of wire to pin plugs and screw the cap of the pin plug into place.
2. Remove the enamel from 2 to 3 mm of both ends of the 1-cm enameled copper wire pieces with the emery cloth or board and blunt the ends.
3. Solder the stripped end of the 1-cm wire to the other end of the 6-foot wire. Repeat steps 1, 2, 3 using the remaining 5- to 6-foot wire.
4. Slide a piece of shrink tubing over each of the newly assembled wires after they have cooled.
5. At this point, you should have two separate 5- to 6-foot-long wires, each terminating at one end with a pin plug, and at the other end with a 2- to 3-mm piece of copper wire from which the enamel has been removed. Put the blunt cannula on the syringe and draw approximately 0.5 cc of mercury into the syringe. (Great care should be used when working with mercury. The work surface should be covered. *Any* mercury that spills should be returned to its container.)
6. Push the cannula into one end of the silastic tubing and then push mercury through the tubing. Be careful not to spill the mercury.
7. While the silastic tubing is attached to the syringe, push the end of one of the wires into the other end of the tubing so that the wire makes contact with the mercury. Be careful not to tear the tubing with the wire. Approximately 1/2 to 3/4 cm of the wire should be carefully inserted into the tubing.
8. Remove the end of the silastic tubing from the syringe. With the mercury-filled tube held upright, cut the tubing at the mercury point and carefully insert the other 1-cm wire into the free end of the silastic tubing until it makes contact with the mercury.
9. Check for electrical continuity with an ohmmeter. If you don't have continuity, the problem could be a broken wire or an air bubble in the column of mercury.
10. Once electrical continuity has been established, apply a small amount of silicone sealer over the tubing/1-cm wire junction. Let it dry, slip the shrink tubing over the junction, and heat the shrink tubing with a soldering iron

*Sleeping and waking disorders: indications and techniques*

or a heat gun until it shrinks around the junction. Apply a small amount of silicone sealer to the end point of the shrink tubing near the silastic tubing.

11. The procedure is complete after a final check with the ohmmeter for electrical continuity. You should also stretch the gauge approximately 2 to 3 cm and confirm corresponding fluctuations in resistance with the ohmmeter.

## Coupler Box

The wire diagrams described above are installed into a project box (available from Radio Shack, part no. 270–222).

Input pin jacks on the coupler box accept the pin plugs of the strain gauges. Input mini phone jacks accept the plugs of the thermistors.

Outputs from the box are pin plugs secured through the box in an appropriate configuration (Figures 8–17 and 8–18). The most useful design is one that allows for input of the three strain gauges and two or three thermistors (provided, of course, that there are the appropriate number of available plugs on the terminal box of the polygraph). The output from two thermistors can be joined by making a "Y" that has two plugs for two thermistors and terminates in one jack that plugs into the coupler box. In this manner you can combine signals from the nostrils and mouth.

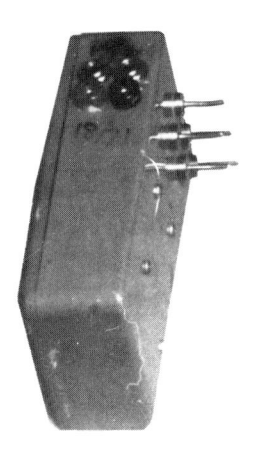

**Figure 8–17.** The coupler box shown on its side to illustrate plugs for strain gauges and thermistors and pins protruding from the back which plug into the terminal box of the polygraph.

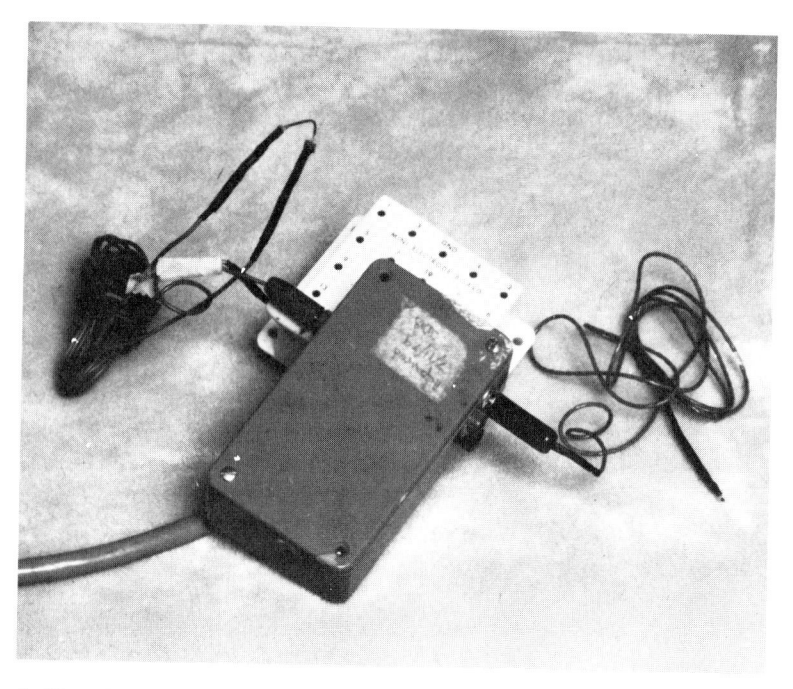

**Figure 8-18.** The coupler box plugged into the terminal box of the polygraph. A strain gauge and thermistor are plugged into the coupler box.

# APPENDIX 8-C

## Oximeter/Polygraph Interface and Calibration

It is essential that the oxygen saturation analog from the Hewlett-Packard ear oximeter be displayed on the polygraphic recordings of sleep apnea patients. This display allows for the crucial correlation between periods of apnea and the decrease in percent oxygen saturation associated with those events.

The interface between the oximeter and polygraph is accomplished easily using a grounded cable of appropriate length, terminating at each end with mini phone jacks. One end of the cable is plugged into the "OS" output jack on the rear panel of the oximeter; the other end is plugged into the J5 input position on the front (or rear) panel of the DC driver amplifier (Figures 8–19 and 8–20.)

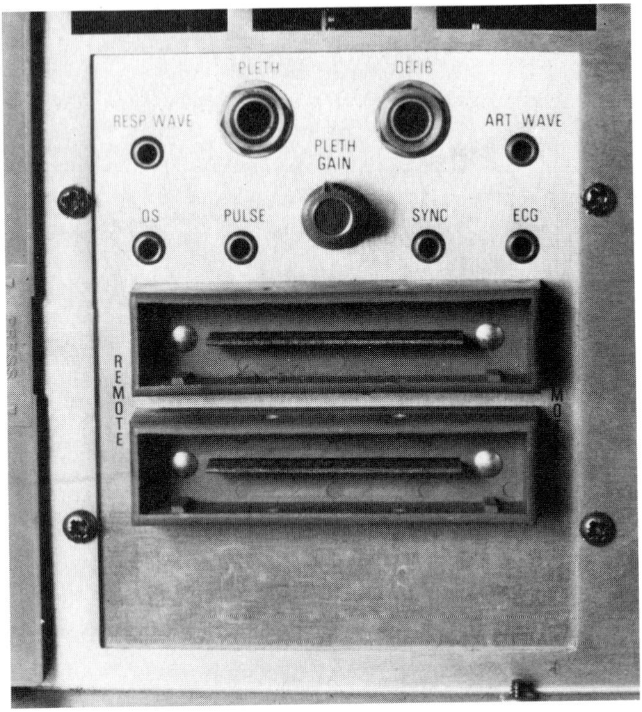

*Sleeping and waking disorders: indications and techniques*

**Figure 8–19.** The rear panel of the oximeter. Note the "OS" position in the upper left corner.

An appropriate channel is one that allows for a 2-inch pen excursion. The recommended scale is 5 mm = 10% oxygen saturation.

## To Calibrate

Calibration is performed with the earpiece in the earpiece cavity.

1. Connect oximeter to polygraph using the grounded cable with mini phone jacks at each end. The output is from the "OS" position on the near panel of the oximeter. The input is the J5 position on the amplifier.
2. Apply power to both oximeter and polygraph and allow normal warm-up time for oximeter.
3. Adjust J5 BLP potentiometer at rear of DC driver amplifier to appropriate zero position of scale on recording chart to correlate with oximeter reading of "00."
4. Standardize oximeter by momentarily depressing "STD" push button switch on front panel of oximeter. This causes the oximeter to store standardization values prior to operation. The standardization process takes approximately 25 seconds to complete.

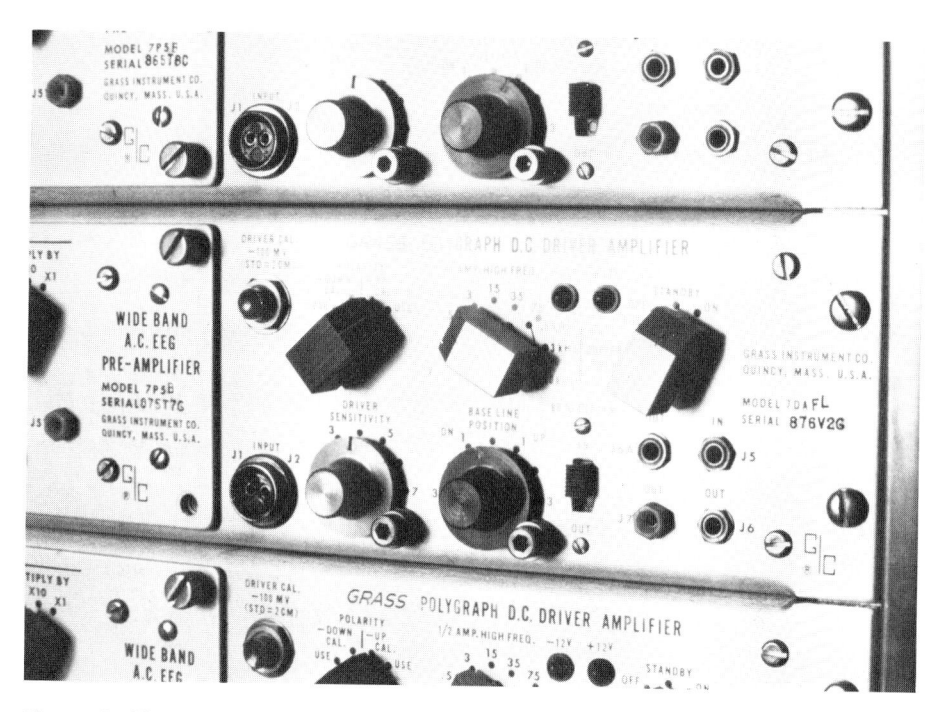

**Figure 8–20a.** A DC driver amplifier. Note "J5 in" position mid-right of photo.

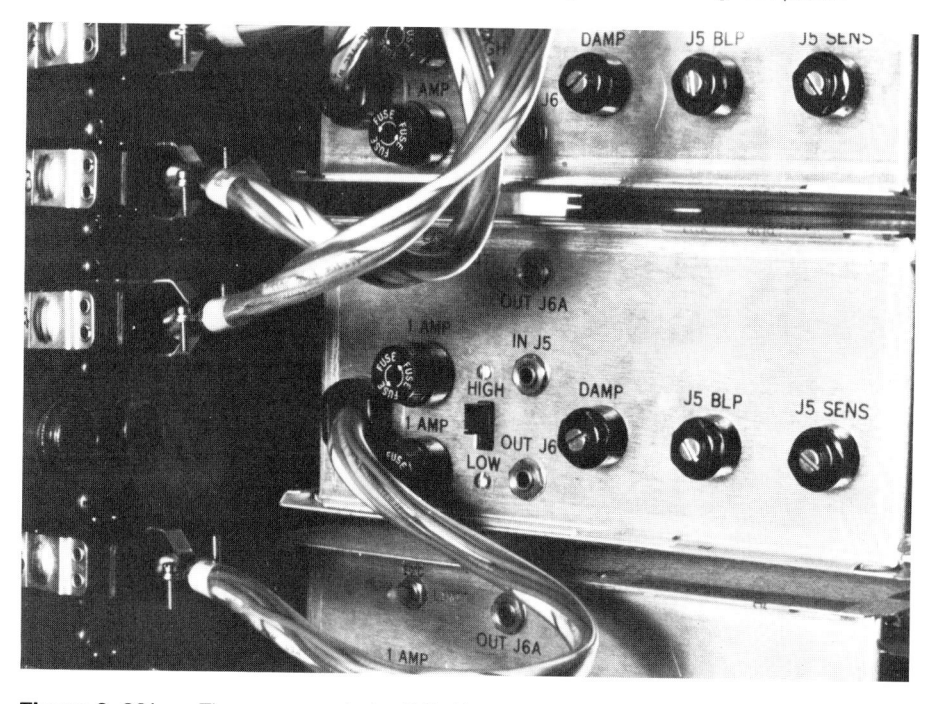

**Figure 8–20b.** The rear panel of a DC driver amplifier. Note the "J5 in" position in the center of the photo.

209

5. Press oximeter test button on front panel of oximeter and hold for approximately 20 seconds until known test figure supplied with each oximeter appears in digital display. Adjust J5 sensitivity potentiometer at rear of DC driver amplifier to correlate with test figure.
6. Move STD/check lever on front of oximeter to check position. This moves a test sample with a known value into the earpiece gap, and the value is displayed. (Check values differ between oximeters, but values are supplied with each instrument.) Adjust J5 sensitivity to correlate with appropriate check value.
7. Repeat procedure until values displayed on oximeter for "00" baseline, TEST, and CHECK correlate with reading on polygraph.

---

My sincere thank-you to Ed Bornstein for providing the photographs for this chapter, to Susan Coons for her editorial comments, and to Lynn Hassler and her staff for their assistance.

# APPENDIX 8–D

## Equipment and Suppliers

| Equipment | Specification | Supplier |
|---|---|---|
| Polygraph<br>AC preamplifier*<br>DC driver amplifier* | Model 7 series<br>Model P511 for EEG<br>Model 7DA | Grass Instrument Company<br>101 Old Colonial Avenue<br>Quincy, Massachusetts 02169<br>(617) 773–0002 |
| Ear oximeters | Model HP–47201A | Hewlett-Packard Company<br>1501 Page Mill Road<br>Palo Alto, California 94305<br>(415) 856–1501 |
|  | 0–600 oximeter | Waters Instruments, Inc.<br>P.O. Box 6117<br>Rochester, Minnesota 55901<br>(507) 288–7777 |
| Respitrace™ |  | Ambulatory Monitoring, Inc.<br>731 Saw Mill River Road<br>Ardsley, New York 10502<br>(914) 693–9232 |
| Holter monitor | AdvanceMed 2600 recorder | AdvanceMed<br>P.O. Box 17401<br>Irvine, California 92713<br>(714) 751–1824 |
| Electrodes for EMG, EOG, ECG | Electrodes–miniature<br>DC 48″ length<br>Part #650437–1 | Beckman Instruments<br>117 California Avenue<br>Palo Alto, California 94305<br>(415) 326–1970 |
| Electrode collars | Part #650454 | Beckman Instruments |
| EEG electrodes | E5H cup disk with hole gold plated | Grass Instrument Company |

*One preamplifier and one DC driver amplifier are needed for each polygraph channel.

# REFERENCES

1. Guilleminault C, Tilkian A, Dement W. The sleep apnea syndromes. Annu Rev Med 1976; 27:465–84.
2. Aserinsky E. Physiological activity associated with segments of the rapid eye movement period. In: Evants E, Ketz D, Williams H, eds. Sleep and altered states of consciousness. Baltimore: Williams & Wilkins, 1967: 35–50.
3. Orem J. Neuronal mechanisms of respiration in REM sleep. Sleep 1980; 3:251–67.
4. Hoppenbrouwers T, Jensen DK, Hodgman GE, Harper RM, Sterman MB. The emergence of a circadian pattern in respiratory rates: comparison between control infants and subsequent siblings of SIDS. Pediatr Res 1980; 14:345–51.
5. Guilleminault C. Sleep apnea syndromes: impact of sleep and sleep states. Sleep 1980; 3:227–34.
6. Guilleminault C, Dement WC, eds. Sleep apnea syndromes. New York: Alan R Liss, 1978.
7. Tilkian AG, Guilleminault C, Schroeder JS, Lehrman KL, Simmons FB, Dement WC. Hemodynamics in sleep induced apnea: studies during wakefulness and sleep. Ann Intern Med 1976; 85:714–9.
8. Guilleminault C, Dement WC. Polysomnography. In: Sackner MA, ed. Diagnostic techniques in pulmonary diseases. New York: Marcel Dekker, 1981:849–60.
9. Guilleminault C, Dement WC. Sleep apnea syndromes and sleep disorders. In: Williams R, Karacan A, eds. Sleep disorders: diagnosis and treatment. New York: John Wiley & Sons, 1978:9–28.
10. Rechtschaffen A, Kales A, eds. A manual of standardized terminology, techniques and scoring for sleep stages of human subjects. Los Angeles: UCLA Brain Information Service/Brain Research Institute, 1968.
11. Guilleminault C, Dement WC. Sleep apnea syndromes. New York: Alan R Liss, 1978:357–63.
12. Shapiro A, Cohen HD. The use of mercury capillary length groups for the measurement of the volume of thoracic and diaphragmatic components of human respiration: a theoretical analysis and practical method. Trans NY Acad Sci 1965, 27:634–49.

# NINE
# RESPIRATORY MONITORING DURING SLEEP: RESPIRATORY INDUCTIVE PLETHYSMOGRAPHY

MARTIN COHN

## Introduction

Use of the respiratory inductive plethysmograph system (Respitrace™)* allows monitoring of changes in rib cage and abdominal compartments that occur with breathing. This system is useful in evaluating patients for the presence of apneic episodes during sleep and for differentiating between central apnea (no airflow and no movement of rib cage or abdomen) and obstructive apnea (no airflow observed, despite rib cage and abdominal effort). Although this system can be used simultaneously with devices designed to detect airflow, such as nasal and oral thermistors, this is not necessary in most patients. It is usually possible to adjust the gain of each compartment signal of the respiratory inductive plethysmograph so that, when the signals are added together electrically, the new summation signal is calibrated for volume. Thus episodes of central apnea are indicated by absence of motion of the rib cage, abdomen, and volume signals (Figure 9–1); and episodes of obstructive apnea are indicated by motion (paradoxic) of the rib cage and abdomen with no significant motion of the sum volume signal (Figure 9–2). The system can also be used to quantitatively measure decreases in tidal volume (hypopnea). When combined with recordings of EEG, EOG, digastric EMG, ECG, and oxygen saturation, the respiratory inductive plethysmograph allows complete assessment of respiration during sleep without the use of additional instruments to measure airflow.

---

*Respitrace Corporation, 731 Saw Mill River Road, Ardsley, New York 10502.

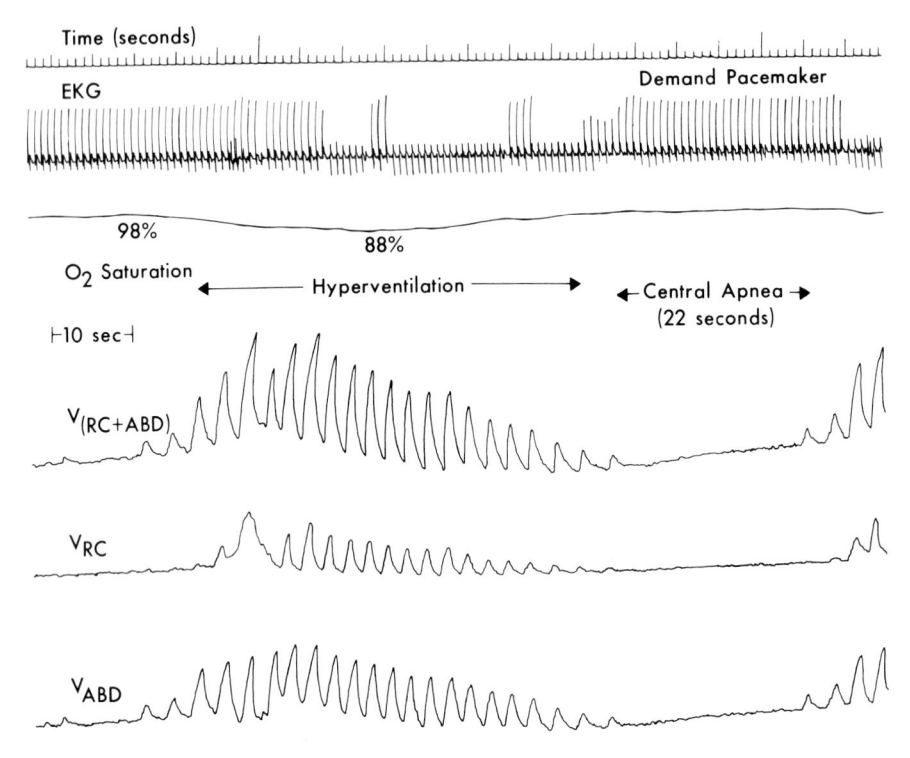

*Sleeping and waking disorders: indications and techniques*

**Figure 9–1.** Absence of motion of respiratory inductive plethysmograph signals from the abdominal ($V_{ABD}$), rib cage ($V_{RC}$), and summation ($V_{RC + ABD}$) channels indicates a central apnea. Note changes in the electrocardiogram (EKG) with cardiac pacemaker firing during the apnea.

## Theory of Operation

For the purpose of determining lung volumes, the respiratory system can be viewed as possessing two degrees of freedom—the independent movements of the rib cage and of the abdomen *(1)*. An inspired volume of air is distributed to these two compartments, with the amount going to the rib cage and to the abdomen varying with position, sleep stage, and other factors. Thus an inspired lung volume will be equal to the sum of the net volume changes in these two compartments. The application of this theory through the use of the respiratory inductive plethysmograph (Respitrace) allows monitoring of respiration over extended periods of time without the use of a mouthpiece *(2,3)*. This is ideal for quantification of apneas and hypopneas occurring during sleep.

The respiratory inductive plethysmograph consists of two coils of wire (respi-

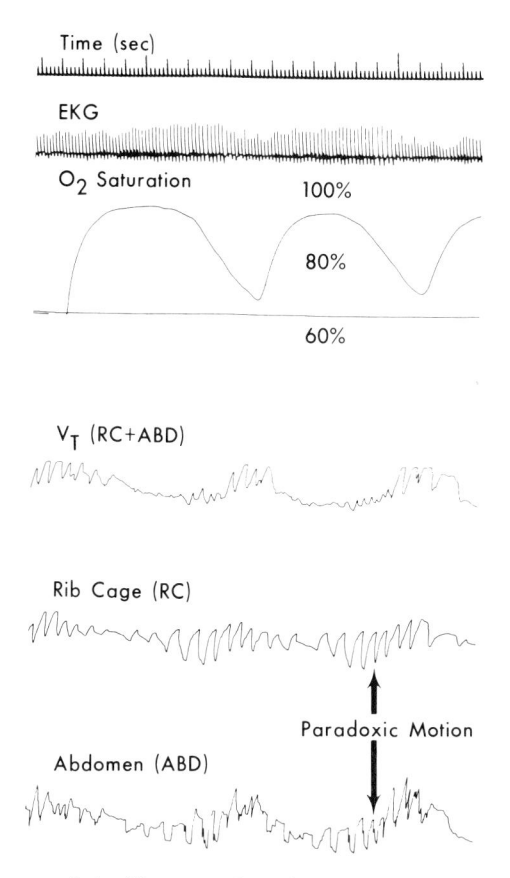

**Figure 9–2.** Absence of significant motion of the respiratory inductive plethysmograph volume signal ($V_T$ (RC + ABD)) along with paradoxic motion of the rib cage (RC) and abdominal (ABD) signals denotes obstructive apneas. Note the associated oxygen desaturation.

bands) encircling the rib cage and abdominal compartments (Figure 9–3). The expansion and contraction of these coils during breathing cause changes in the oscillating frequency of circuits within the electronic system. These frequency changes are demodulated to produce output voltage signals. After these signals are calibrated for volume, their sum will be equivalent to the volume inspired and expired. An analysis of the rib cage, abdominal, and summation signals allows a quantification of apneas (cessation of airflow) and hypopneas (decrease in tidal volume), as well as a determination of whether their origin is central (decreased respiratory center output) or obstructive (oropharyngeal obstruction impairing airflow despite presence of effort to breathe).

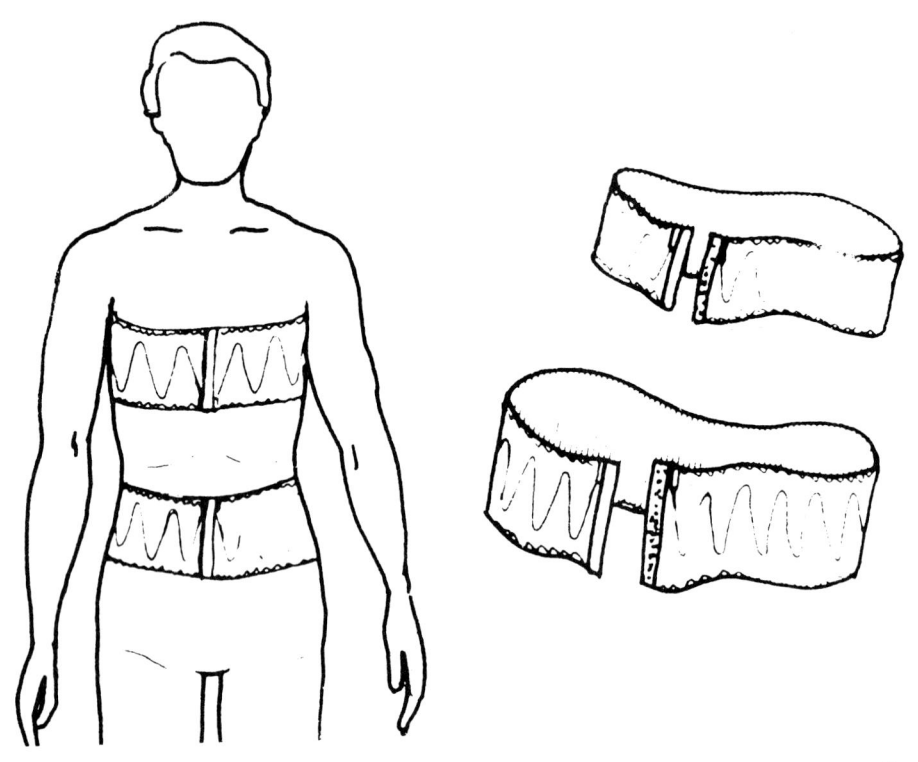

*Sleeping and waking disorders: indications and techniques*

**Figure 9–3.** Illustration of the respiratory inductive plethysmograph transducer coils (respibands) correctly positioned around the rib cage and abdomen.

## Calibration

For the summation signal (formed by adding the rib cage and abdominal signals together) to reflect tidal volume, the rib cage and abdominal signals must be amplified by rib cage and abdominal calibration factors, respectively, so that

$$\text{Equation 1} \quad (RC)(X) + (ABD)(Y) = VOL$$

where $RC$ is the rib cage signal deflection, $ABD$ is the abdominal signal deflection, $X$ is the rib cage calibration factor, $Y$ is the abdominal calibration factor, and $VOL$ is the sum of the volume changes of these compartments, or the tidal volume *(4)*.

To determine $X$ and $Y$, one takes advantage of the observation that, while standing, most subjects breathe predominantly with rib cage compartment expansion; whereas, while supine, breathing is accomplished primarily by abdominal expansion. Thus by recording the rib cage and abdominal signal outputs in these two positions along with a known volume (either via a spirometer or spirobag), one may determine $X$ and $Y$ using one of two methods. The first requires solving Equation 1 for $X$ and $Y$ so that:

**Equation 2**   $X = (ABD)(vol) - (abd)(VOL) / (rc)(ABD) - (RC)(abd)$

and

**Equation 3**   $Y = (RC)(vol) - (rc)(VOL) / (RC)(abd) - (rc)(ABD)$

where uppercase letters represent volumes obtained from a standing patient and lowercase letters represent those from a supine one. The second method is based on rearranging Equation 1 to

**Equation 4**   $(RC)(X) / (VOL) + (ABD)(Y) / (VOL) = 1$

which, when plotted with *RC/VOL* on the *y*-axis and *ABD/VOL* on the *x*-axis, should have a slope of $-1$ and intercepts at 1.0 on both axes. From the *VOL*, *RC*, and *ABD* values obtained while breathing in the supine and standing positions before calibration, a best-fit (or least-squares) line is produced that is "distorted" from the ideal. The reciprocal of the *y*-axis intercept of this line will be *X*, the rib cage calibration factor, and the reciprocal of the *x*-axis intercept will be *Y*, the abdominal calibration factor. This second method usually provides the most accurate calibration of the respiratory inductive plethysmograph (5).

After determining the rib cage and abdominal calibration factors, the electronic amplifiers of the respiratory inductive plethysmograph channels are appropriately adjusted. This is simplified by using an internal reference calibration voltage in the electronic device. When the calibration factors are entered into each of the channels, the derived summation channel will provide a spirogram reflecting tidal volume.

The following steps summarize the above calibration method:

1. **Placement of Respibands.**   Place one transducer coil evenly around the rib cage, just under the armpits. Place the other coil evenly around the abdomen, with its upper edge below the lowest rib (Figure 9–3). The coils may be fixed in position by wrapping each with a wide Ace bandage using the least required snugness. Alternately, an elastic mesh (Surgifix) may be worn over the torso to minimize slippage of the coils. Connect the oscillators to each coil and attach them to the Respitrace amplifier unit.
2. **Match Rib Cage and Abdominal Signal Amplifier Gains of Respitrace System.**   Using an internal reference voltage, equalize the gains of the rib cage and abdominal amplifiers of the Respitrace unit so that the signal outputs

*Sleeping and waking disorders: indications and techniques*

    read 1.0 volt each on the digital voltmeter. The summation channel (volume) will then read 2.0 volts.

3. **Calibrate Rib Cage, Abdominal, and Volume Channels of Recorder.** Input these rib cage, abdominal, and volume calibration signals from the Respitrace unit into a recorder, and adjust the recorder amplifiers so that the excursion of each channel is appropriate. By convention, a 1.0-volt signal is made to equal a 1.0-liter volume; therefore, a full-channel deflection need only be approximately 5.0 volts, i.e., 5.0 liters. Figure 9–4A shows the pen deflec-

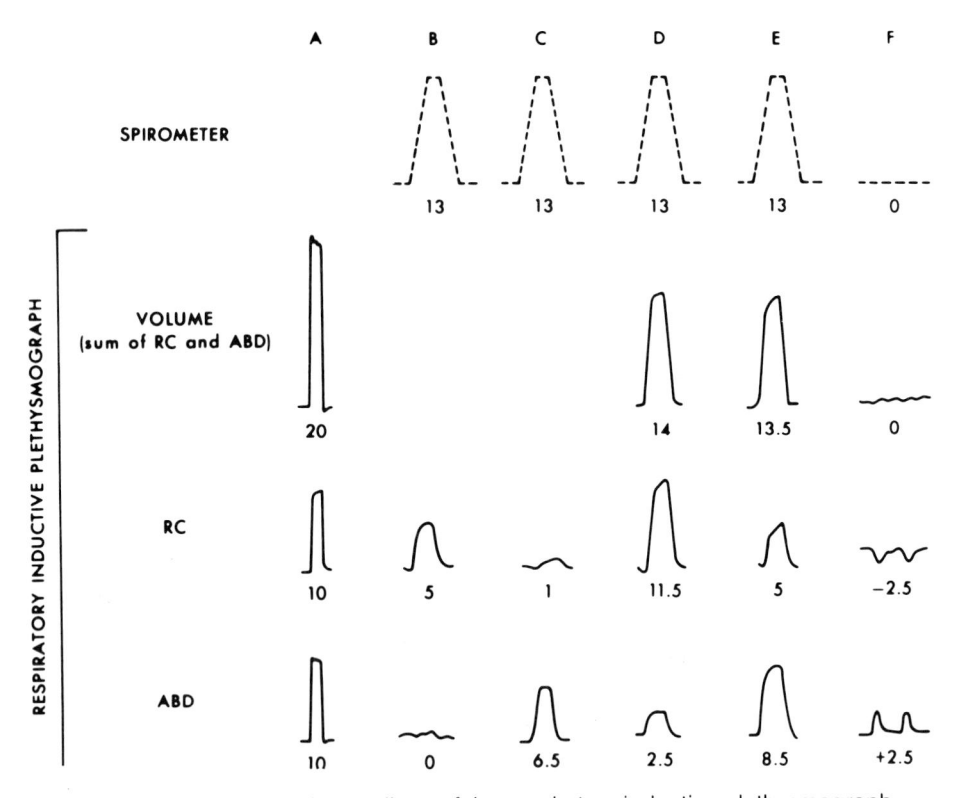

**Figure 9–4.** Examples of recordings of the respiratory inductive plethysmograph. (RC = rib cage, ABD = abdomen, RC + ABD = volume, 1.0 volt = 10 linear-excursion units.)
    A: while breathing in and out of the spirobag for calibration.
    B: standing position, during calibration.
    C: supine, during calibration.
    D: standing position, during validation.
    E: supine, during validation.
    F: while attempting to breathe during upper-airway obstruction.
(The dotted line illustrates what the signal would have looked like if a spirometer had been used.)

218

tions of the voltage-output calibration signals of the rib cage, abdominal, and volume channels after such adjustment.

4. **Collection of Respitrace Signals for Determining Calibration Factors Using a Spirometer or Spirobag.** If using a standard spirometer, calibrate so that a 1.0-volt signal equals a 1.0-liter volume, and record five to ten quiet breaths while the subject is standing (Figure 9–4B). Repeat while the subject is supine (Figure 9–4C). For each position, select one or more representative breaths and measure the linear excursions of the rib cage, abdominal, and spirometer signals.

   If using a spirobag (Figure 9–5), determine what the linear excursion from a spirometer would be for the calibrated volume of the spirobag. For example, if the spirobag's capacity is 1.3 liters, the corresponding spirometer signal would be 1.3 volts, or a linear deflection of 13 units (if 1.0 volt produced 10.0 linear-excursion units). Have the subject, while standing, completely fill and empty the spirobag five or six times as the rib cage and abdominal output signals are being recorded. Repeat while the subject is supine. Select one or more representative breaths in each position and measure the linear excursions of the rib cage and abdominal signals (Figures 9–4B and 9–4C).

5. **Compute the Calibration Factors.** Using the measured values (rib cage, abdomen, and either spirometer or spirobag excursions in both positions), compute the rib cage and abdominal calibration factors, $X$ and $Y$, respectively, using one of the following methods.

## Method I

Use Equation 2 to calculate $X$, the rib cage gain factor, and Equation 1 rearranged to

**Equation 5**  $Y = vol - (rc)(X) / abd$

to calculate $Y$, the abdominal calibration factor.

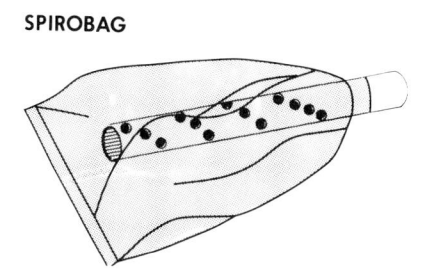

**SPIROBAG**

**Figure 9–5.** Illustration of spirobag. When the subject completely inflates and deflates the bag, the tidal volume will equal the known calibrated volume of the spirobag.

A T155 programmable calculator (Texas Instruments) may be used as follows:
a. To program, press *LRN, RCL 2, x, RCL 6, −,*
   *RCL 5, x, RCL 3, =, ÷,*
   *RCL 7, =, R/S, x, RCL 4,*
   *−, RCL 6, =, ÷, RCL 5,*
   *=, +/−, R/S, Rst, LRN,*
   *Rst.*
b. Enter *RC*, press *STO 1*.
   Enter *ABD*, press *STO 2*.
   Enter *VOL*, press *STO 3*.
   Enter *rc*, press *STO 4*.
   Enter *abd*, press *STO 5*.
   Enter *vol*, press *STO 6*.
c. Press *RCL 4, x, RCL 2, −, (RCL 1, x, RCL 5), = , STO 7*.
d. Press *R/S*. The display reads *X*, the rib cage calibration factor.
e. Press *R/S* again. The display reads *Y*, the abdominal calibration factor.

For example, using Figures 9–4B and 9–4C, $RC = 5$, $ABD = 0$, and $VOL = 13$ while standing; and $rc = 1$, $abd = 6.5$, and $vol = 13$ while supine. These values are entered into the program, step 3 is performed, and the program is run, displaying $X = 2.6$ and $Y = 1.6$.

## Method II

Since *X* and *Y* have been set to equal unity, one may calculate *RC/VOL* and *ABD/VOL* for one or more breaths in each position. Then, using the *RC/VOL* values for the y-axis determinant and the *ABD/VOL* values for the x-axis determinant for each breath, one may determine the x-axis and y-axis intercepts of a best-fit or least-squares regression line either graphically or by using a calculator with linear-regression capabilities. The reciprocal of the y-axis intercept will be the rib cage calibration factor, *X*; and the reciprocal of the x-axis intercept will be the abdominal calibration factor, *Y*.

For example, after three or more breaths are analyzed for both the standing and supine positions, *VOL*, *RC*, and *ABD* are determined, and *RC/VOL* and *ABD/VOL* are calculated for each breath as shown in the following table:

|         | Standing |      |      | Supine |      |      |
|---------|------|------|------|------|------|------|
| VOL     | 13   | 13   | 13   | 13   | 13   | 13   |
| RC      | 5    | 4.7  | 4.2  | 1    | 1    | 1    |
| ABD     | 0    | 1.3  | 0.8  | 6.5  | 7.3  | 5.5  |
| RC/VOL  | 0.38 | 0.36 | 0.32 | 0.08 | 0.08 | 0.08 |
| ABD/VOL | 0    | 0.1  | 0.06 | 0.5  | 0.56 | 0.42 |

*Respiratory monitoring during sleep: respiratory inductive plethysmography*

Using *ABD/VOL* as the *x*-ordinate and *RC/VOL* as the *y*-ordinate, points are determined and plotted on graph paper as shown in Figure 9–6. A line is drawn to best fit the points, and the *y*-axis intercept (0.38) is determined. Its reciprocal (2.6) is *X*, the rib cage calibration factor. The *x*-axis intercept (0.64) is determined, and its reciprocal (1.6) is *Y*, the abdominal calibration factor.

Alternately, one may use a programmable calculator with linear regression functions (such as TI55) as follows:

a. To program, press ÷, Const, *R/S*, =, *STO* 0,
   *R/S*, =, ⇄ *Y, RCL* 0, Σ +,
   *R/S, Rst, LRN, Rst*.
b. Enter *VOL*, press *R/S*.
c. Enter *RC*, press *R/S*. Display reads *RC/VOL*.
d. Enter *ABD*, press *R/S*. Display reads number of breaths entered.
e. Repeat steps 2–4 for each breath, then:
f. Enter 0, press *y′*, 1/*x*. Display reads *X*, the rib cage calibration factor.
g. Enter 0, press *x′*, 1/*x*. Display reads *Y*, the abdominal calibration factor.
h. To start over, enter 0, press *STO* 1, *STO* 2, . . . *STO* 7 (to clear linear-regression memories).

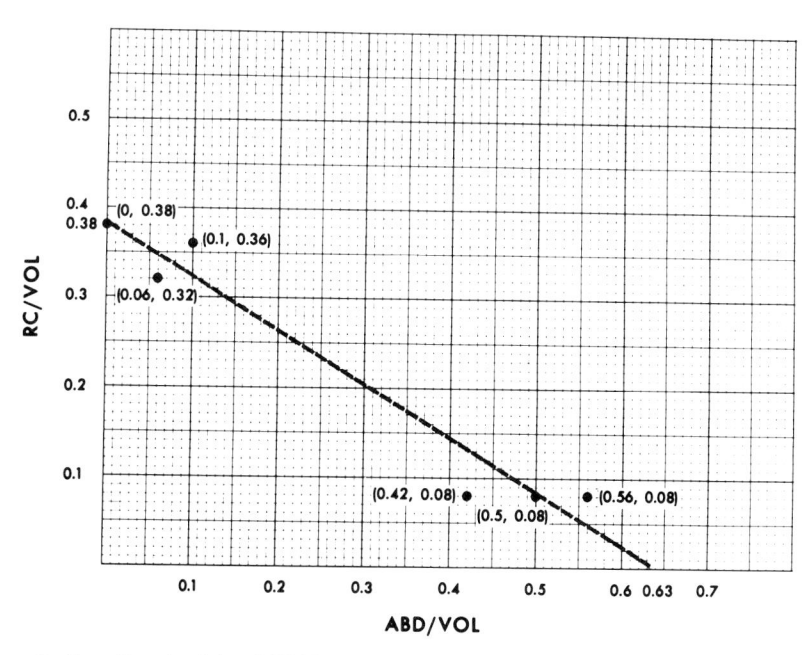

**Figure 9–6.** Graph of the *RC/VOL* and *ABD/VOL* values along with the best-fit line. The reciprocal of the *y*-axis intercept is *X*, the rib cage calibration factor; the reciprocal of the *x*-axis intercept is *Y*, the abdominal calibration factor. (See text for discussion.)

For example, enter *VOL*, press *R/S*, enter *RC*, press *R/S*, enter *ABD*, press *R/S* for the six sets of values from the above table. Enter 0, press y', 1/x, and the display reads 2.6, which is X, the rib cage calibration factor. Enter 0, press x', 1/x, and the display reads 1.6, which is Y, the abdominal calibration factor.

6. **Input the Calibration Factors into the Respitrace Amplifiers.** Using the internal reference voltage of the Respitrace amplifier unit, increase or decrease the rib cage and abdominal amplifier gains so they equal the calibration factors X and Y, respectively. For example, if X is 2.6 and Y is 1.6, the voltage outputs should be adjusted to read 2.6 volts on the rib cage channel and 1.6 on the abdominal channel.

7. **Validate the Accuracy of the Calibration Procedure.** Validate this calibration procedure by comparing the volume signal from the respiratory inductive plethysmograph with either simultaneous spirometry or the expected spirometry excursion based on the calibrated volume of the spirobag. In general, the respiratory inductive plethysmograph volume should be within 10% of the actual volume measured by simultaneous spirometry or spirobag. If it is not, the calibration procedure should be repeated. For example, Figure 9–4D shows the Respitrace signals after calibration while the standing subject breathes in and out of the spirobag. The Respitrace volume of 14 units is within 10% of the expected value of 13. Likewise, while supine (Figure 9–4E), the Respitrace volume of 13.5 units is within 10% of the expected value of 13.

8. **Analysis of the Rib Cage, Abdominal, and Volume Signals of the Respiratory Inductive Plethysmograph.** Because the volume signal represents a calibrated spirogram, it may be analyzed for the determination of tidal volume, breathing frequency, and the time components (inspiratory and expiratory times) of respiration. Absence of signal movement represents an apneic period (no airflow), and a decrease in tidal volume represents a hypopnea.

An analysis of the rib cage and abdominal signals allows an assessment of the contribution and phase relationship of each to breathing. This is important in the recognition of apneas and hypopneas due to upper-airway obstruction. During complete upper-airway obstruction, a diaphragmatic contraction during attempted inspiration produces an increase in the abdominal compartment size and consequently a positive abdominal signal output. At the same time, the rib cage compartment decreases in size by an equal amount, producing a negative rib cage signal output. Since the two signals are equal and opposite in direction, their sum is 0 (Figure 9–4F). Thus obstructive apneas are easily recognized by the combination of absent tidal volume associated with paradoxic rib cage and abdominal motion (Figure 9–2).

# REFERENCES

1. Konno K, Mead J. Measurement of the separate volume changes of rib cage and abdomen during breathing. J Appl Physiol 1967; 22:487–522.
2. Cohn MA, Watson H, Weisshaut R, Stott F, Sackner MA. A transducer for non-invasive monitoring of respiration. In: Stott FD, Raftery EB, Sleight P, Goulding L, eds. ISAM 1977: Proceedings of the Second International Symposium on Ambulatory Monitoring. London: Academic Press, 1978: 119–28.
3. Cohn MA, Rao BVA, Davis B, et al. Measurement of tidal ventilation and forced vital capacity in normals and patients with obstructive lung disease with a respiratory inductive plethysomograph. In: Stott FD, Raftery EB, Goulding L, eds. ISAM 1979: Proceedings of the Third International Symposium on Ambulatory Monitoring. London: Academic Press, 1980: 355–65.
4. Watson H. The technology of respiratory inductive plethysomography. In: Stott FD, Raftery EB, Goulding L, eds. ISAM 1979: Proceedings of the Third International Symposium on Ambulatory Monitoring. London: Academic Press, 1980: 537–58.
5. Watson HL, Birch SJ, Gruen WG, Cohn MA, Schneider AW, Sackner MA. Comparison of calibration techniques for respiratory inductive plethysmography in humans and sheep. Am Rev Respir Dis (abstract) 1981;123:181.

# TEN
# EVALUATING DISORDERS OF INITIATING AND MAINTAINING SLEEP (DIMS)

PETER J. HAURI

## Prevalence

Difficulties in falling and staying asleep are common. Indeed, Ware *(1)* estimates that in the United States alone, 75 million people feel that their sleep is not what it should be.

Numerous surveys during the last two decades have attempted to document incidence rates for insomnia. In 1962, McGhie and Russel *(2)* surveyed 2400 British subjects from age 15 to 75. They found that 5%–10% of males and 5%–30% of females had difficulties falling asleep. A surprising 35% of the entire group reported frequent nocturnal arousals. A more extensive study was carried out in 1964 in the U.S. *(3)*. It involved more than one million people and found that 13% of the men and 36% of the women over the age of 30 complained of poor sleep. Similarly, in another U.S. study *(4)* done during 1970–71 and involving 2552 people, 11% of the men and 17% of the women reported "a lot of trouble" getting to sleep or staying asleep, whereas an additional 19% of the sample reported minor problems with sleep.

It is sometimes said that urban stress may cause an excessive amount of insomnia. However, in a study carried out in a central-Florida county *(5)* in 1969–70 involving 1645 adults, 22% "sometimes" had trouble getting to sleep or staying asleep, whereas fully 13% claimed they "often" had such problems. The overall total of 35% with at least occasional sleep difficulties in the central-Florida sample compares closely with the 32% who complained of sleep difficulties in a survey of the Los Angeles metropolitan area *(6)* involving 1000 adults. In both studies, females reported more sleep problems than males, and the incidence rates increased with age.

Based on these and other studies, a recent Institute of Medicine Report *(7)* estimated that about one-third of the adult population reports some sleep disturbance in any given year. About 15%–20% of those reporting a problem—that is, about 6% of the total adult population—bring these sleep complaints to the attention of a physician who prescribes a sleeping pill for about half of them, or for about 3% of the adult population. Similar prescription patterns are also reported for other countries, for example in Great Britain *(8)* and Australia *(9)*.

In the studies quoted above, the exact percentages of people with sleep disturbances vary somewhat, probably depending on the population sample and on the way the question was phrased. Nevertheless, nobody disputes the fact that disorders of initiating and maintaining sleep are widespread. Obviously, all these people could not be evaluated with polysomnography at a sleep disorders center, nor should they be. This chapter discusses how most patients with sleep disturbances should be evaluated, when a referral to a sleep disorders center is appropriate, how such an evaluation is carried out, and what kinds of diagnoses can be expected. At the end of the chapter, some technical issues concerning sleep evaluations are then discussed for those who are actually doing such work.

# Evaluation of a DIMS Complaint Outside of the Sleep Disorders Center

Although not diagnostic, a serious and chronic complaint of insomnia indicates that something is wrong with the patient and should always be taken seriously. Evaluating the complaint of chronic insomnia is initially much more important than eliminating one symptom with hypnotics. In this sense, insomnia is like chronic fever, a condition that should not be treated lightly with antipyretics unless the condition that is causing the fever has been diagnosed.

## Sleep History

Taking a thorough sleep history is the first step toward understanding the complaint of insomnia. The following issues are usually explored:

1. Chief sleep complaint, including its development over time, its fluctuations with stress, and the events that surround its initial occurrence.
2. Procedures used so far for dealing with this complaint, including medication and nondrug therapies that have been tried, and the patient's past compliance with such treatment.
3. Daytime performance and mood, both after adequate sleep and after poor nights.
4. Associated sleep complaints and their development over time.
5. Sleep before the complaint, i.e., a detailed evaluation of sleep as a child, an adolescent, and a young adult.
6. The patient's view of the sleep problem and what it means to him, speculations about etiology, and hopes for the future.

## Sleep Diaries

It is often useful to "fortify" the initial sleep history with a sleep log. This means having patients write down for one or two weeks when they went to bed, how long it took them to fall asleep, how often they awakened at night, how long they slept each night, when they got up, and how they felt upon awakening. They should also write down their drug intake during the day and whether any naps were taken. Discrepancies between this sleep log and the patient's reported "average" sleep at home are often quite striking and may lead to diagnostic insight. Similarly, a sleep log documents the regularity of a patient's sleep habits, a crucial issue. Finally, this log is later used to assess progress that may be made once different interventions have started.

## Sleep Questionnaires

Instead of eliciting an oral sleep history, one may use a sleep questionnaire to get the process started. Such a questionnaire has the advantage of efficiency. The patient answers most of the sleep-history questions before the interview with a physician, who can then skim the questionnaire, skip some areas, and spend more time on others, depending on clinical judgment.

## Interview with Bed Partner

Bed partners are often better sources of sleep information than the patients themselves. The partner might be queried intensively about the patient's sleeping habits, about drug intake before sleep, about possible psychologic problems, changes in sleep habits over time, and possible stress at home or on the job. As is typical for many psychosomatic diseases, such stresses may often be more apparent to the partner than to the patient. In addition, the bed partner should be questioned about repetitive kicking or abnormal breathing patterns to evaluate possible nocturnal myoclonus or sleep apnea. If either of these problems is reported by the partner, referral to a sleep disorders center seems indicated.

## Psychiatric Evaluation

While taking a sleep history, the interviewer should be alert for possible signs of psychopathology. These are then carefully followed up in an effort to decide whether a psychiatric consultation seems indicated. Specifically, personality traits, situational and behavioral factors, and possible stresses at home and at work are explored as possible contributors to the insomnia.

If the sleep complaint seems associated with a psychiatric condition, that condition is treated first. Many disorders of initiating and maintaining sleep are psychiatric in origin, and they wax and wane with the amount of psychiatric or environmental stress. Treating the psychiatric problem that causes the sleep problem is usually much more effective than treating the sleep disturbance that the patient complains about.

## Physical Exam

Sleep disorders may stem from medical problems such as endocrine, neurologic, or allergic disorders and pain or discomfort from other diseases. If a physical exam or laboratory workup suggests problems in these areas, a referral to the appropriate specialist is usually much more effective than the direct treatment of the insomnia secondary to the medical problem.

# Treatment of DIMS Complaints

## Treatment with Hypnotics

Arguments have been carried out over the last 20 years concerning the treatment of insomnia with hypnotics. The following guidelines seem to represent a consensus of many sleep disorder specialists.

1. Although most hypnotics are initially effective, most lose efficacy when used chronically. When abruptly withdrawn, sleep is then often quite seriously disturbed for a few days or weeks. The time course of this habituation-withdrawal curve is varied. A patient may become habituated to secobarbital within one week, whereas flurazepam has been shown to remain somewhat effective even after an entire month of chronic use. Other medications may lie somewhere in between these two extremes. Similar differences may be expected for the "rebound" insomnia, which may be immediate and brief after some drugs, prolonged and/or delayed after others.
2. Hypnotics often seem indicated in transient situational insomnia, which may last for up to three weeks. Rarely are they indicated for chronic, long-term use. Indeed, the chronic use of some hypnotics may in itself contribute to insomnia.
3. Because of the initial effectiveness of most hypnotics, combined with the rebound insomnia after withdrawal, insomniacs should be informed that they can only "borrow" sleep with hypnotics, they cannot "buy" it. Thus, it seems appropriate to use hypnotics in times of stress, but only if one plans hypnotic withdrawal ahead of time and is willing to undergo the expected withdrawal insomnia at that time.
4. Episodic use of hypnotics, not more than once or twice per week, would seem to be appropriate in most chronic, serious insomnias to occasionally break the helpless panic of a sleepless night.
5. Warn patients about the interaction between hypnotics and alcohol.
6. Use care when prescribing hypnotics for heavy snorers because hypnotics depress respiratory centers.

7. It is almost never indicated to increase a hypnotic dose that was previously adequate. If habituation has occurred, withdrawal is recommended to restore potency.
8. Withdraw patients gradually if they have been on heavy doses of hypnotics.

## Nondrug Treatment

1. *Sleep hygiene* is crucial to people who are prone to insomnia. This means regular arousal times, no naps during the day, moderate amounts of exercise, no coffee after lunch, no alcohol in the evening, adequate time for unwinding, and possibly a light bedtime snack *(10,11)*.
2. *Relaxation training* seems indicated if the patient is tense *(12)*. The type of relaxation seems to be less important than a thorough, competent training in the technique. One-hour "how-to-do-it" sessions will rarely be adequate.

# Guidelines for Referral of Patients to a Sleep Disorders Center

## Cost-Effectiveness Considerations

The decision to refer to a patient to a sleep disorders center basically relates to cost-effectiveness considerations. One weighs concern about the patient's long-range health and the potential benefits of the evaluation against its cost. The Dartmouth Sleep Disorders Center recently did a nine-month follow-up study of about 100 chronic and severe insomniacs who had gone through the evaluation as discussed in this chapter. We found that about one-fourth to one-third of such patients derived major benefits from an evaluation, and that an additional group derived some, but not major, benefits.

## Criteria for Judging the Seriousness of the Sleep Problem

Referral to a sleep disorders center seems indicated only if the following three conditions are met:

1. The insomnia is *chronic* and *serious,* clearly interfering significantly with daytime functioning, performance, and mood.
2. The insomnia is *not secondary* to an ongoing, diagnosed medical or psychiatric problem. However, should the insomnia remain long after the known psychiatric or medical problem has been adequately treated, a referral might then be considered.
3. Best efforts to deal with the insomnia have been rigorously pursued along the lines outlined above for *at least six months,* with little effect.

# Evaluation for DIMS at a Sleep Disorders Center

Although most sleep disorders centers have their own approach, the following seems to present a consensus of what is done by most.

## Referral

A detailed understanding of the referral is necessary. Why is the patient being referred at this time? What has been done so far to treat the DIMS, and with what effects? Associated medical and psychologic problems and their current status are of interest, laboratory data should be included, and the referring physician's understanding of the patient's home and work situation needs to be explored. This can be done either in a referral letter to the sleep disorders center or by telephone.

## Intake Interview

The intake interview follows the outline for a sleep history, discussed earlier, but may be much more detailed. The interviewer needs to be very sensitive to psychologic factors such as covert depression, anxiety, or stress. It is usually indicated that the intake interview be followed by a detailed psychiatric evaluation that may include psychologic testing and neuropsychologic evaluations. Many centers have each patient answer at least some psychologic questionnaires (such as the MMPI) to be used as a guide to decide whether a patient needs referral to a psychiatrist or a psychologist.

## Physical Exam

Although most patients have had physical examinations in the past, a physician who knows about sleep disorders usually performs a more detailed examination while the patient is evaluated at the center. This may include laboratory tests or referrals for neurologic, allergic, endocrine, and/or cardiac evaluations, as indicated. Some abnormalities are difficult to diagnose without an evaluation of physiologic changes during sleep. For example, the patient's pulmonary performance may be adequate during waking, but disturbed during sleep. Similarly, frequent nocturnal arousals may be secondary to EEG abnormalities, which may be either absent on a waking EEG or termed "benign" during wakefulness.

Following the collection of this information, a staff conference decides whether polysomnography seems indicated in a given case.

# Polysomnographic (PSG) Recording

1. **Purposes of PSG** Depending on the question to be settled, one or several nights of recording may be necessary. PSG is used to clarify the following issues:
   a. Rule out DIMS associated with sleep-induced respiratory impairment, sleep-related myoclonus, or sleep-related epileptic phenomena.
   b. Document the actual amount of EEG-defined sleep, sleep latency, and general sleep architecture (REM latency, percentage of different stages, and sleep-stage changes).
   c. Document atypical polysomnographic features such as poor spindles, alpha intrusion into sleep, unusual muscle tension when trying to sleep or when sleeping, and frequent "mini" arousals.
   d. Compare the EEG measures obtained from the polysomnogram, such as sleep latency and sleep efficiency, with the subjective evaluation of these measures given by the patient in the morning.
   e. Assess the first-night effect to evaluate such factors as generalization of learning from the bedroom to the lab and the patient's reaction to stress and novelty.
   f. Observe the behavior of the patient around sleep onset and during the night. These observations are often crucial for a clinical understanding of a patient's insomnia. To achieve this goal, it is mandatory that the nighttime observer be sensitive and trained in clinical observations, and that this person participate actively in staff meetings during which the patient is discussed.

2. **Issues Regarding PSG**
   a. *Recording With or Without Medication?* Many patients referred to a sleep disorders center are taking numerous medications, such as hypnotics, antidepressants, tranquilizers, stimulants, and antihypertensives. These medications disturb and distort sleep. Should the patient be recorded while on drugs or after withdrawal?

   If small doses are involved, especially if they are taken intermittently, patients should be asked to refrain from taking them and should be recorded drug-free, after appropriate periods of abstinence. These abstinence periods vary with individual drugs and depend on the half-life of the active components. Required abstinence periods of one to three weeks are common.

   If the patient is referred while on heavy, chronic doses of medication, it often seems preferable to record sleep both while on drugs and while off. Recording the patient while on drugs indicates what the medications are doing to sleep. Recording the patient while off drugs, after appropriate withdrawal periods, indicates to what extent the drugs were contributing to the sleep problem and, once withdrawn, whether some other disorder of initiating and maintaining sleep emerges.

Withdrawing patients from heavy doses of CNS depressants is not easy. In addition to the problems of psychologic dependence on sleeping pills and the rebound insomnia that occurs when withdrawing from such medications, precipitous withdrawal from hypnotics may have serious medical side effects, including life-threatening seizures. Advice about withdrawal from medication should be in the hands of the sleep center physician. Withdrawal often requires an inpatient setting and should follow established procedures, such as described in Wilker *(13)* or Shader et al. *(14)*. Basically, the patient is first stabilized on a steady dose of the medication from which he is then gradually withdrawn. Major therapeutic work is usually necessary, both during withdrawal and afterward, in an effort to prevent readdiction as soon as the patient leaves the hospital.

Most insomniacs on heavy doses of CNS depressants are extremely reluctant to withdraw from their medicine but may be willing to go along with withdrawal if it is an absolute prerequisite for a polysomnographic evaluation. For these patients, the crucial treatment may actually occur *before* the patient is evaluated drug-free at the center!

b. *How Many Nights of Polysomnography?* Webb *(15)* found that at least five nights of evaluation may be necessary, even for normal sleepers, to assess adequately the time spent in various sleep stages. Insomniacs would most likely need even more nights because their sleep fluctuates more from night to night than that of normal sleepers. Running that many nights would make the clinical evaluation of insomniacs prohibitively expensive. Fortunately, it is rarely necessary, from a clinical point of view, to know accurately the variables with which Webb had been concerned.

To rule out such possibilities as sleep apnea, myoclonus, and atypical polysomnographic features, *one night* of polysomnography may be enough. Even though sleep is disturbed and curtailed during that first night, the atypical features will be apparent anyway, as long as the patient obtains at least a few hours of adequate sleep.

Should the amount of sleep and its pattern be at issue, for example, in a suspected insomnia complaint without objective findings, a minimum of *two or three nights* of polysomnography are usually required. Similarly, should the first night in the lab suggest a problem, such as sleep apnea or nocturnal epilepsy, follow-up nights may be needed to evaluate it further. For example, if possible spike and wave discharges are observed on the one EEG lead during the first night, but a routine clinical waking EEG is normal, additional nights are required to study the EEG during sleep with a full montage of electrodes, at standard clinical speeds. Additional nights may also be indicated to evaluate the first-night effect or to gain some sleep information if the first night in the laboratory was extremely atypical.

3. **Special Problems.**
   a. *Children* are often frightened by the sleep lab technology. Many seem to need a much wider range of movement to fall asleep than the standard electrodes allow. We have found it best to ask a parent to accompany the child to the lab and to sleep there as well. After set-up, the parent goes through the usual bedtime routine with the child, including storytelling, toothbrushing, etc. This parent-child interaction around bedtime often yields significant clues concerning the etiology of the child's problem. The parent may then remain with the child until sleep onset, or a technician may observe the child through a one-way mirror. Electrodes are not plugged in until after the child has fallen asleep for at least a few minutes.
   b. *The elderly* present the clinician with the problem of separating normal effects of aging from sleep pathology. With age, sleep typically fragments: there are more and longer awakenings at night and more naps during the day. The EEG amplitude decreases. Although EEG waves with frequencies in the delta range are often observed, they do not have the required amplitude to be scored as "delta" according to the Rechtschaffen-Kales system.

   According to a recent study by Coleman et al. at Stanford *(16)*, 39% of their patients over 60 years of age showed a sleep apnea syndrome and 18% showed nocturnal myoclonus and restless legs syndrome. Thus older patients show these syndromes in significantly larger numbers than younger patients. It is impossible at present to decide which of these changes are due to normal aging, and which are due to pathologic processes. Clinically, it seems best to treat only those problems that lead to significant complaints or problems, but not those that are incidentally found. For example, observing some sleep apneas in an elderly patient without awakenings and without significant oxygen desaturation is cause for little concern unless the patient also shows hypertension, cardiac problems, or excessive sleepiness during the day.

# Confirmation of DIMS Diagnoses by Polysomnography

The following discussion is based on the Diagnostic Classification of Sleep and Arousal Disorders published recently by the ASDC *(17)*. Table 10–1 summarizes the disorders of initiating and maintaining sleep (DIMS) according to that classification. For details on each category, consult the original publication. In the following, each category is briefly characterized for recognition. In addition, certain aspects of each category are highlighted if their understanding contributes significantly to adequate diagnosis and management.

*Sleeping and waking disorders: indications and techniques*

**Table 10-1**  DIMS: Disorders of Initiating and Maintaining Sleep (Insomnias)

|  | Recommended ICD-9-CM Code | See Footnote |
|---|---|---|
| 1. Psychophysiological | | |
|    a. Transient and situational | 307.41-0 | |
|    b. Persistent | 307.42-0 | |
| 2. Associated with psychiatric disorders | | |
|    a. Symptom and personality disorders | 307.42-1 | 1 |
|    b. Affective disorders | 307.42-2 | 2 |
|    c. Other functional psychoses | 307.42-3 | 3 |
| 3. Associated with use of drugs and alcohol | | |
|    a. Tolerance to or withdrawal from CNS depressants | 780.52-0 | 4 |
|    b. Sustained use of CNS stimulants | 780.52-1 | 5 |
|    c. Sustained use of or withdrawal from other drugs | 780.52-2 | 6 |
|    d. Chronic alcoholism | 780.52-3 | 7 |
| 4. Associated with sleep-induced respiratory impairment | | |
|    a. Sleep apnea DIMS syndrome | 780.51-0 | |
|    b. Alveolar hypoventilation DIMS syndrome | 780.51-1 | |
| 5. Associated with sleep-related (nocturnal) myoclonus and "restless legs" | | |
|    a. Sleep-related (nocturnal) myoclonus DIMS syndrome | 780.52-4 | 8 |
|    b. "Restless legs" DIMS syndrome | 780.52-5 | 9 |
| 6. Associated with other medical, toxic, and environmental conditions | 780.52-6 | 10 |
| 7. Childhood-onset DIMS | 780.52-7 | |
| 8. Associated with other DIMS conditions | | |
|    a. Repeated REM-sleep interruptions | 307.48-0 | |
|    b. Atypical polysomnographic features | 307.48-1 | |
|    c. Not otherwise specified* | 780.52-9 or 307.42-9 | 11 |
| 9. No DIMS abnormality | | |
|    a. Short sleeper | 307.49-0 | |
|    b. Subjective DIMS complaint without objective findings | 307.49-1 | |
|    c. Not otherwise specified* | 307.40-1 | |

1. Use additional code to identify:
   anxiety (300.00–300.09)
   personality disorder (301.0–301.9)
   symptom disorders (306.0–306.9, 307.0–307.3, 307.5–307.9, 316).
2. Use additional code to identify:
   major affective disorder (296.0–296.9, 296.82, 298.0)
   minor affective disorder (300.4, 301.10–301.13, 311).

## A.1.a. Transient and Situational Psychophysiologic DIMS

This category represents a brief period of sleep disturbance (less than three weeks), usually provoked by acute emotional arousal or conflict. Patients with this problem rarely reach sleep disorders centers. Hypnotics often seem indicated to help patients get over the acute crisis, but these should be prescribed only after it has been established that the problem is truly situational, not the beginning of a more serious disturbance. Care should be taken to make sure that situational DIMS does not develop into a persistent psychophysiologic problem.

## A.1.b. Persistent Psychophysiologic DIMS

According to the ASDC description, this type of insomnia develops as a result of the mutually reinforcing factors of chronic, somatized anxiety/tension and negative conditioning to sleep.

To focus the evaluation of such patients, some initial theoretical comments seem indicated. As explained in detail elsewhere *(18)*, during periods of situational insomnia due to stress, most of us develop two types of learned, maladaptive behavior. First, we try harder to sleep, and this trying in itself interferes with the process of falling asleep. Second, the stimuli surrounding bedtime, such as the bedroom, darkness, and tooth-

---

3. Use additional code to identify:
schizophrenia (295.0–295.9)
other functional psychosis (297.0–298.9).
4. Use additional code to identify barbiturate, sedative, or hypnotic:
dependence (304.1)
withdrawal (292.0)
5. Use additional code to identify:
amphetamine or other psychostimulant abuse (305.7).
6. Use additional code to identify:
drug withdrawal (292.0)
tranquilizer dependence (304.1)
unspecified drug dependence (304.9)
7. Use additional code to identify:
alcohol amnestic syndrome (291.1)
alcohol dementia (291.2)
chronic alcoholism (303.9)
8. Use additional code to identify:
abnormal involuntary movements (781.0).
9. Use additional code to identify:
restless legs (333.99).
10. Code also underlying condition, as:
Cushing's syndrome (255.0)
Use additional code for environmental condition, as:
exposure to noise (E928.1).
11. This category is set aside for DIMS that are as yet undesignated and undescribed; use codes 307.44–9 if the disorder is functional and 780.52–9 if it has organic etiology.

brushing, become associated with (conditioned to) arousal and frustration, rather than being experienced as harbingers of sleep. Just going to the bedroom or brushing teeth may then trigger feelings of tension and frustration.

In good sleepers, these learned, maladaptive habits extinguish after the stress has abated. The occasional nights of insomnia that occur in a poor sleeper, however, reinforce these maladaptive habits and prevent their extinction. Whether these occasionally occurring poor nights of sleep are based on somatized anxiety/tension, on hyperarousal, or on some defect in the neuronal sleep circuitry will depend on the individual, but all will claim that their sleep had been somewhat tenuous even before their actual insomnia developed.

Polysomnography helps in the diagnosis of this problem by first establishing that there is, indeed, a sleep problem. Careful comparisons of home versus lab sleep give clues concerning the role of learning factors. For example, a patient may sleep much better in the lab than at home and know that the lab sleep was better. This may indicate that maladaptive conditioning factors did not generalize from the home to the lab, or that the patient, hoping to have the insomnia clearly documented in the lab, did not try so hard to fall asleep and therefore slept more easily in the lab. Similarly, the measurement of EMG tension (to be discussed below) during bedtime might give clues about the amount of somatized tension surrounding insomnia. It is important to observe the progression of EMG tension during prolonged times spent awake in bed. One often finds patients who show more and more EMG tension as they lie in bed awake, becoming increasingly frustrated as they are unable to fall asleep.

## A.2. DIMS Associated with Psychiatric Disorders

Once the sleep problem has been clearly associated with a diagnosable and classifiable psychiatric disorder, that disorder should be treated according to standard psychiatric practice rather than dealing with the sleep disturbance. Polysomnographic evaluation is only indicated if the insomnia remains after the psychiatric disturbance has waned. Behavioral factors learned during the psychiatric disturbance may maintain the insomnia in those cases (see discussion above).

## A.3. DIMS Associated with Use of Drugs and Alcohol

The diagnosis of this problem requires two polysomnographic recordings: one on medication and one after appropriate withdrawal. If this category fits the patient, insomnia will disappear once adequate withdrawal is achieved.

## A.4. Sleep-Induced Respiratory Impairment

This condition is described in Chapter Seven and will not be discussed here.

## A.5. Sleep-Related (Nocturnal) Myoclonus and "Restless Legs"

These conditions are described in Chapter Twelve and will not be discussed here.

## A.6. DIMS Associated with Other Medical, Toxic, and Environmental Conditions

This category covers known medical (including neurologic), toxic, and environmental conditions that are associated with DIMS. The onset, time course, and termination of the insomnias that are classified here are closely tied to the state of the related condition. Polysomnography is only indicated if the insomnia does not wane after the presumed etiologic condition has disappeared.

## A.7. Childhood-Onset DIMS

This type of insomnia is characterized by a distinctive history of unexplained problems with insomnia before puberty and by their persistence into adulthood. Hauri and Olmstead *(19)* have demonstrated that the sleep disturbance in this condition is usually quite severe and that it may be associated with some as yet undetermined neurologic dysfunctioning, possibly akin to minimal brain dysfunction or hyperkinesis.

Polysomnographic evaluations in childhood-onset insomnia are indicated to assess the severity of the problem. However, psychologic/behavioral assessments are also necessary. Having to live with chronic insomnia since childhood apparently affects psychologic and physiologic functioning quite differently in different patients. For example, learned behavioral and psychologic reactions to the problem may aggravate the insomnia. The sleep-lab evaluation may indicate the amount of somatized tension, as assessed by frontalis EMG, or it may indicate that the problem has resulted in excessive anxiety or depression. Such findings may become crucial guides to the sensitive treatment of an otherwise mostly organic problem.

## A.8.a DIMS Associated with Repeated REM-Sleep Interruptions

This is a sleep-maintenance insomnia with a characteristic pattern of awakenings mainly from REM periods. Obviously, it can only be diagnosed by polysomnography. Awakenings longer than three minutes must occur from at least three-fourths of all REM periods, and less than one-fifth of the awakenings must come from NREM sleep. The diagnosis is important because it has some implications for treatment *(20)*.

Although some DIMS associated with repeated REM sleep interruptions may be based on the fact that REM sleep is very light in humans or on the fact that seriously disturbing dreams might awaken the sleeper, others seem rooted in the characteristic physiology of REM sleep. For example, sleep apneas occurring only in REM sleep may awaken the patient (Guilleminault, personal communication).

## A.9.b. Subjective DIMS Complaint without Objective Findings

In this condition, sleep is experienced as frequently interrupted and "nonrestorative," and the polysomnogram is marked by abnormal features. It appears that some insomniacs have extremely poor spindles, show a highly atypical sleep architecture, may display many short arousals, or exhibit sudden unexplained drops in EMG recordings. If this happens in the absence of drug-induced changes and in the absence of either medical or psychiatric disturbances, one might speculate that the sleep disturbance is associated with these atypical features. However, little research has been published on this type of insomnia.

A subtype of the above is "alpha-delta" sleep, the intrusion of high-amplitude alpha waves into NREM sleep *(21,22)*. This pattern is often secondary to use of drugs or to withdrawal from them and should then be so classified. If not drug-related, alpha intrusions into NREM seem associated with "non-restorative" sleep: patients showing much alpha during sleep often suffer from vague aches, pains, malaise, and stiffness upon awakening. Many are diagnosed as having "fibrositis."

## A.9.a. Short Sleeper

Short sleepers are those who require substantially *less* sleep per 24 hours than is average for their age gorup. Although they may be concerned about their "insomnia," they are usually diagnosed by the fact that they feel and function relatively well throughout waking, despite chronically decreased sleep. Polysomnography is not usually required.

## A.9.b. Subjective DIMS Complaint without Objective Findings

This is the designation for a convincing and honest complaint of "insomnia" that cannot be substantiated in the laboratory but is made by an individual lacking in apparent psychopathology. Different from the persistent psychophysiologic insomniac, who may sleep well in the lab and know the next morning that sleep was good, the patient with a subjective DIMS complaint sleeps well in the lab according to polysomnography but still complains of having slept poorly.

Originally, it had been assumed that people who showed this pattern were basically chronic complainers, hypochondriacs, patients in search of attention, etc. However, most patients whose complaint of insomnia cannot be substantiated in the lab do *not* show the expected psychopathology *(23)*.

Because patients classified here show no medical or psychiatric pathology, have apparently adequate sleep, but still complain about insomnia, one is forced to speculate that the problem may lie somewhere within sleep itself. Maybe the essence of sleep is not reflected in the brain waves or in the way we record and score these waves. Maybe a much more detailed analysis is required to find the abnormality in these people.

A polysomnographic evaluation covering at least two to three nights is usually necessary to classify patients into this category. Careful psychiatric interviewing and psychologic testing is also crucial to separate those to be classified here from those who *do* show a psychologic reason for their complaint.

# Technical Issues

Most technical issues concerning polysomnography are discussed in Chapter One. Included here are only topics that are issues specific to the diagnosis of DIMS.

## Minimal Number of Channels Required for Polysomnography

Practices vary from center to center, depending mainly on whether insomniacs typically spend one or more nights in the lab.

If more than one night is typically planned, the first night in the lab should include recording of at least the four channels required by the Rechtschaffen-Kales method plus one channel of airflow (combined thermistors in front of nose and mouth), two channels of bipolar anterior tibialis EMG (right and left), one channel of ECG, plus one channel of integrated frontalis EMG. The first night's record is scored immediately upon awakening the patient, and atypical findings can then be evaluated during subsequent nights. For example, if the record shows irregular breathing patterns of *any* kind, the recording for the second night should include separate nasal and oral airflow thermistors, measures of chest movement (either intercostal EMG or strain gauges), and ear oximetry in an effort to diagnose the problem. Similarly, if some atypical EEG waves are noted on the record of the first night, a full 8- to 12-channel EEG montage might be used on the second night to further identify the problem.

If the center traditionally runs only one night of evaluation of insomniacs, a more elaborate montage is needed. McGregor et al. *(24)* suggest a minimum of 12 channels, including one EEG ($C_4/A_{1,2}$), three channels of eye movements, one chin EMG, two anterior tibialis EMGs (left and right), three measures of airflow (oral and right and left nasal thermistors), one measure of thoraco-abdominal movements, and one ECG. Although this constellation certainly diagnoses sleep apnea and is sensitive to all kinds of deviations in eye movements, abnormal EEG features can only be found if they manifest themselves on the $C_4$ electrode. Their spread over the entire cortex cannot be followed by McGregor's montage. Similarly, it is hard to assess muscle tension in the insomniac from a chin lead alone.

If only one night can be obtained from an insomniac on a 12-channel polygraph, I would suggest the following montage:

Four channels EEG (including $C_3/A_2$ and temporal leads).
Two channels eye movements (EOG).
One channel chin EMG.
One airflow measure (nasal/oral thermistor combined in series).
One measure of chest effort (intercostal EMG).
Two anterior tibialis EMGs (left and right).
One integrated frontalis EMG.

In such a setup, the nighttime observer would have to be very astute. If atypical EEG waves were observed, the paper would have to be switched to clinical speed. If sleep apneas were observed, an ear oximeter might be applied during the second half of the night, replacing the integrated frontalis EMG.

## Scoring

Ever since different sleep stages have been described, the tendency has been to squeeze any and all sleep into these five EEG-defined stages. While this may be justified for research studies, for clinical evaluation it is often more important to notice that the patient shows atypical waves or atypical combinations of waves rather than knowing exactly how much stage 2 or delta sleep is obtained. Indeed, one of the most sensitive indicators of abnormal sleep patterns is often the time it takes an experienced technician to score an artifact-free record or the number of pages that such a scorer cannot classify with certainty.

Atypical polysomnographic features have not been quantified for clinical evaluations. For research purposes, hybrid detectors of sleep spindles, K complexes, etc. have been built by individual labs. Others have filtered certain frequency bands (e.g., alpha) from the EEG and quantified the strength of these bands either by reset integrators or by computer techniques. No diagnostically useful norms have been published. Once again, the diagnostician is usually dependent on the technician who scores the records, a person who should be trained to watch for the specific waves and wave forms that might be of interest in work on insomnia.

## Recording Frontalis EMG

The existence of excessive somatized tension is an important parameter to be considered in the diagnosis of persistent psychophysiologic insomnia. It also has important implications for treatment *(12)*. Furthermore, it may be important to know why muscle tension changes as the patient lies in bed, trying to sleep. A chronically tense patient may need different behavioral treatments than one who is relaxed throughout the day but who tenses markedly as bedtime approaches.

Muscle tension is usually assessed in the frontalis because it is very easy to measure there. Also, at least according to biofeedback tradition, EMG recordings from this area are sensitive indicators of somatized tension, and they correlate relatively well with tension in other parts of the musculature.

For a crude evaluation of a tense versus a relaxed frontalis EMG, a standard EEG cup electrode is applied about one inch above each eyebrow. After appropriate amplification and filtering, the output is quantified by reset integrators. The main problem in this setup is the 60-cps artifact, which cannot be easily rejected when recording EMG and cannot be easily detected from the reset integrator. Very sharp notch filters for 60 cps are therefore needed.

During sleep, especially during REM sleep, frontalis EMG tension decreases to levels close to cable noise. A low-noise amplifier might have to be placed close to the patient's bed if EMG during sleep is of interest, as has been described elsewhere (25).

## Subjective Evaluation of Laboratory Sleep

A detailed interview with the insomniac is required after each laboratory night, before the diagnostician or the patient knows the polysomnographic findings. This interview often yields the best information toward an adequate diagnosis. Besides asking for such items as subjective sleep latency, number of awakenings, and depth of sleep, one inquires carefully about any possible differences between the laboratory night that has just passed and typical sleep at home. If the lab night was different, the patient's speculations about this difference often contain clues to understanding the problem. Was the different sleep in the lab caused by a lack of environmental noise in the lab, by the lack of a bedside clock, by being away from trouble with children and family, by feeling safe here, or by not trying so hard to sleep, possibly in an unconscious effort to demonstrate how seriously one is suffering? Psychosomatic patients are notoriously poor at sensing and understanding broad psychologic issues. Dealing with the concrete issue of why they slept differently in the lab than at home often yields more insight for such insomniacs than dealing with the same issues on a more abstract, psychiatric level.

## Home Recordings

Laboratory recordings are expensive. In addition, sleep in the laboratory may be atypical. Although the difference between laboratory sleep and home sleep is of diagnostic interest in persistent psychophysiologic insomnia, other types of poor sleep might be better diagnosed if we knew the patients' typical sleep at home rather than their laboratory sleep.

A number of home recording devices have been developed over the years. They are listed here in order of increasing complexity. It seems likely that the next few years will see important developments in home recording, as electronic technology and miniaturization advance.

1. *Movement detectors* attached to the bed are actually refinements of the old Szymanski Actographs (26). Piezoelectric crystals may be used (27), or the difference in electric potential may be measured between two plates of a condensor placed underneath a mattress (28). Bed movements are recorded

on tape, together with actual clock time. Remarkably accurate estimates of sleep time can be obtained in most insomniacs because they toss and turn in bed. However, this method will overestimate the amount of sleep that is obtained in depressive insomniacs and others who lie in bed awake for hours without moving.
2. *Wrist actographs* have been advocated by Kupfer and by Kripke's group *(29)*. Their output is again recorded on tape, together with the actual clock time. Kripke reported very accurate estimates of sleep time when comparing the data from wrist actographs with the data obtained by standard polysomnography. However, patients have to wear the wrist actograph, and they are tied to a tape recorder. This makes wrist actographs more cumbersome than the piezoelectric crystals of the earlier methods.
3. *Periodic photos of the bed* (e.g., every 15 minutes) have been advocated by Hobson et al. *(30)* as a means of assessing home sleep. Insomniacs can be distinguished from normals using this technique, but many patients find the periodically occurring flashes quite bothersome.
4. *Analog recording of the EEG* into a tape recorder at home was advocated by Wilkinson et al. as early as 1973 *(31)*. Although these investigators record information on tape, to be transcribed later in the lab, others *(32,33)* obtain a real-time writeout over regular telephone wires from the home to the lab. These systems require that the technician visit the home at bedtime to apply the electrodes before the patient retires.
5. *Digital recording of polysomnography* is currently being explored at Stanford (personal communication). It may be a method of the future, if the storage of that much digitized data can be handled economically.

# Summary

This chapter first discussed the evaluation and treatment of patients with a complaint of insomnia, as it can be performed by a private physician. Indications for referral to a sleep disorders center were then enumerated, and techniques were discussed for evaluation of such patients at a center. This included specifying the role of polysomnography in evaluating disorders of initiating and maintaining sleep (DIMS). Different types of insomnia were then discussed, together with possible ways to diagnose them. Some comments concerning the technical aspects of the evaluation of disorders of initiating and maintaining sleep concluded the chapter.

# REFERENCES

1. Ware JC. The symptom of insomnia: causes and cures. Psychiatr Ann 1979; 9:27–49.
2. McGhie A, Russel SM. The subjective assessment of normal sleep patterns. J Ment Sci 1962; 108:642–54.
3. Hammond EC. Some preliminary findings on physical complaints from a prospective study of 1,064,004 men and women. Am J Public Health 1964; 54:11–23.
4. Balter MB, Bauer ML. Patterns of prescribing and use of hypnotic drugs in the United States. In: Clift AD, ed. Sleep disturbance and hypnotic drug dependence. New York: Excerpta Medica, 1975:261–93.
5. Karacan I, Thornby JI, Anch M, et al. Prevalence of sleep disturbance in a primarily urban Florida county. Soc Sci Med 1976; 10:239–44.
6. Bixler EO, Kales A, Soldatos CR, Kales JD, Healey S. Prevalence of sleep disorders in the Los Angeles metropolitan area. Am J Psychiatry 1979; 136:1257–62.
7. Institute of Medicine. Sleeping pills, insomnia, and medical practice. Washington, DC: National Academy of Sciences, 1979.
8. Clift AD. Sleep disturbance in general practice. In: Clift AD, ed. Sleep disturbance and hypnotic drug dependence. New York: Excerpta Medica, 1975:155–77.
9. Whitlock FA. Hypnotics, sedatives and tranquillisers—prescribing trends in Australia. In: Clift AD, ed. Sleep disturbance and hypnotic drug dependence. New York: Excerpta Medica, 1975:295–310.
10. Hauri P. The sleep disorders. Kalamazoo, Michigan: The Upjohn Company, 1977.
11. Regestein QR. Practical ways to manage chronic insomnia. Med Times 1979; 107:19–23.
12. Hauri P. Treating psychophysiological insomnia with biofeedback. Arch Gen Psychiatry, in press.
13. Wikler A. Diagnosis and treatment of drug dependence of the barbiturate type. Am J Psychiatry 1968; 125:758–765.
14. Shader RI, Caine ED, Meyer RE. Treatment of dependence on barbiturates and sedative-hypnotics. In: Shader RI, ed. Manual of psychiatric therapeutics. Boston: Little, Brown and Company, 1975:195–202.
15. Webb WB. The reliability of sleep stages: theoretical and clinical implications. Paper presented at the 12th annual meeting of the APSS, San Diego, California, May 3–6, 1973.

16. Coleman RM, Miles LE, Guilleminault C, Zarcone VP, van den Hoed J, Dement WC. Sleep-wake disorders in the elderly: a polysomnographic analysis. J Am Geriatr Soc, in press.
17. Association of Sleep Disorders Centers. Diagnostic classification of sleep and arousal disorders. 1st ed. Prepared by the Sleep Disorders Classification Committee, HP Roffwarg, chairman. Sleep 1979; 2:1–137.
18. Hauri P. Behavioral treatment of insomnia. Med Times 1979; 107:36–47.
19. Hauri P, Olmstead E. Childhood-onset insomnia. Sleep 1980; 3:59–65.
20. Greenberg R. Dream interruption insomnia. J Nerv Ment Dis 1967; 144:18–21.
21. Hauri P, Hawkins DR. Alpha-delta sleep. Electroencephalogr Clin Neurophysiol 1973; 34:233-7.
22. Moldofsky H. Musculoskeletal symptoms and non-REM sleep disturbance in patients with "fibrositis syndrome" and healthy subjects. Psychosom Med 1975; 37:341–51.
23. Piccione P, Zorick F, Roth T, Stepanski E. Sleep and personality in subjective insomniacs. Paper presented at the 20th annual meeting of the APSS, Mexico City, Mexico, March 25–29, 1980.
24. McGregor PA, Weitzman ED, Pollak CP. Polysomnographic recording techniques used for the diagnosis of sleep disorders in a sleep disorders center. Am J EEG Technol 1978; 18:107–32.
25. Bliwise D, Coleman R, Bergmann B, Wincor MZ, Pivik RT, Rechtschaffen A. Facial muscle tonus during REM and NREM sleep. Psychophysiology 1974; 11:497–508.
26. Szymanski JS. Eine Methode zur Untersuchung der Ruhe und Aktivitätsperioden bei Tieren. Pflügers Arch 1914; 158:343–385.
27. Muzet A, Becht J, Jacquot P, König PA. A technique for recording human body posture during sleep. Psychophysiology 1972; 9:660–2.
28. Alihanka J, Vaahtoranta K. A static charge sensitive bed. A new method for recording body movements during sleep. Electroencephalogr Clin Neurophysiol 1979; 46:731–734.
29. Mullaney DJ, Kripke DF, Messin S. Wrist actograph measures sleep duration. Sleep Res 1979; 8:266.
30. Hobson JS, Prokop J, Spagna T. Time-lapse photography distinguishes good and poor sleep. Sleep Res 1978; 7:291.
31. Wilkinson RT, Herbert M. A "pocket" portable EEG recorder: adapting the Stott Miniature Analog Tape Recording System to record sleeping EEG on trains. Paper presented at the 12th annual meeting of the APSS, San Diego, California, May 3–6, 1973.
32. Hanley J, Zweizig JR, Kado RT, Adey WR, Rovner LD. Combined telephone and radiotelemetry of the EEG. Electroencephalogr Clin Neurophysiol 1969; 26:323–4.
33. Coates TJ, Rosekind MR, Thoresen CE. All night sleep recording in clients' homes by telephone. J Behav Ther & Exp Psychiatry 1978; 9:157–62.

# ELEVEN
# DEPRESSIVE PATIENTS AND THE SLEEP LABORATORY

CHARLES F. REYNOLDS III
PATRICIA A. COBLE
DAVID J. KUPFER
DAVID H. SHAW

## Introduction

This chapter will present the current status of EEG sleep technology as applied to the diagnosis and treatment of affective states, particularly depressive disorders. The recently published *Diagnostic Classification of Sleep and Arousal Disorders (1)* recognizes depression as a cause of both disorders of initiating and maintaining sleep (DIMS) and disorders of excessive sleepiness (DOES). Our own clinical experience supports this: affective disorder is the major diagnosis in 35%–40% of patients seen in our Sleep Evaluation Center. EEG sleep studies have been performed on depressed patients since the late 1940s, but relatively few studies prior to 1976 showed sufficient attention to such methodological problems and confounding variables as selection of homogeneous patient samples, drug status of patients, age, and laboratory setting. These few studies were reviewed by Kupfer and Foster in *Sleep Disorders: Diagnosis and Treatment,* edited by Williams and Karacan *(2)*. The six pre-1976 studies cited report the EEG sleep characteristics of 119 drug-free patients with "depression": one of the most consistent findings is a shortened REM-sleep latency. Other findings, which are more variable, include a prolonged sleep latency, impaired sleep efficiency, and diminished slow-wave sleep.

We present here our own protocol for performing EEG sleep studies in depressed patients, followed by a summary of results from a series of recent studies (since 1976) and an exposition of issues for further research (current limitations of procedure).

# Protocol for EEG Sleep Studies in Depressed Patients

Our protocol for EEG sleep studies of depressive patients, as set forth in Table 11–1, consists of a series of technical steps or "demands": *(a)* We perform a diagnostic assessment by using the structured format of the Schedule for Affective Disorders and Schizophrenia *(3)*. This provides a standardized evaluation of present state and longitudinal course of the patient's illness. It also facilitates selection of a homogenous clinical sample for research purposes. *(b)* Concurrently, we perform an extensive medical evaluation of depressive patients, including a thorough physical and neurological examination and a series of laboratory investigations: CBC, SMA-15, thyroid function tests, VDRL, urinalysis, urine for drug screening, ECG, and EEG. Additional laboratory studies are ordered as indicated. We have found that depression may mask serious underlying medical illnesses, including various endocrinopathies, malignancies, and neurological illnesses. Moreover, these medical-affective syndromes have EEG sleep characteristics very different from those found in primary depression *(4)*. *(c)* We insist upon an observation period of 14 days, during which patients are kept free of psychotropic drugs and alcohol. The purpose of this demand is to establish the diagnosis and to minimize drug effects on EEG sleep characteristics. *(d)* Inpatients on our Clinical Research Unit for affective disorders have sleep studies in their own rooms, to minimize any need for adaptation associated with sleeping in a different location. Outpatients are given a tour of the laboratory before the study to minimize anticipatory anxiety. *(e)* All patients are told to avoid ingestion of caffeine after 1800 on the nights of studies. *(f)* Patients are instructed not to change their daytime nap schedules; thus, when sleep studies are performed, the patient is in "steady-state," i.e., his sleep-wake cycle is as regular as possible and entrained to ward schedule (in the case of inpatients). *(g)* Concurrent with the drug-free observation period and medical workup, patients' symptoms are evaluated serially with self- and observer-rating scales, principally the Hamilton Rating Scale for Depression *(5)* and the KDS self-rating scales *(6)*.

**Table 11–1** Technical Demands for the Performance of EEG Sleep Studies in Depression

1. Rigorous, standardized, and serial diagnostic assessment (SADS, Hamilton, KDS scales).
2. Physical and laboratory evaluation.
3. Drug-free observation period of 14 days.
4. Reduction of anticipatory anxiety.
5. Avoidance of caffeine after 1800 on night of studies.
6. Maintenance of daytime nap schedule.
7. Two consecutive baseline nights of EEG sleep studies.
8. Visual and automated analysis of EEG sleep data.

rating scales, principally the Hamilton Rating Scale for Depression *(5)* and the KDS self-rating scales *(6)*.

At the end of the 14-day drug-free observation period, we perform two consecutive all-night recordings. Our routine four-channel montage consists of EEG ($C_3/A_2$), left and right monopolar electro-oculogram (EOG), and submental electromyogram (EMG). An appropriate montage is added if there is clinical evidence of sleep-associated ventilatory disturbance or myoclonus. However, on the basis of data to be presented, we recommend that routine polysomnographic screening for sleep apnea and nocturnal myoclonus not be performed in patients meeting Research Diagnostic Criteria (RDC) for affective disorders because the yield of significant findings is very low.

We use the Grass model 78-B polygraph for recording sleep, with a calibration of 50 $\mu$V = 7 mm pen deflection, and with all electrode impedances less than 5,000 ohms. Paper speed is 10 mm/sec. Records are scored with modified Kales-Rechtschaffen criteria *(7)*, maintaining inter-rater scoring reliability of 0.9. We also tape records for purposes of automated analysis on the PDP-11 microcomputer. Figure 11–1 presents a flowchart of our automated data analysis procedures. These consist of two main pathways: REM analysis (REMA) and delta wave analysis (DELA). Each night of sleep is played back at high speed into a PDP-11 microcomputer (20–30 minutes to process each night). REM analysis uses both EOG channels to produce five variables for each minute of the night between calibration signals: count per minute, maximum height/REM, duration/REM, area/REM, and binocular synchrony. Delta analysis utilizes the EEG channel recorded on tape and can examine any of 16 bins selected, each with different frequency and amplitude parameters. The standard delta setting of 0.5–2.0 Hz and 75–200 $\mu$V is collected in bin 1. The EEG channel is sampled at a rate of 200 times per second, stored until 2000 samples are collected, averaged, and adjusted for baseline drift, and then sent to a baseline crossing detector and to an amplitude (peak) detector. With each baseline crossing, the period of the preceding half wave is computed from the prior crossing, with the peak noted and checked against the 16 bins. If a particular cycle matches the requirements for a bin, the counter for that bin is incremented. (More than one bin can be incremented owing to individual parameters set for each bin.) Following each minute of sampling, each bin count is written in a file sequentially.

After coding the visually staged sleep into a minute-by-minute form, all three files are merged into one file with the three data types in parallel. Each night of sleep can then be analyzed for structure by visual and automated analysis. The visually scored portion allows us to detect and delete awake minutes from the REM and delta as well as to eliminate movement artifacts. We have found a very high positive correlation between visually scored REM activity and the count measure in REMA; in addition, height, duration, and area also show positive correlations. Delta counts from bin 1 are highly correlated (positive) with visually scored delta minutes. Delta waves are detected most often in stage 4 sleep, somewhat less often in stage 3, still less often in stage 2, and only occasionally in stage 1. A very high inverse correlation exists between REM periods and delta periods; thus, when there is REM, there is seldom any delta detected and vice versa (Figure 11–2). These automated techniques permit an in-depth study of

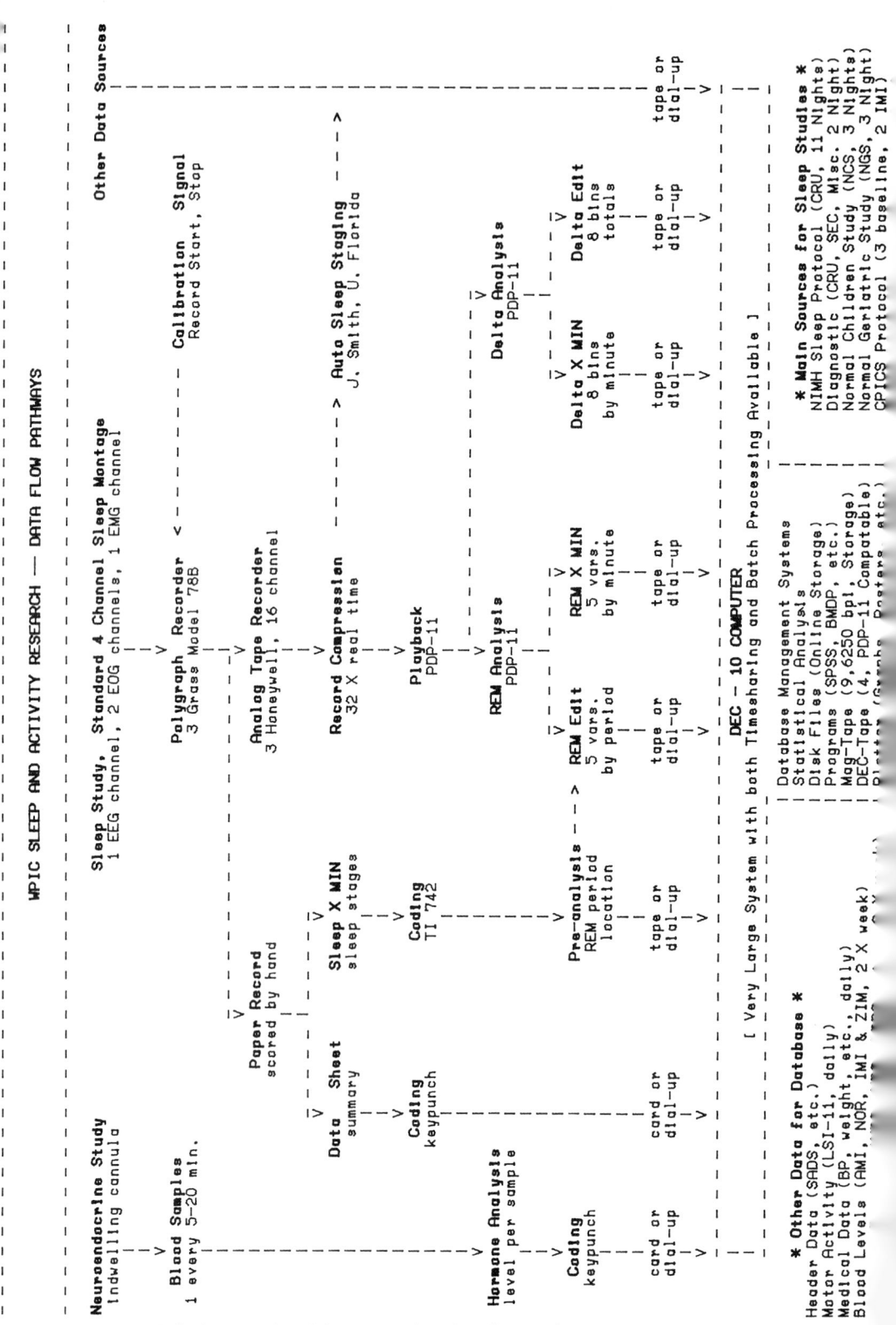

**Figure 11–1.** WPIC sleep and activity research—data flow pathways.

*Depressive patients and the sleep laboratory*

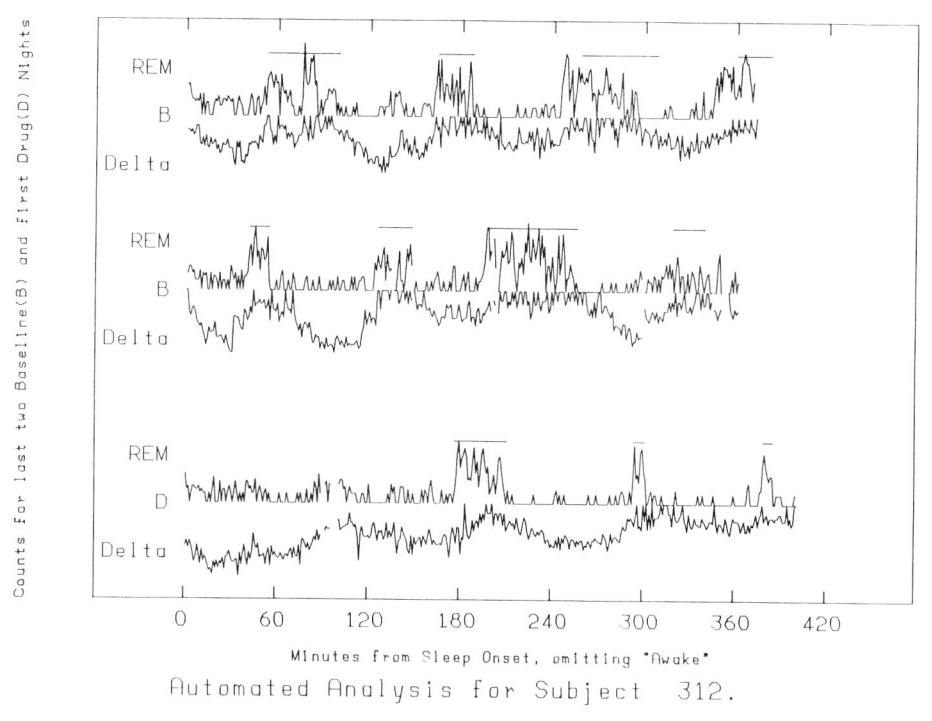

**Figure 11–2.** Demonstration of automated analysis of two nights of drug-free sleep preceding one night of 50 mg amitriptyline. Bars indicate visually scored REM sleep. The areas above each midline reflect REM count per minute; the areas below the midline reflect delta wave count per minute. This figure reflects the finding that REM activity and delta activity are generally mutually exclusive. The figure also shows a drug-induced increase in REM latency and an "anticipating pause" in delta activity at approximately baseline REM latency, which corresponds to the baseline delta cycle.

overall sleep structure and patterning and provide a method to examine minute-by-minute changes occurring within a REM period or delta period.

Concurrent with automated analysis, we divide the hand-scored EEG sleep variables into three groups for purposes of further analysis: *(a)* sleep continuity; *(b)* sleep architecture; and *(c)* REM sleep indexes (Table 11–2). Sleep continuity indexes include *total recording period* (TRP); *time spent asleep* (TSA), or net sleep time; *sleep efficiency,* a ratio of TSA/TRP ($\times$ 100); *sleep latency* (SL), the time from the beginning of the recording to the onset of stage 2 sleep (at least ten uninterrupted minutes); *intermittent wakefulness* (A), time spent awake which is bounded by sleep; and *early morning awakening* (EMA), time spent awake after the last sleep occurrence and before

249

*Sleeping and waking disorders: indications and techniques*

**Table 11-2**  EEG Sleep Variables

*Sleep continuity*
1. Total recording period (TRP): Minutes of total recording
2. Sleep latency (SL): Time from lights-out until the appearance of stage 2 sleep
3. Awake (A): Time spent awake after sleep onset and before the final morning awakening
4. Early morning awakening (EMA): Time spent awake from the final awakening until the patient gets out of bed; (SQEMA): square root of EMA
5. Time spent asleep (TSA): Time spent asleep less any awake (A) time during the night after sleep onset and prior to EMA
6. Sleep efficiency (TSA/TRP): Time spent asleep (TSA) divided by total recording time (TRP) times 100
7. Sleep maintenance (SM): TSA/TRP with SL and EM removed. (SSM): Normalized SM

*Sleep architecture*
1. Percentage of each stage of sleep expressed as a ratio to TSA (stage 1 %, stage 2 %, stage 3 %, stage 4 %)
2. Minutes of each stage of sleep (stage 1 min, etc.)
3. Percent delta (delta %): Combined percentage of stage 3 and stage 4 sleep
4. REM percent (RT/TSA): Ratio of REM sleep time to TSA
5. 2-REM percent (PC 2R): Percentage of minutes of stage 2 sleep presenting rapid eye movements

*REM measures*
1. REM latency (RL): Number of minutes of sleep until the first REM period; (SQRL): square root of RL
2. REM activity (RA): Each minute of REM sleep is scored on a 9-point scale (0-8) for REM patterns, the sum for the whole night providing RA
3. Average REM activity (RA/TSA): Ratio of RA to TSA
4. REM density (RA/RT): Ratio of RA to RT
5. Number of REM periods (NUMR): Number of REM periods throughout the night

the end of the recording period. Sleep architecture indexes are *percentages of net sleep time* (TSA) spent in the different stages of sleep: These are conventionally designated stages 1, 2, 3, 4, REM, and 2-REM. Further, *delta sleep* is the sum of stages 3 and 4; *stage 2 REM* is stage 2 sleep with rapid eye movement intrusions. REM-sleep indexes include *REM-sleep time* (RT); *REM-sleep activity* (RA), an integrative measure of the frequency and intensity of rapid eye movements per minute of REM sleep, scored visually on a scale of 1-8; *REM density* (RA/RT); *average REM activity* (RA/TSA); and *REM-sleep latency* (RL), the time between sleep onset and the first REM-sleep period, minus awakening between sleep onset and first REM period. Since we have not generally found in our laboratory large or important first-night effects *(8)*, we average the two nights of sleep data from each subject for purposes of analysis.

# Results of Recent Studies

## Primary versus Secondary Depressives

Table 11–3 shows EEG sleep characteristics of primary and secondary depressives (2). The distinction between primary and secondary depression is made on the basis of RDC criteria (3): "primary" means that there is no antecedent history of psychiatric disorder, other than affective disorder per se, whereas "secondary" means that the patient has had a history of some other psychiatric disorder, such as alcoholism. The group of 47 primary depressives consisted of 18 men and 29 women, with a mean age of 45.7 years. The group of 48 secondary depressives consisted of 11 men and 37 women, with a mean age of 37.0 years. The primary depressives differed from the secondary depressives particularly in terms of shorter REM sleep latency (38.6 versus 72.3 minutes, $p < 0.001$), greater REM sleep percentage (21.7 versus 17.8, $p < 0.01$), greater phasic

**Table 11–3** EEG Sleep Characteristics of Primary and Secondary Depressives, 1978

|  | Primary Depressives (N = 47) | Secondary Depressives (N = 48) | Probability |
|---|---|---|---|
| *Sleep continuity* | | | |
| Sleep latency (min) | 49.0 ± 6.8 | 45.0 ± 5.9 | NS* |
| Early morning awakening (min) | 19.7 ± 4.2 | 6.1 ± 2.3 | < .01 |
| Awake (min) | 37.1 ± 5.7 | 22.5 ± 4.6 | < .05 |
| Time spent asleep (min) | 304.4 ± 8.8 | 336.2 ± 8.3 | < .01 |
| Awake/time spent asleep (%) | 14.3 ± 2.6 | 8.1 ± 2.0 | < .05 |
| TSA/total recording period | 74.7 ± 2.3 | 82.2 ± 1.9 | < .01 |
| *Sleep architecture* | | | |
| Percent of stage 1 sleep | 11.0 ± 1.03 | 9.3 ± 0.70 | NS |
| Percent of stage 2 sleep | 63.7 ± 3.2 | 67.5 ± 2.9 | NS |
| Percent of delta sleep | 2.8 ± 0.53 | 4.4 ± 0.98 | NS |
| Percent of stage 1 REM | 21.7 ± 0.77 | 17.8 ± 0.82 | < .01 |
| Percent of stage 2 REM | 1.0 ± 0.20 | 1.0 ± 0.24 | NS |
| *REM measures* | | | |
| REM latency (min) | 38.6 ± 3.2 | 72.3 ± 4.3 | < .001 |
| REM activity (units) | 126.3 ± 7.9 | 83.8 ± 8.0 | < .001 |
| REM activity/time spent asleep | 0.43 ± 0.03 | 0.24 ± 0.02 | < .001 |
| REM activity/REM time | 1.95 ± 0.09 | 1.31 ± 0.08 | < .001 |

*Not significant.

REM activity (126.3 versus 83.8 units, $p < 0.001$), more impaired sleep efficiency (74.7% versus 82.2%, $p < 0.01$), and greater early morning awakening (19.7 versus 6.1 minutes, $p < 0.01$). In a separate study, using regression and discriminant analyses, Coble et al. showed that EEG sleep variables correctly classified by diagnosis 85% of a sample of 40 outpatient primary and secondary depressives *(9)*. This level of discrimination is comparable to that of Gillin et al., who found that EEG sleep variables could correctly classify 82% of a sample of age-matched normal subjects, inpatient depressives, and primary insomniacs *(10)*.

A second large-scale investigation recently completed in our laboratory on 87 patients with primary depression confirms the findings of the earlier study of 95 patients *(11)*. The replication study group consisted of 54 females and 33 males with a mean age of 36.9 years and with a mean Hamilton depression-rating score of 38. As shown in Table 11–4, their overall sleep pattern showed an average sleep-onset latency of 40 minutes, a reduced sleep efficiency of 81%, and both intermittent wakefulness and early morning awakening. Stage 1 sleep was elevated to approximately 10%, whereas slow-wave sleep was reduced to approximately 2%. This group also showed a reduced mean REM latency of 47 minutes and a REM activity of 108 units.

**Table 11–4**  Selected Sleep Characteristics in 87 Primary Depressives, 1980

|  | Mean | SD |
|---|---|---|
| *Sleep continuity* |  |  |
| Sleep latency (min) | 39.4 | (23.7) |
| Early morning awakening (min) | 18.4 | (34.3) |
| Awake (min) | 19.5 | (21.8) |
| Time spent asleep (min) | 327.2 | (50.5) |
| Awake/time spent asleep (%) | 7.2 | (10.4) |
| Sleep efficiency (%) | 81.0 | (12.4) |
| Sleep maintenance (%) | 89.7 | (12.4) |
| *Sleep architecture* |  |  |
| Percent of stage 1 sleep | 9.6 | (4.0) |
| Percent of stage 2 sleep | 62.8 | (7.4) |
| Percent of delta sleep | 1.0 | (4.1) |
| Percent of stage 1 REM | 24.0 | (62) |
| Percent of stage 2 REM | 1.7 | (1.9) |
| *REM sleep measures* |  |  |
| REM latency (min) | 47.5 | (26.2) |
| REM time (min) | 78.6 | (23.7) |
| REM activity (units) | 107.9 | (61.0) |
| REM activity/time spent asleep | 33.8 | (19.6) |
| REM activity/REM time | 134.8 | (56.1) |
| Number of REM periods | 3.5 | (0.8) |

We have also recently compared EEG sleep findings in 18 outpatients and 18 inpatients, all of whom met criteria for primary depressive disorders and who were matched for age, sex, and symptom severity as measured by the KDS 1 and 2 self-rating scales *(12)*. The mean age of the outpatients was 39.6 years and that of the inpatients, 39.2 years. Both groups contained 11 women and 7 men. Using paired *t* tests, there were no significant differences between groups on any of the EEG sleep variables, except for a longer total recording period in the outpatients ($p < 0.005$) and a longer sleep latency in the outpatients ($p < 0.1$). These data support the argument that EEG sleep data can be used in the diagnosis of both outpatients and inpatients with affective disorders.

When primary depressives are compared to age-matched normals from data published by Williams et al. *(13)*, both sleep continuity and sleep architecture measures are different at the 0.001 level *(2)*. REM latency is also significantly reduced in the primary depressives (38.6 versus 77.3 minutes, $p < 0.001$), but is not significantly reduced in the secondary depressives compared to age-matched normals (72.3 versus 82.0 minutes).

In a comparison of delusional versus nondelusional primary depressives, as shown in Table 11–5, the delusional depressives show greater impairment in sleep continuity indexes, with less sleep efficiency ($p < 0.001$), less TSA (net sleep time) ($p < 0.05$), and more early morning awakening ($p < 0.05$) *(2)*. Delusional patients also show significantly lower REM and delta sleep percentages ($p < 0.05$).

We recently compared the EEG sleep characteristics of 29 delusional depressed patients with those of 12 patients diagnosed to have a schizoaffective disorder *(11)*. Interestingly, it was not possible to distinguish schizoaffective illness from psychotic depression on the basis of major EEG sleep parameters. No significant differences in measures of sleep continuity, sleep architecture, or REM sleep emerged except for the amount of REM time in the first REM period ($8.0 \pm 2.2$ minutes in the schizoaffective group versus $13.0 \pm 8.6$ minutes in the delusional depressives, $p < 0.05$).

An earlier study of EEG sleep findings in bipolar depressives showed that these patients also have a short REM latency. The contrast with unipolar depressives is evident in the sleep-continuity indexes, where unipolars tend to be hyposomnic and bipolars tend to be hypersomnic *(14)*.

When patients with medical diseases concurrent with a depressive syndrome (medical-depressives) are compared with patients who have primary depression, while controlling for age and symptom severity, it is particularly the reduction in phasic REM activity indexes that distinguishes the former group from the latter (Table 11–6) *(2,4)*. The medical-depressive syndromes do not appear to be characterized by a reduced REM-sleep latency in contrast to primary depression.

In summary, we have found that EEG sleep measures significantly discriminate between depressed and normal subjects and among subtypes of depression (primary versus secondary, primary unipolar versus bipolar, primary delusional versus nondelusional, and primary versus medical-depressive). Our data indicate the importance of sleep discontinuity in 80%–85% of all depressed patients (inpatients and outpatients), with the remaining 15%–20% (bipolars) showing features of hypersomnia. Another

**Table 11–5**  EEG Sleep Characteristics of Primary Psychotic and Nonpsychotic Depressives

|  | Psychotic Depressives (N = 17) | Nonpsychotic Depressives (N = 30) | Probability |
|---|---|---|---|
| *Sleep continuity* | | | |
| Sleep latency (min) | 64.82 ± 14.5 | 40.00 ± 6.4 | NS* |
| Early morning awakening (min) | 31.11 ± 8.1 | 13.20 ± 4.5 | < .05 |
| Awake (min) | 54.18 ± 11.0 | 27.40 ± 5.7 | NS |
| Time spent asleep (min) | 278.59 ± 14.6 | 319.07 ± 10.2 | < .05 |
| Awake/time spent asleep (%) | 21.51 ± 5.5 | 10.19 ± 2.5 | NS |
| TSA/total recording period | 64.87 ± 3.5 | 80.28 ± 2.6 | < .001 |
| *Sleep architecture* | | | |
| Percent of stage 1 sleep | 13.64 ± 2.4 | 9.48 ± 0.8 | NS |
| Percent of stage 2 sleep | 63.7 ± 2.8 | 63.7 ± 2.0 | NS |
| Percent of delta sleep | 1.68 ± 0.39 | 2.93 ± 0.8 | < .05 |
| Percent of stage 1 REM | 19.61 ± 1.4 | 22.95 ± 0.9 | < .05 |
| Percent of stage 2 REM | 1.38 ± 0.40 | 0.82 ± 0.2 | NS |
| *REM measures* | | | |
| REM latency (min) | 36.29 ± 5.3 | 39.97 ± 4.1 | NS |
| REM activity (units) | 113.76 ± 13.4 | 133.40 ± 9.7 | NS |
| REM activity/time spent asleep | 0.42 ± 0.04 | 0.44 ± 0.3 | NS |
| REM activity/REM time | 2.10 ± 0.20 | 1.87 ± 0.1 | NS |

*Not significant.

common feature of depression has been the reduction in delta sleep, although this does not seem to be specific for affective states. The most prominent feature to be found in most types of affective disorders, including both inpatients and outpatients with primary depression, has been the shortened REM-sleep latency. A fourth sleep feature reported in depression has been the presence of increased REM activity at the beginning of the night. We have found that for many depressed patients, especially those more than 40 years old, not only does the first REM period occur very early in the night, but it also appears to be associated with a higher density of REM activity than is seen in age-matched normal controls. In one investigation of 35 depressed inpatients, using the automated REM analyzer, we found an increased number of rapid eye movements in the first REM period relative to subsequent REM periods *(15)*.

**Table 11-6** Comparison Between Patients with Medical Diseases Concurrent with a Depressive Syndrome and Patients with Primary Depression on Selected REM-Sleep Measures

|  | Primary Depression (N = 12) | Medical Patients (N = 12) | Probability |
|---|---|---|---|
| *REM measures* | | | |
| REM latency (min) | 42.2 ± 6.1 | 71.8 ± 8.9 | < .05 |
| Total REM time (min) | 73.9 ± 5.4 | 44.2 ± 4.4 | < .01 |
| Total REM activity (units) | 150.5 ± 19.6 | 46.8 ± 6.1 | < .001 |
| REM density (RA/RT) | 2.0 ± 0.1 | 1.1. ± 0.1 | < .001 |
| *First REM period* | | | |
| REM cycle length (first–second) | 116.3 ± 12.0 | 125.0 ± 13.8 | NS* |
| Length—first REM period (min) | 24.0 ± 2.3 | 12.3 ± 2.8 | < .01 |
| Activity—first REM period (units) | 44.5 ± 7.2 | 12.4 ± 3.3 | < .001 |
| Density—first REM period (RA/RT) | 1.85 ± 0.1 | 1.0 ± 0.1 | < .001 |
| *Second REM period* | | | |
| REM cycle length (second–third) | 99.7 ± 5.1 | 91.5 ± 9.7 | NS |
| Length—second REM period (min) | 16.0 ± 2.4 | 14.4 ± 1.8 | NS |
| Activity—second REM period (units) | 28.1 ± 5.3 | 18.3 ± 3.7 | NS |
| Density—second REM period (RA/RT) | 1.75 ± 0.2 | 1.27 ± 0.2 | NS |

*Not significant.

## Relationship of Depressive Psychopathology to Specific EEG Sleep Variables

We have observed relationships between the severity of depression and specific EEG sleep variables in both observer ratings and self-ratings. For example, severity of depression as measured by the Hamilton rating scale or the KDS self-rating scales correlates inversely to a significant extent with shortening of REM latency and decrease in sleep efficiency *(16)*. We have observed this to be the case in both middle-aged and elderly depressives. In a group of 18 hospitalized elderly patients (mean age 64.3 years) with major depressive disorders, a significant correlation was found between sleep efficiency

*Sleeping and waking disorders: indications and techniques*

and the Hamilton depression rating ($r = -0.55$, $p < 0.05$) *(17)*. Similarly, the REM latency correlated inversely with the severity of depression as measured by the KDS scales ($r = -0.59$, $p < 0.01$). In this same group, sleep efficiency and sleep latency were also significantly related to the degree of cognitive disorder that the patients reported ($p < 0.05$).

We have examined a group of 29 primary psychotic depressives for relationships between EEG sleep and particular delusional states *(11)*. When the 29 patients were classified according to type of delusion, 16 patients had primarily delusions of guilt or sin. A comparison of the sleep of this group with that of the remaining 13 patients showed that sleep continuity was much more disturbed in those patients who had delusions of guilt. Similar differences were also observed in the total number of REM minutes. Using a discriminant analysis, only two sleep variables (REM time of the first REM period and sleep efficiency) successfully discriminated 79% of the patients ($\kappa = 0.58$, $p < 0.001$; 14 of the 16 patients with delusions of guilt and 9 of the 13 with other delusions). In contrast, patients with somatic delusions showed higher REM

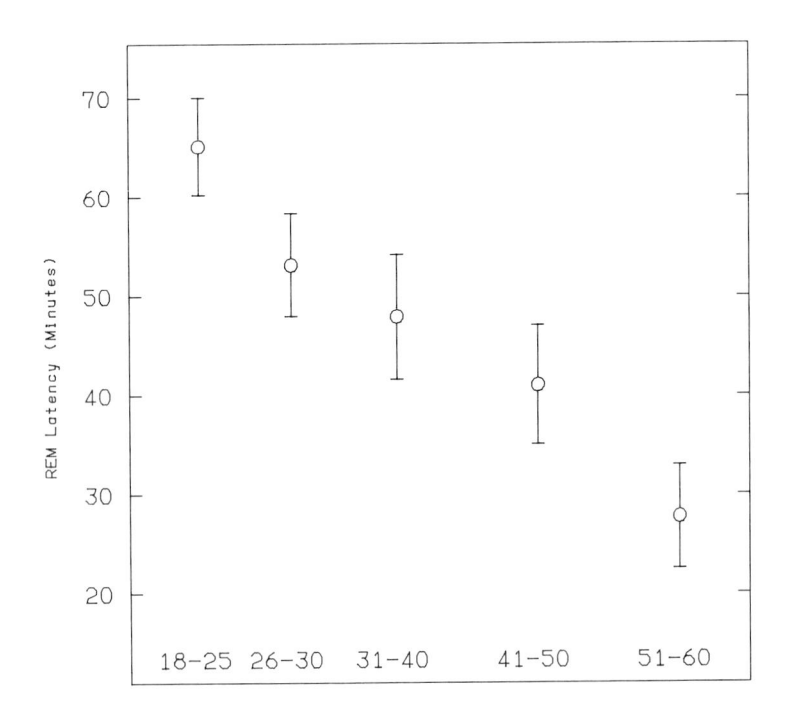

**Figure 11-3.** REM latency findings in depressed patients as a function of age.

*Depressive patients and the sleep laboratory*

activity, particularly in the first REM period. When we compared the 7 patients with somatic delusions to the 13 with only delusions of guilt, three sleep measures (sleep efficiency, total REM activity, and REM activity in the first REM period) discriminated correctly 75% of the patients ($p < 0.007$). In summary, these recent studies of depressed patients with delusions have established that other specific sleep variables, in addition to sleep discontinuity, may be related to various types of delusions.

## Relationship of Age to EEG Sleep Variables

We have found that age, as well as type and severity of psychopathology, correlates with specific EEG sleep variables in depression. The several major sleep characteristics that typify primary depression are inversely related to age, including short REM latency, low sleep efficiency, and reduced delta sleep *(18)*. REM latency changes considerably throughout the age continuum (Figure 11–3). For the most part, there is some support for the speculation that EEG sleep in the majority of primary depressives mirrors "premature" aging, although better data are needed on REM latency in older normals.

Table 11–7 shows the age-related decrease in REM-sleep latency that we have found in patients with major depressive disorders of the primary type, both delusional and nondelusional. In using REM-sleep latency as an objective correlate of depression, one must be careful to take into account the patient's age; thus, a REM-sleep latency of 50 minutes will have more implication for a diagnosis of depression in a 25-year-old than in a 70-year-old, when age-related variance is taken into account. Again, since similar changes in sleep continuity and sleep architecture indexes have been reported as a function of age in normals *(19)*, this underscores the importance of controlling for age in interpreting EEG sleep changes found in affective illness.

**Table 11–7** REM Latency Estimates
(Time in Minutes)

|  | Age Groups | | | | |
|---|---|---|---|---|---|
| Percentiles | 18–25 | 26–30 | 31–40 | 41–50 | 51–60 |
| 85% | 97 | 81 | 71 | 3 | 46 |
| 70% | 80 | 66 | 58 | 49 | 34 |
| 50% | 64 | 51 | 44 | 37 | 24 |
| 30% | 49 | 38 | 32 | 26 | 16 |
| 15% | 37 | 28 | 23 | 18 | 9 |
| Average age (in years) | 22 | 28 | 36 | 46 | 54 |

NOTE: Sample percentile estimates for REM latency generated within each age group. All patients (N = 87) meet major depression, primary type criterion with Hamilton Rating Scale score of 18 or higher.

## Relationship of EEG Sleep Findings in Depression to ASDC Nosology

We recently applied the ASDC nosology for the classification of sleep and arousal disorders (1) to a sample of 174 patients seen in our Sleep Evaluation Center (20). In our sample there were over twice as many disorders of initiating and maintaining sleep (DIMS) as there were disorders of excessive sleepiness (DOES). We found that 68% of diagnoses in DIMS were psychiatric, particularly affective disorders. Among the total of 61 patients with affective disorders, 46 (75%) had DIMS, whereas the remaining 15 (25%) had DOES. This finding is consistent with earlier clinical observations that about 80% of primary depressives are hyposomnic, whereas 20% are hypersomnic when ill (14,16). We also observed that only 58% of the entire sample of 174 patients could be adequately classified with one diagnosis and that substance abuse was the most common of the secondary DIMS diagnoses (59.1%). In contrast, medical disorders (e.g., hypertension) were the most common secondary diagnoses among DOES (51.8%). We think that these findings attest to the complexity of sleep disorders generally and to the importance of a thorough medical and psychiatric workup, particularly in conjunction with the EEG sleep evaluation of depressed patients.

## Relationship of Depressive Psychopathology to Sleep Apnea and Nocturnal Myoclonus

Our laboratory has reported a case of delusional depression in a man with severe mixed sleep apnea syndrome who improved clinically and polysmnographically when treated with methylphenidate and thioridazine (21). Since sleep disturbance (either hyposomnia or hypersomnia) is frequent in affective disorders and since the presence of undiagnosed sleep apnea or nocturnal myoclonus can complicate treatment, we performed screening polysomnography on a series of 86 consecutive inpatients who met RDC criteria form major affective disorders (22). The most common diagnosis (N = 40) was primary, unipolar, and nondelusional depression, but the sample also included 22 secondary depressives, 8 bipolars, 10 delusionals, and 2 schizoaffectives. All patients were psychotropic drug-free for 10–12 days at the time of sleep studies. We found that 13 patients (15.1%) had sleep apneas and that 1 patient had nocturnal myoclonus (without sleep apnea). It deserves emphasis that the apnea tended to be extremely mild, with an average of 27.8 episodes per patient and with a mean duration per episode of 15.0 seconds. The apnea was obstructive or mixed and was accompanied by mild and insignificant cardiac arrhythmia in all cases. Only 4 of the 13 patients had apnea indexes greater than five, and even here the total apnea was considered mild. Much of the apnea occurred during REM sleep (68.3%). There was no association of apnea with gender, but apneic patients were significantly older than nonapneic patients ($p < 0.005$).

We have also examined the relationship of depressive psychopathology to the sleep apnea syndrome (23). In a group of 12 patients with sleep apnea syndromes, we found significant correlations between depression self-rating scores on the KDS 1 and

2 scales and severity of sleep apnea as measured by a number of apneic episodes ($r = 0.74$, $p < 0.01$) and percentage of sleep time spent without airflow ($r = 0.71$, $p < 0.01$). Patients with obstructive sleep apnea reported significantly more depressive symptomatology than patients with central sleep apnea ($p < 0.05$). The more depressed patients invariably had obstructive sleep apnea. We found a marked similarity of the EEG sleep characteristics of depressed apneics to those of other patients with medical-depressive syndromes, particularly in reduced REM-sleep density. We believe that this finding supports the concept that depression in sleep apnea syndromes may be medical-depressive in nature, rather than primary-depressive.

# Issues for Further Research

## State, Trait, or Both

Whether EEG sleep changes associated with affective disorders reflect the patient's actual state, a vulnerability to affective states, or a combination of both, deserves further investigation. The relative lack of *longitudinal* EEG sleep data (before, during, and after affective episodes), as distinguished from *cross-sectional* studies, makes the issue difficult to resolve at present. Another approach to the problem would be to perform EEG sleep studies in the first-degree family members of patients with affective disorders to test the hypothesis that 10%–20% of such relatives might show a reduced REM latency, implying that the latter is a biological marker of the vulnerability to develop clinically apparent affective disorders. Our observations that REM latency correlates inversely with the severity of depression and that increased sleep continuity is found in delusional depressives provide support for the argument that EEG sleep variables are also a sensitive indicator of the patient's actual state. We are currently involved in longitudinal EEG sleep studies of depressed patients during and between attacks.

## Sensitivity versus Specificity

To establish more conclusively that EEG sleep changes seen in depression are specific to affective disorders, it would be desirable to have EEG sleep data on other homogeneous groups of well-diagnosed psychiatric patients, such as schizophrenics or patients with anxiety disorders. In an early report on six acute schizophrenic patients (medication-free), Kupfer et al. observed significantly elevated REM latencies in association with severe sleep-continuity disturbances *(24)*. Later studies of schizoaffective patients by Reich et al. *(25)* showed short REM latencies in comparison with acute schizophrenics, particularly in patients who eventually needed antidepressant medication. In a recent review of the literature on sleep in schizophrenia, Mendelson et al. concluded that no specific abnormalities of sleep have emerged from cross-sectional studies of schizophrenic patients *(26)*. There are also very few data on EEG sleep changes in anxiety disorders. We are currently investigating a group of patients who meet Research Diagnostic Criteria for generalized anxiety disorder. On preliminary analysis, it appears that these patients do not show shortening of REM latency in contrast to patients with primary depressive disorders.

Although a statistically inverse relationship exists between clinical severity and short REM latency, the application of a cutoff of 50 minutes for REM latency has demonstrated that 70%–75% of patients diagnosed with primary depression are accurately identified *(27)*. When we examined the diagnostic performance of short REM latency (under 50 minutes) in a manner similar to that used for describing sensitivity and specificity for neuroendocrine determinations of the dexamethasone suppression test *(28)*, the reanalysis of 43 patients from a 1976 study demonstrated an 83% sensitivity and a 74% specificity.

## Treatment Response Prediction

There is now some evidence that early drug-induced changes in the sleep EEGs of depressed patients can predict which patients will respond satisfactorily to antidepressant medication *(29)*. For example, patients who show a good response to amitriptyline also have significantly greater prolongation of REM-sleep latency than do poor responders in response to challenge doses of the medication. Similarly, good responders show a significantly greater suppression of REM sleep and REM-sleep activity than do poor responders. We have used four sleep variables from the first drug nights (REM latency, sleep-onset difficulty, sleep efficiency, and stage 2–REM percentage) to generate a multiple regression equation highly correlated with the final clinical response as measured by the Hamilton score ($r = 0.75$). Thus, patients whose immediate response to amitriptyline included lengthening of REM latency, reduction of sleep-onset difficulty and stage 2–REM sleep, and increased sleep efficiency showed the best clinical response four weeks later. We are currently investigating the relationship of these drug-induced changes to plasma antidepressant levels, particularly plasma levels of amitriptyline and nortriptyline.

## Differential Diagnosis of Depression and Dementia in Old Age

Our studies of elderly depressives to date have indicated that these patients also show shortened REM latency, reduced sleep time, and high REM density *(17,30)*. This has prompted us to hypothesize that EEG sleep findings may help in the difficult differential diagnosis of depression, dementia, and depressive pseudo-dementia in old age. Feinberg et al *(31)* and Prinz *(32)* have observed diminished amounts of REM sleep and REM-sleep activity in relation to chronic organic brain syndromes, including Alzheimer disease. Their observations, together with our own findings of diminished phasic REM activity and density in medical-depressive syndromes *(4)*, raise the possibility that elderly patients with Alzheimer disease can be distinguished from depressives on the basis of both REM-latency and REM-activity findings in conjunction with a thorough neuropsychiatric workup.

# Summary

There is growing evidence that EEG sleep studies provide useful and predictable psychobiologic correlates for the diagnosis of primary and secondary affective states (including medical-depressive syndromes), of delusional and nondelusional primary depression, and of bipolar and unipolar primary depression. These findings also support the ASDC classification of depression both as a disorder of initiating and maintaining sleep (DIMS) and as a disorder of excessive sleepiness (DOES). EEG sleep changes in affective states must be viewed in relation to other variables known to affect sleep, such as age, medication, and type and severity of psychopathology (e.g., presence and type of delusions).

In screening patients with major affective disorders, we have not found a clinically significant incidence of sleep apnea or nocturnal myoclonus. Accordingly, we do not recommend routine screening of depressed patients for these disorders unless there is specific clinical symptomatology indicating polysomnography, such as longstanding or severe excessive daytime sleepiness or refractory insomnia. There is evidence that depression associated with sleep apnea syndromes is related to the severity of the syndromes and is a medical-depressive syndrome rather than a form of primary depression.

Further research into the following issues is needed: *(a)* Are EEG sleep changes in affective illness state- or trait-related, or both? *(b)* Are the EEG sleep changes seen in depression specific to this disorder, as distinguished from other well-defined psychiatric disorders such as schizophrenia, generalized anxiety disorder, or Alzheimer disease? *(c)* Can EEG sleep changes in depression predict satisfactory response to antidepressant drug therapy? We believe that current data indicate that EEG sleep changes in depression are related to both state and trait, but that family and longitudinal studies are necessary to answer the question conclusively; that EEG sleep changes in depression will be shown to be specific to affective states, as well as sensitive to the severity of affective symptoms; and that EEG sleep studies will prove useful in predicting satisfactory response to antidepressant medication.

# REFERENCES

1. Association of Sleep Disorders Centers. Diagnostic classification of sleep and arousal disorders. 1st ed. Prepared by the Sleep Disorders Classification Committee, HP Roffwarg, chairman. Sleep 1979; 2:1–137.
2. Kupfer DJ, Foster FG. EEG sleep and depression. In: Williams RL, Karacan I, eds. Sleep disorders: diagnosis and treatment. New York: John Wiley and Sons, 1978:163–204.
3. Spitzer RL, Endicott J, Robins E. Research diagnostic criteria: rationale and reliability. Arch Gen Psychiatry 1978; 35:773–82.
4. Foster FG, Kupfer DJ, Coble P, et al. Rapid eye movement sleep density: an objective indicator in medical-depressive syndromes. Arch Gen Psychiatry 1976; 33:1120–3.
5. Hamilton M. A rating scale for depression. J Neurol Neurosurg Psychiatry 1960; 23:56–62.
6. Wogan M, Amdur M, Kupfer DJ, et al. The KDS-1: validity, reliability, and independence among symptom clusters for clinic and normal samples. Psychol Rep 1973; 32:503–6.
7. Rechtschaffen A, Kales A, eds. A manual of standardized terminology, techniques and scoring system for sleep stages of human subjects. Los Angeles: Brain Information Service/Brain Research Institute, 1968. (Also available as NIH Publ 204, US Government printing office, Washington, DC, 1968.)
8. Coble PA, McPartland RJ, Silva WJ, et al. Is there a first-night effect? (A revisit). Biol Psychiatry 1974; 9:215–9.
9. Coble PA, Foster FG, Kupfer DJ. Electroencephalographic sleep diagnosis of primary depression. Arch Gen Psychiatry 1976; 33:1124–7.
10. Gillin JC, Duncan W, Pettigrew KD, et al. Successful separation of depressed, normal, and insomniac subjects by EEG sleep data. Arch Gen Psychiatry 1979; 36:85–90.
11. Kupfer DJ. Sleep disorder in depression. In: Friedman E, Mann J, Gershon S, eds. Depression and antidepressants. New York: Raven Press, in press.
12. Reynolds CF, Newton TF, Shaw DH, et al. Electroencephalographic sleep findings in outpatients with primary non-delusional depression. (In preparation.)
13. Williams RL, Karacan I, Hursch CJ. Electroencephalography (EEG) of human sleep. New York: John Wiley and Sons, 1974.
14. Kupfer DJ, Himmelhoch JM, Swartzberg M, et al. Hypersomnia in manic-depressive disease. Dis Nerv Syst 1972; 33:720–4.
15. McPartland RJ, Kupfer DJ, Coble PA, et al. REM sleep in primary depression: a computerized analysis. Electroencephalogr Clin Neurophysiol 1978; 44:513–7.

16. Kupfer DJ, Foster FG, Detre TP. Sleep continuity disturbance in depression. Dis Nerv Syst 1973; 34:192–5.
17. Kupfer DJ, Spiker DG, Coble PA, et al. Electroencephalographic sleep recordings and depression in the elderly. J Am Geriatr Soc 1978; 26:53–7.
18. Ulrich RF, Shaw DH, Kupfer DJ. Effects of aging on EEG sleep in depression. Sleep 1980; 3:31–40.
19. Feinberg I. Functional implications of changes in sleep physiology with age. In: Terry RD, Gershon S, eds. Neurobiology of aging. New York: Raven Press, 1976:23–41.
20. Reynolds CF, Shubin RS, Coble PA, et al. Diagnostic classification of sleep disorders: implications for psychiatric practice. J Clin Psychiatry, in press.
21. Neil JF, Spiker DG, Reynolds CF, et al. The myth of one illness: a patient with psychotic depression and mixed sleep apnea responsive to methylphenidate and thioridazine. Sleep Res 1978; 7:244.
22. Reynolds CF, Coble PA, Spiker DG, et al. Polysomnographic screening for sleep apnea and nocturnal myoclonus in affective disorders. (Submitted.)
23. Reynolds CF, Coble PA, Black RS, et al. Sleep architecture correlates of depression in sleep apnea. (Submitted.)
24. Kupfer DJ, Wyatt RJ, Scott J, et al. Sleep disturbance in acute schizophrenic patients. Am J Psychiatry 1970; 126:1213–23.
25. Reich L, Weiss BL, Coble P, et al. Sleep disturbance in schizophrenia. Arch Gen Psychiatry 1975; 32:51–5.
26. Mendelson WB, Gillin JC, Wyatt RJ, eds. Human sleep and its disorders. New York: Plenum Press, 1977.
27. Kupfer DJ, Coble PA, Spiker DG, et al. REM sleep and depression. Presented at the American Psychiatric Association Meeting, San Francisco, California, 1980.
28. Carroll BJ, Feinberg M, Steiner M, et al. Diagnostic application of the dexamethasone suppression test in depressed outpatients. In: Mendelwics J, ed. Advances in biological psychiatry. Amsterdam: Elsevier, 1980.
29. Kupfer DJ, Spiker DG, Coble PA, et al. Depression, EEG sleep, and clinical response. Compr Psychiatry 1980; 21:212–20.
30. Reynolds CF, Coble P, Black RS, et al. Sleep disturbances in a series of elderly patients: polysomnographic findings. J Am Geriatr Soc 1980; 28:164–70.
31. Feinberg I, Koresco RL, Heller N. EEG sleep patterns as a function of normal and pathological aging in man. J Psychiatr Res 1967; 5:107–44.
32. Prinz PN. Sleep patterns in the healthy aged: relationship with intellectual functions. J Gerontol 1977; 32:179–86.

# TWELVE
# PERIODIC MOVEMENTS IN SLEEP (NOCTURNAL MYOCLONUS) AND RESTLESS LEGS SYNDROME

RICHARD M. COLEMAN

## Introduction

Periodic movements in sleep (PMS) are stereotyped, repetitive movements of the lower extremities that occur during sleep (Figure 12–1). These movements are triggered by sleep, and although sometimes associated with awakenings, they are not accompanied by abnormal EEG activity. The term PMS was adopted because the previously used term, nocturnal myoclonus, has been used to refer to a variety of phenomena and is a source of confusion. However, nocturnal myoclonus will be used in this chapter whenever a previous author's usage of this term was equivalent to PMS.

## Historical Background

In 1953, Sir Charles Symonds introduced the term nocturnal myoclonus to refer to involuntary clonic movements of the lower extremities during sleep *(1)*. Because he did not perform nocturnal polygraphic monitoring and did not distinguish PMS from sleep starts and epilepsy, Symonds erroneously concluded that these movements were an epileptic variant. A careful review of Symonds's five cases suggests that he studied an assortment of distinct phenomena including restless legs syndrome, sleep starts, seizure disorders, and possibly periodic movements in sleep *(2)*.

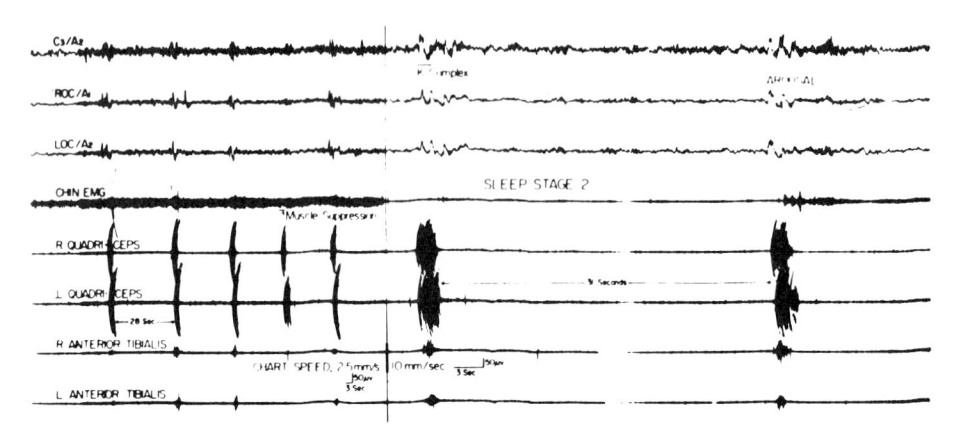

*Sleeping and waking disorders: indications and techniques*

**Figure 12–1.** Criteria for scoring PMS. The left side of the figure shows five consecutive stereotypic movements with an inter-event interval of 28 seconds. This demonstrates the minimum requirement for scoring PMS used by Coleman et al. *(50)*. The right side of the figure shows a K complex and, later, a brief arousal in association with the leg movements.

However, other studies provide a basis for distinguishing these different movement disorders. As early as 1685, Willis described restless legs syndrome: "Wherefore to some, on being a bed, they betake themselves to sleep, presently in the arms and legs, leapings and contractions of the tendons, and so great a restlessness and tossings of their members ensue that the diseased are no more able to sleep than if they were in the place of the greatest torture" *(3)*. All-night polygraphic sleep recordings of patients with restless legs syndrome were first performed in 1965 by Lugaresi and his collaborators. In addition to motor restlessness prior to sleep onset, they reported that many of these patients had periodic leg movements during sleep *(4,5)*. These leg movements were initially described as "involuntary clonic contractions" and were easily detected during sleep with electromyographic (EMG) recordings of the anterior tibialis muscles. In 1966, Lugaresi et al. also polygraphically recorded the first cases of periodic leg movements during nocturnal sleep in the absence of restless legs syndrome *(6)*. They reported that the movements in these patients occurred after sleep onset, primarily in NREM stages 1–2, and were frequently accompanied by K complexes or sleep spindles. The leg movements typically repeated at regular intervals of 25–30 seconds.

In 1959, Oswald clearly identified and differentiated "hypnic myoclonus" (sleep starts) from PMS in polygraphic recordings and concluded that they were a normal phenomenon and unlikely to be epileptic *(7)*. These brief extremity movements generally occurred during the transition from wakefulness to sleep, were not periodic, and only rarely caused subjective sleep complaints. This result was confirmed by Gastaut and Broughton in 1965 *(8)*. They further described "hypnic myoclonus" (sleep starts) associated with sleep onset in normal volunteers. "Hypnagogic partial myoclonic jerks" were defined as brief (20–100 msec), spontaneous, aperiodic EMG activity without displacement of extremities. "Hypnagogic massive myoclonic jerks" were evidenced by spontaneous, aperiodic EMG activity of ≥ 1 second in duration involving displacement of the extremities. Both types of movements occurred most frequently in stage 1 sleep and could be clearly distinguished from myoclonic epilepsy, psychomotor seizures, and restless legs.

In most neurologic conditions associated with myoclonus (i.e., brief, vigorous, jerking movements) *(9)*, the movements disappear during sleep or, if they persist, are present in both sleep and wakefulness. Myoclonic epilepsy, which has been confused with PMS, rarely persists during sleep. Lugaresi and his collaborators, however, studied the nocturnal sleep of patients with myoclonic epilepsy whose movements persisted during sleep *(10)*. They reported that the muscle contractions in the extremities occurred sporadically, were more clonic than periodic leg movements, and were accompanied by cortical spike activity. In early studies, Lundborg in 1904 *(11)* and Clark in 1912 *(12)* used the term "nocturnal myoclonus with epilepsy" to describe myoclonic epilepsy patients whose strong movements during nocturnal sleep resulted in awakenings.

# Differentiation of Terminology

It is evident from this historical review that a variety of distinct phenomena have been subsumed under the term nocturnal myoclonus. Furthermore, it is clear from clinical experience that centers treating sleep-wake disorder patients encounter two distinct syndromes: periodic movements in sleep (PMS) and restless legs syndrome (RLS). For these reasons, plus the finding that the durations of periodic leg movements in sleep are not truly myoclonic, the preferred term is PMS. It is ironic that Symonds subsequently realized that his use of the term nocturnal myoclonus was inaccurate "since the occurrence (of movements) is related to sleep whether nocturnal or diurnal" *(13)*. In addition, he recognized that these sleep-related movements were distinct from myoclonus epilepsy.

## Restless Legs Syndrome (RLS)

Restless legs syndrome (RLS) may occur alone or with PMS. This syndrome is characterized by the occurrence of "unpleasant creeping sensations," primarily in the legs, that appear only at rest and produce an "irresistible need to keep the limbs in motion" *(14)*. These sensations usually are not painful but are sufficiently uncomfortable to produce severe chronic insomnia in many patients. Affected individuals must rub and kick their legs or walk about to relieve symptoms, often delaying sleep onset for several hours. There has been some confusion in differentiating PMS from restless legs syndrome. For example, Symonds's case #4 ("nocturnal myoclonus") appears to be a typical case of RLS *(1,2)*. Restless legs can be characterized as being primarily a problem of wakefulness; whereas, as we have seen, PMS is primarily a phenomenon related to sleep *(15)*. Although the two syndromes frequently occur together, patients with RLS may not have periodic leg movements upon falling asleep.

*Review of the Literature*   There is much more extensive literature on restless legs syndrome than on PMS, probably because it occurs during wakefulness. Good historical reviews of the literature can be found in works by Ekbom *(14)*, Coccagna et al. *(16)*, and Coleman *(17)*. Although both Ekbom *(18)* and Willis *(3)* referred to myoclonic jerks in their descriptions of the restless legs syndrome, only Allison *(19)*, Tuvo *(20)*, and Bornstein *(21)* distinguished involuntary muscle jerks (most likely PMS) and the voluntary movements used by patients to eliminate unpleasant sensations. Ekbom *(18)* was the first to organize and describe the clinical findings in a comprehensive manner. He reported that the symptoms are exclusively subjective and, in addition to a peculiar paresthesia, may include sensations of pain, cold, and weakness in the legs. Ekbom suggested that the prevalence of RLS may be 5% in the general population. Murray reported this figure is accurate only when patients are questioned intensively, and even then most report only a mild complaint *(22)*.

Lugaresi and his collaborators were the first investigators to carry out nocturnal polygraphic recordings in patients with RLS and to emphasize that it was a fairly common cause of insomnia *(5,23,24,25)*. They confirmed the findings of Murphy *(26)* and Bornstein *(21)* that in severe cases, depression and suicidal ideation may be present. Typical paresthesias and motor restlessness were present in all cases, and the following trends were noted: *(a)* Restless leg movements were most frequent in the first part of the night and during wakefulness. *(b)* Sleep was interrupted by numerous awakenings. *(c)* Total sleep time was markedly reduced, including some nights of complete wakefulness. *(d)* Not surprisingly, the number of sleep cycles and percentages of sleep stages 3–4 and REM were reduced in comparison with normal subjects. *(e)* PMS occurred primarily with the transition into sleep and continued during sleep. The movements diminished slightly during stage 2 sleep, disappeared in stages 3–4 sleep, and rarely reappeared during REM sleep.

*Etiologic Hypotheses*   The etiology of restless legs syndrome remains undetermined, although many hypotheses have been advanced *(17)*. Cases studied by Roth et al. *(27)* and Frankel et al. *(28)*, utilizing nocturnal polysomnography and clinical electromyography, suggest that a distal neuropathy or lower motor neuron disease could be responsible for RLS. However, Harriman et al. *(29)* performed muscle biopsies on the peroneus brevis muscle of ten patients with RLS and ten age-matched controls, and found no evidence of organic pathology.

*Relationship to Other Disorders*   A high prevalence of RLS has been found in patients with various diseases. Norlander described three RLS patients whose symptoms developed with the onset of anemia and disappeared with iron treatment *(30)*. Behrman also noted an association of anemia with restless legs *(31)*, as did Ekbom who found that 25% of a randomly selected group of severe RLS cases had iron deficiency anemia *(32)*. Iron deficiency anemia is a common sequel to partial gastrectomy, and Ekbom found that 12.6% of 317 patients followed up after partial gastrectomy had restless legs syndrome *(32)*. Upmark and Meurling found restless legs syndrome in 8 of 24 partially gastrectomized patients *(33)*. Aspenstrom *(34)* reported that 42% of 80 patients with sideropenia had restless legs syndrome, and Norlander *(30)* studied six female patients, including three familial cases, who had RLS associated with folate deficiency; folic acid therapy relieved the symptoms better than placebos in many of their patients. Several other studies have noted a familial pattern in RLS *(24,35)*. Restless legs syndrome has also been described as occurring in the following conditions: avitaminosis in prisoners of war *(36)*, primary amyloidosis with peripheral neuropathy *(37)*, carcinoma *(38)*, uremia *(39,40,41)*, diabetic neuropathy *(42)*, normal pregnancy *(18)*, and acute poliomyelitis *(43)*.

*Treatment of RLS*    Despite many descriptive studies of RLS, there is still no well-defined or reliable treatment. Few controlled, double-blind studies have been performed. Coleman *(17)* summarized treatments recommended over a 32-year period and found that a wide variety of drugs have been used with varying degrees of success; no treatment was judged clearly effective. Currently, clinical success has been claimed with carbamazepine *(15)*, 5-hydroxytryptophan *(44)*, folic acid *(36)*, vitamin E *(45)*, and caffeine withdrawal *(46)*.

In summary, RLS is frequently associated with PMS. It is one of two subjective complaints that may be predictive of the presence of PMS. (The other is a bed-partner's complaint of being kicked excessively or periodically during the night.) Because the subjective complaint of restless legs typically occurs just prior to sleep onset, patients are aware of their motor restlessness. However, they are usually unaware of periodic leg movements once they fall asleep. Thus RLS serves as an indication of the probable presence of PMS.

## Periodic Movements in Sleep (PMS or "Nocturnal Myoclonus")

Both Symonds *(1)* and Lugaresi *(23)* noted the association between subjective complaints of insomnia and restless legs. Dement and Guilleminault *(47)* emphasized that nocturnal myoclonus without restless legs could be an important cause of insomnia. This group also noted that periodic leg movements were often associated with changes to lighter sleep states or full arousal *(48)*. In the first large case-series study, Guilleminault et al. *(49)* reported that 16 of 140 patients complaining of chronic insomnia had nocturnal myoclonus. Only 2 of the 16 had restless legs syndrome. Using polygraphic and cinematographic techniques, they reported that movements consisted of "a rapid partial flexion of the foot at the ankle, extension of the big toe, and partial flexion of the knee and hip." They also noted that movements were easily distinguishable from other sleep-related movements by their periodic occurrence (every 20–40 seconds) and stereotyped pattern.

In a case series of 441 consecutive patients, Coleman et al. found that periodic leg movements occurred in a wide variety of sleep disorders besides insomnia *(50)*. The prevalence of PMS (defined as $\geq$ 40 movements per night) was not statistically different among the following diagnostic groups: insomnia, narcolepsy, sleep apnea, and other miscellaneous diagnoses. This finding held true for severe cases—patients averaging greater than 50 movements per hour of NREM sleep. This study raised the possibility that, in a certain number of cases, PMS may result from a chronic sleep-wake disturbance rather than be a cause of it. Another important finding was that the prevalence of PMS showed a statistically significant increase with age (Figure 12–2).

Bixler et al. reported that 7.7% of 78 normal subjects and 9.4% of 106 insomniacs "showed signs of myoclonus activity" without specifying a definition of the movements they studied *(51)*. They suggested that asymptomatic PMS may be fairly common and that PMS cannot be routinely considered to cause sleep-wake disorders. Other studies have reported cases of PMS in the absence of a sleep-wake complaint *(7,50)*. Carskadon et al. have found a high percentage of PMS in elderly subjects without sleep complaints but with objective daytime sleepiness *(52)*, which indicates that the concept of having a sleep-wake complaint is very subjective. Tauber et al. *(53)* found no cases of PMS in 14 normal volunteers and 4 patients with various neurologic diseases.

*Relationship to Other Disorders*   In addition to the association with restless legs syndrome and insomnia, PMS has been polygraphically studied during nocturnal sleep

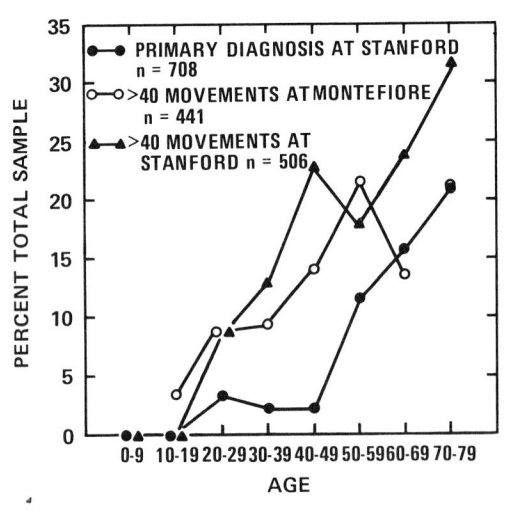

**Figure 12–2.** Age-related prevalence of PMS. The age-related prevalence of PMS in patients seen at two large sleep centers is shown. The criterion used for defining PMS was $\geq$ 40 leg movements per night, which is roughly equivalent to a Movement Index of 5. Additionally, clinical diagnoses of PMS-insomnia and PMS-hypersomnia syndrome combined are shown for the Stanford Sleep Disorders Center. The diagnostic criterion for PMS syndrome was the broad ASDC nosology definition.*

in patients with the following conditions: uremia and hemodialysis *(54,55)*, chlorimipramine hydrochloride treatment of narcoleptics *(56)*, stiff-man syndrome *(57)*, narcolepsy *(50,58)*, sleep apnea *(50,59)*, nocturnal epilepsy *(50,57)*, delayed sleep phase syndrome *(50)*, hypersomnia *(50,60)*, and drug withdrawal *(61)*. Therefore, it is clear that PMS occurs in a wide variety of sleep-wake disorders *(2)*.

*Diagnosing PMS with Polysomnography*   One of the major problems in evaluating the clinical findings is clearly defining when a PMS syndrome should be considered pathologic and when it should be considered a parasomnia, i.e., an associated finding during polysomnography that does not cause either insomnia or daytime sleepiness. Similarly, in assessing the results of PMS studies, it is important to distinguish between scored movement (myoclonus) events and the clinical diagnosis of PMS or nocturnal myoclonus. According to the Association of Sleep Disorders Centers's (ASDC) nosology,* a clinical diagnosis of nocturnal myoclonus is reserved for patients whose movements are "consistently followed by a partial arousal or awakening" *(61)*; more exact criteria have not been specified to date. In these patients, nocturnal myoclonus is considered to be the cause of the patient's sleep-wake complaint. However, no studies have explicitly demonstrated that PMS actually causes insomnia or excessive sleepiness, i.e., by experimentally producing or inhibiting PMS and quantifying changes in subjective complaints.

Diagnosing PMS can be quite complex. Table 12–1 lists some combinations of patient complaints and polygraphic results that are commonly seen in sleep disorders centers. In addition, the suggested ASDC nosology diagnosis is given.

*Clinical Criteria*   Table 12–1 shows that it is possible to have PMS with or without a sleep complaint and that PMS may or may not be associated with arousals. Once the clinician has confirmed the presence of PMS by a polysomnogram, a diagnostic decision is made. A diagnosis of PMS-insomnia syndrome or PMS-hypersomnia syndrome appears justified only when the movements are associated with arousals.

*Scoring Criteria*   Compounding the difficulty of making the clinical diagnosis of PMS is the lack of established standards for scoring the movements themselves. Even in those studies where PMS has been clearly differentiated from other conditions, scoring rules often have not been specified. Ideally, to accurately define PMS, a three-dimensional histogram of the duration, amplitude, and interval between consecutive movements should be plotted for all leg-EMG activity in a group of controls and well-known cases. This analysis would enable investigators to define PMS empirically and distinguish it from other movements during sleep.

Two previous studies have begun preliminary work in defining PMS. Coleman et al. *(17,50)* defined movement events as stereotyped episodes of EMG activity lasting

---

*Association of Sleep Disorders Centers. Diagnostic classification of sleep and arousal disorders. 1st edition. Prepared by the Sleep Disorders Classification Committee, HP Roffwarg, chairman. Sleep 1979; 2:1–137. This source currently uses the term "Sleep-related (Nocturnal) Myoclonus" to describe PMS.

*Sleeping and waking disorders: indications and techniques*

**Table 12–1**  Diagnosing PMS (Nocturnal Myoclonus)

| Patient Complaint | Results of Polysomnogram (PSG) | ASDC Diagnosis | |
|---|---|---|---|
| Insomnia | PMS with arousal | PMS-insomnia syndrome | (A.5.a) |
| Insomnia | PMS without arousal | PMS-parasomnia syndrome | (D.4.n.) |
| Excessive sleepiness | PMS with arousal | PMS-hypersomnia syndrome | (B.5.a) |
| Excessive sleepiness | PMS without arousal | PMS-parasomnia syndrome | (D.4.n.) |
| No patient complaint | PMS without arousal | PMS-parasomnia syndrome | (D.4.n.) |

0.5–4.0 seconds when they occurred as part of a rhythmic train of five or more events with an inter-event interval of 20–40 seconds (4–60 seconds in rare instances). Movements occurring synchronously (within 4 seconds) in the right and left legs were counted as one movement event. Using these definitions, a detailed analysis of ten PMS patients (15 PSGs in all) found the grand mean for over 6500 inter-event intervals was 26 seconds. The period length in individual patients ranged from 20 ± 8 seconds to 43 ± 20 seconds. Clusters of successive movements (myoclonic epochs) typically lasted anywhere from 10 to 75 minutes, and these epochs sometimes recurred every 90 minutes.

Guilleminault et al. *(49)* defined somewhat different criteria: three or more separate EMG discharges with a duration of 5–10 seconds and an inter-event interval < 120 seconds (usually 20–40 seconds). Recently, this definition has been revised so that the duration of movements is 0.5–5.0 seconds and the inter-event interval must be 5–120 seconds. Similar to the criteria described by Coleman et al. *(17,50)*, movements are only counted if they are part of a series of three or more consecutive movements. Isolated, individual leg movements are not counted.

At the Stanford Sleep Disorders Center, all patients with a diagnosis of nocturnal myoclonus syndromes from 1978–1979 have been compared to all patients with PMS (at least three movements, according to the revised criteria of Guilleminault) but without a clinical diagnosis of nocturnal myoclonus syndrome. Each underwent an all-night polysomnogram with leg-EMG recordings. Diagnoses were made by each patient's sleep clinic physician, who was blind to the reported analysis. A diagnosis of nocturnal myoclonus syndrome was made when the physician judged that movements were consistently associated with arousals (i.e., using the broad ASDC nosology criteria). Table 12–2 is a comparison of leg movements in these two patient groups.

**Table 12-2** Comparison of Patients with PMS Syndromes versus PMS Events

|  | PMS Syndromes (62 Patients) | | PMS Events without Diagnosis (163 Patients) | | |
| --- | --- | --- | --- | --- | --- |
| Parameter | Mean | SD | Mean | SD | Level of Significance |
| # PMS | 185.3 | 155.4 | 31.7 | 44.0 | .001 |
| # PMS with arousal | 86.0 | 112.9 | 15.5 | 23.8 | .001 |
| # PMS with awakening | 4.6 | 6.0 | 1.3 | 3.0 | .05 |
| Movement index | 32.0 | 18.3 | 3.1 | 5.8 | .001 |
| PMS arousal index | 14.5 | 5.3 | 2.3 | 3.1 | .001 |

NOTE: Movement index is the average number of PMS per hour of sleep. PMS arousal index is the average number of periodic leg movements associated with arousals (i.e., alpha events, K complexes, and < 15-second awakenings) per hour of sleep. Wilcoxon test used for mean differences.

Table 12–2 demonstrates that despite great interpatient variability, there are significant differences between patients judged to have nocturnal myoclonus syndrome and those with PMS but without a clinical diagnosis. Analysis of the distribution of PMS and the indexes suggests that guidelines for making the diagnosis of nocturnal myoclonus can be established.

Although there is no consensus, the following definitions are an integration of previous research, the ASDC nosology, and research in progress at Stanford:

1. An all-night polysomnogram (PSG) is needed, including EMG recordings from both legs.
2. A movement is scored when it occurs as part of a series of four consecutive movements that are separated by at least 4 but not more than 90 seconds. In most instances, however, the movements should be separated by 20–40 seconds.
3. The duration of the movements should be between 0.5 and 5.0 seconds.
4. The amplitude of the movements should be at least one-half the pen deflection of the leg-EMG activity recorded in the presleep testing period.
5. A patient is considered to have PMS or nocturnal myoclonus when the myoclonus index (number of periodic leg movements per hour of sleep) is ≥ 5. This number of movements is considered sufficient for diagnosing nocturnal myoclonus as a parasomnia.
6. A diagnosis of nocturnal myoclonus syndrome (A.5.a or B.5.a) should be reserved for patients who average at least five arousals with PMS per hour of sleep.

*Sleeping and waking disorders: indications and techniques*

These conservative definitions should be sufficient to describe and differentiate the majority of patients with PMS. However, there will continue to be borderline cases. For example, cases of PMS where only one or two movements result in sustained awakenings may exist. Such cases should be identified and classified as variants of PMS.

*Prevalence of Diagnoses of PMS ("Nocturnal Myoclonus")*  Table 12–3 shows the prevalence of primary diagnoses of nocturnal myoclonus and restless legs syndrome associated with insomnia and disorders of excessive sleepiness (DOES) in certified sleep disorders centers (in most instances covering the two-year period from January 1978 to December 1979). These results are based upon polygraphic recordings and follow the diagnostic definitions of the ASDC nosology *(61)*.

These cases represent 148 of 1231 insomniac primary diagnoses (12.2%) and 70 of 1983 DOES primary diagnoses (3%). Nocturnal myoclonus ranked fourth in frequency for insomnia diagnoses and seventh for DOES disorders. The wide range in prevalence among centers (3%–26%) may reflect the lack of exact criteria for differentiating other types of leg movements from the diagnosis of "nocturnal myoclonus." Additionally, sleep disorders centers differ in the patient population they treat. For example, although 18% of insomnia patients at Montefiore had a significant number of periodic leg movements (≥ 40), only 4% had a diagnosis of nocturnal myoclonus.

**Table 12–3**  Prevalence of Diagnoses of PMS (Nocturnal Myoclonus)

| Hospital (City) | % of Insomnia Cases with Diagnoses of PMS | % of DOES Cases with Diagnoses of PMS |
|---|---|---|
| Baylor (Houston) | 12.9% | 2.0% |
| Baptist Memorial (Memphis) | 6.5 | 2.5 |
| Western Psychiatric (Pittsburgh) | 2.9 | 1.5 |
| Presbyterian (Oklahoma City) | 8.9 | 0.0 |
| Ohio State University (Columbus) | 11.7 | 1.2 |
| Montefiore (New York) | 4.0 | 0.9 |
| Henry Ford (Detroit) | 20.0 | 6.6 |
| Mt. Sinai (Miami) | 25.0 | 0.0 |
| Stanford University (Palo Alto) | 9.9 | 2.5 |
| Univ. California (Irvine) | 26.3 | 13.9 |
| Holy Cross (Mission Hills) | 14.7 | 11.9 |

NOTE: These data are from a cooperative case series in progress carried out by the Association of Sleep Disorders Centers.

However, it is evident from the overall findings that nocturnal myoclonus syndrome is a major clinical finding in a substantial number of patients presenting with complaints of insomnia at sleep disorders centers.

*Sleep Patterns in PMS*   Small but significant negative correlations have been reported between myoclonic indexes (number of movements per hour of sleep) and both total sleep time and number of REM minutes *(50)*. Patients with regularly recurring movements (i.e., small deviations in period length) had less sleep disturbance than those whose movements repeated irregularly. An analysis of variance between PMS patients (those with ≥ 40 movements) and controls matched for age, sex, and sleep-wake diagnosis found only one significant difference: Patients with PMS had a lower sleep-efficiency percentage (time asleep divided by time in bed) of 69% in comparison with 74%. Except for a decreased sleep efficiency, which may be a result of multiple brief arousals, the sleep of PMS patients showed disturbances similar to those of other sleep disorder patients.

*Personality Patterns Associated with PMS*   Two studies have investigated personality patterns of PMS patients using the Minnesota Multiphasic Personality Inventory (MMPI). Kales et al. *(62)* reported that only the psychasthenia scale was significantly different (greater) in 10 PMS insomniacs compared to 96 non-PMS insomniacs. Coleman *(17)* compared the MMPI scores of 46 PMS patients with those of 46 non-PMS patients who were matched for age, sex, and sleep-wake diagnosis (e.g., insomnia, sleep apnea, narcolepsy, miscellaneous). PMS patients scored higher than controls on the hypochondriasis and hysteria scales, and lower on the social introversion scale. There were no significant differences in the percentages of patients with scores in the pathologic range (61% PMS versus 70% for controls). Both studies concluded that PMS should not routinely be considered an independent physiologic cause of sleep complaints because personality patterns are generally similar to patients with psychogenic insomnia.

*Etiologic Hypotheses*   Although the etiology of PMS is unknown, several hypotheses have been advanced: epilepsy *(1)*, spinal cord pathology *(23)*, biologic abnormalities *(54,55)*, brainstem oscillator *(63,64)*, phasic activity dissociation–pontine geniculate spike activity *(56,48,65)*, hyperactivity of alpha motor neurons *(66)*, sleep-wake rhythm disturbance *(50)*, and disruption of inhibitory neurotransmitters *(31,49)*. Several studies in man during sleep and coma have noted the similarity of the periodicity in PMS to other central nervous system functions, including periodic sleep apnea *(67)*, periodic breathing in acute brain trauma *(68)*, heart rate *(63,67)*, spinal fluid pressure *(69)*, spasms in comatose patients *(64)*, and arterial blood pressure *(63,67)*. It has been suggested that a central nervous system pacemaker may be responsible for the remarkable periodicity of these phenomena. Two essential etiologic questions must be answered: *(a)* Why is PMS, unlike most movement disorders, initiated rather than inhibited by sleep? *(b)* What mechanism regulates the remarkable periodicity of the movements?

*Treatment of PMS*  Clinicians treating patients with PMS are hindered by the scarcity of controlled drug studies. Most reports have been based upon subjective follow-up without objective polygraphic data. In one of the few polygraphic studies, Guilleminault et al. obtained negative results with 5-HTP *(49)*. Lioresal (baclofen) did not decrease the number of leg movements but did produce an increase in total sleep time and a decrease in the duration of individual movements *(66)*.

Oshtory and Vijayan *(70)* reported that 1 mg of clonazepam (a benzodiazepine also used in treating myoclonic epilepsy) was effective in eliminating movements and improving sleep in two cases. Assessment of clonazepam treatment in 15 nocturnal myoclonus insomnia patients at the Stanford Sleep Disorders Center, based on subjective follow-up, indicated that the drug had a variable effect and was completely successful only in a few cases. Several patients reported that clonazepam lost its effectiveness after long-term usage. Coleman *(17)* reported that clonazepam was effective in reducing movements in only one of three cases studied polygraphically. Many patients will report improvements in their sleep-wake functioning, even though the movements are still seen in polygraphic recording. This result suggests that clonazepam may be having a placebo effect, or perhaps it reduces the arousing effect of PMS.

Treatment with conventional sleeping pills and muscle relaxants has also been ineffective, as judged by the number of symptomatic patients who have tried these drugs without success prior to consulting a sleep disorders center *(15,50)*. In fact, it has been suggested from clinical experience that cases of PMS may be induced or made worse by tricyclic antidepressants and withdrawal from hypnotic medications *(61)*. However, a careful drug history of 53 patients indicated that PMS did not result as a side effect of any particular class of medications *(17)*.

In summary, there is no definitive treatment for PMS at the present time. In some cases where PMS is not considered the primary sleep-wake pathology, treatment should focus on other aspects of sleep-wake functioning, such as circadian rhythms, depression, etc. In nocturnal myoclonus insomnia syndrome, clonazepam is currently the most widely prescribed treatment and appears to benefit some patients.

# Technical Preparation for Recording PMS in Sleep Clinics

## Placement of Electrodes

The most common electrode placement for recording PMS is on the anterior tibialis muscles. Recordings are also frequently made from the quadriceps femoris muscles. It is important to record activity from both legs because many patients show movements in one leg only, or switch from one leg to the other throughout the night. Without recording both legs, cases of PMS can be completely missed, and both the severity and number of movements can be greatly underestimated (Figure 12–3).

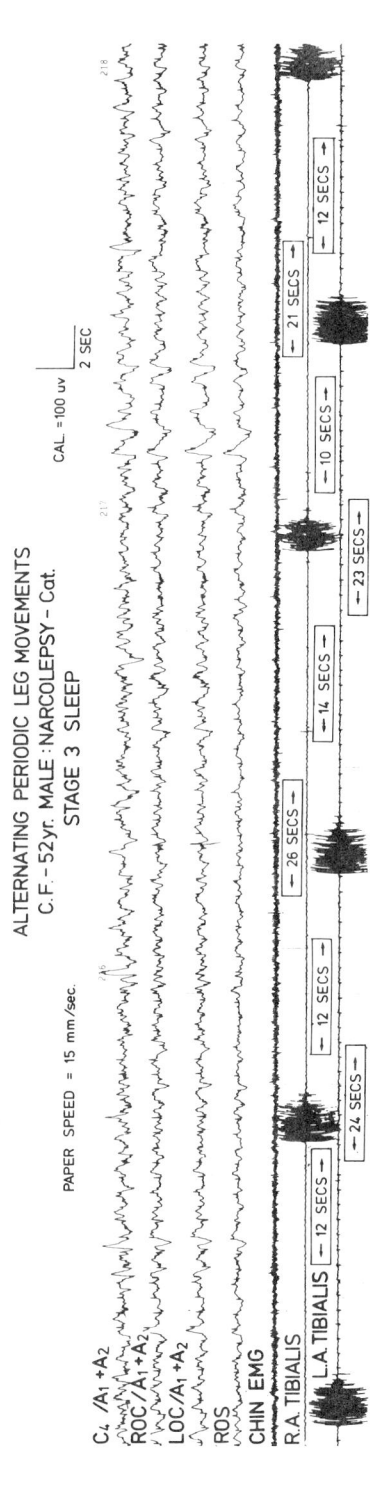

**Figure 12–3.** Alternating PMS. Movement-event intervals are calculated for each leg alone and by viewing the leg channels as one oscillating system. This figure demonstrates the complex relation between left-leg and right-leg movements. It also illustrates the importance of recording both legs.

The normal action of the anterior tibialis muscle is dorsiflexion of the ankle joint and assistance in inversion of the joint. To locate this muscle for electrode placement, the patient should be in a supine or sitting position while the examiner supports the leg above the ankle joint. While the examiner applies pressure against the medial side and dorsal surface of the joint, the patient dorsiflexes the ankle and inverts the foot (Figure 12–4). Two electrode sites are selected on the belly of the muscle from each leg. The electrodes are placed about 2 cm apart on the long axis of the muscle. Because the primary objective of the recording technique is to detect the presence or absence of movements, exact electrode placement is not crucial if movements are reliably reproduced on the polygraph.

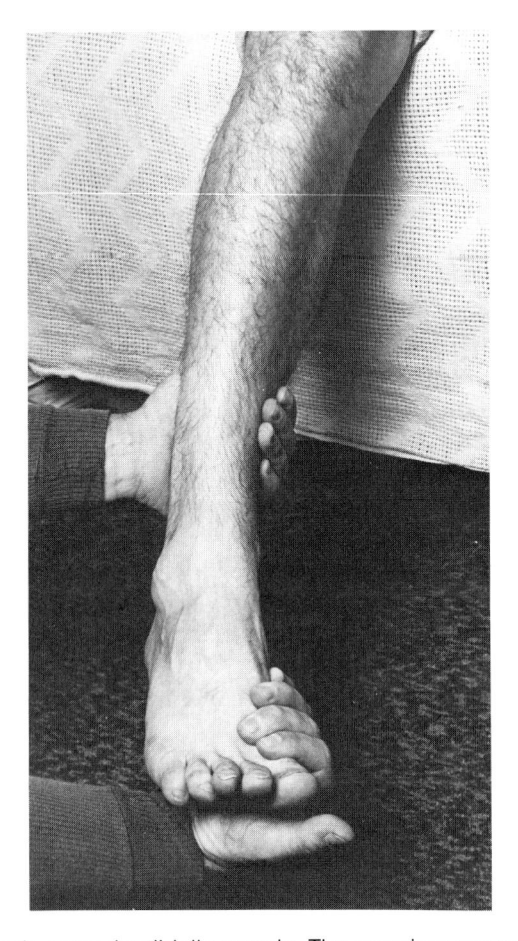

**Figure 12–4.** Testing anterior tibialis muscle. The examiner supports the patient's lower leg and applies pressure to the medial side and dorsal surface. The patient dorsiflexes the ankle and inverts the foot.

## Application of Electrodes

In most diagnostic tests, silver–silver chloride miniature disk electrodes (Beckman) are used (Figures 12–5 and 12–6). The skin is prepared by rubbing it with a sterile alcohol pad and gently making a short, superficial scratch with a sterile hypodermic needle. A drop of electrode paste is applied to the scratch and the electrode is applied with a sterile adhesive collar. A piece of adhesive tape helps keep the surface electrode and collar attached to the skin. Slack electrode wire is coiled and taped gently near the electrode sites or on the lateral portion of the knee, allowing enough play for the knee to extend and flex fully. This stress loop allows the coil to expand when large movements occur, thus preventing electrode displacement. The remaining wire is attached to the subject's side or shoulder and plugged into the terminal box with other recording electrodes. These techniques usually result in a DC-electrode resistance of 2000 ohms or less. A resistance less than 3000 ohms is considered satisfactory, but $> 5000$ ohms usually necessitates reapplication of the electrodes.

Two other types of electrodes can be utilized in recording leg-EMG activity. Fine-wire electrodes and needle electrodes (both bipolar and unipolar) have the advantage of localizing EMG activity from specific muscle sites and can record individual motor

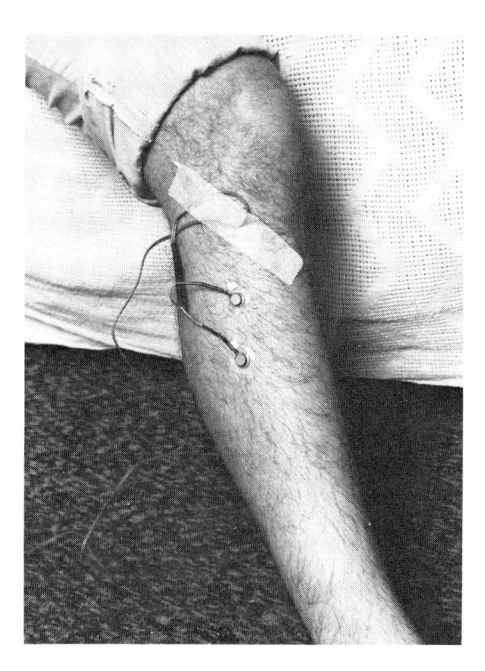

**Figure 12–5.** Electrode placement. Two miniature surface electrodes are placed 2–4 cm apart on the belly of the anterior tibialis. A safety (stress) loop of electrode wire is gently taped above the recording sites.

units. These techniques are more important in research studies because clinical investigations are typically concerned with the presence or absence of large leg movements. Fine-wire electrodes give the most accurate assessment of activity from single motor units. Needle electrodes have the advantage of rapid and easy application in all-night sleep studies *(53)*. A complete description of EMG techniques with needle and fine-wire electrodes is given by Basmajian *(71)*.

## Calibration of the Polygraph

The EMG signal from each pair of electrodes is amplified and displayed on recording paper using a standard polygraph. The output from each pair of electrodes appears on a separate polygraphic channel, allowing the investigator to compare left and right leg movements. While lying awake in bed, patients are asked to dorsiflex and extend each foot (plantar flexion). The EMG pattern is compared during periods of flexion and relaxation to validate the technical procedures described. The polygraphic settings for recording PMS are selected with a preference for normal EMG activity, which typically ranges in frequency from 20–200 Hz *(71)*. Some polygraphs (e.g., Mingograph) with ink-jet galvanometers can reliably reproduce signals up to 700 Hz. However, the limitations of a standard pen writing polygraph may necessitate a maximum high-frequency setting of 75 Hz. The amplification should be the maximum that allows a good signal-to-noise ratio; in a standard pen-writing polygraph, the preamplifier gain is set at 20 $\mu$V/cm. The sensitivity should be adjusted as necessary to produce a baseline signal about 0.5 cm in amplitude.

## Artifacts

Several types of artifacts can occur in recording periodic movements in sleep:

1. *Respiratory artifact* is seen as slow, rolling background movements on the leg channel of the polygraph. This is usually caused by the long leg-electrode wires, which extend from the leg to behind the subject's head, passing over the abdomen or chest. This artifact is eliminated by relocating the electrode wires so they do not touch the patient's body near the abdomen or chest or by adjusting the low-frequency filter to decrease the time constant.
2. *Cable-movement artifact* is occasionally found when the leg-electrode wires are touching the subject. Other movements, such as head turning, can be reflected in the leg channel.
3. *ECG artifact* will also occasionally appear on the leg channel but does not usually interfere with interpreting EMG activity. ECG artifact can sometimes be eliminated by repositioning the electrodes, bringing them closer together or moving them away from a prominent blood vessel.
4. *Faulty electrodes,* electrodes that are ripped off or have great increases in resistance, are the major causes of poor recordings. Reapplication of electrodes is necessary in such instances.

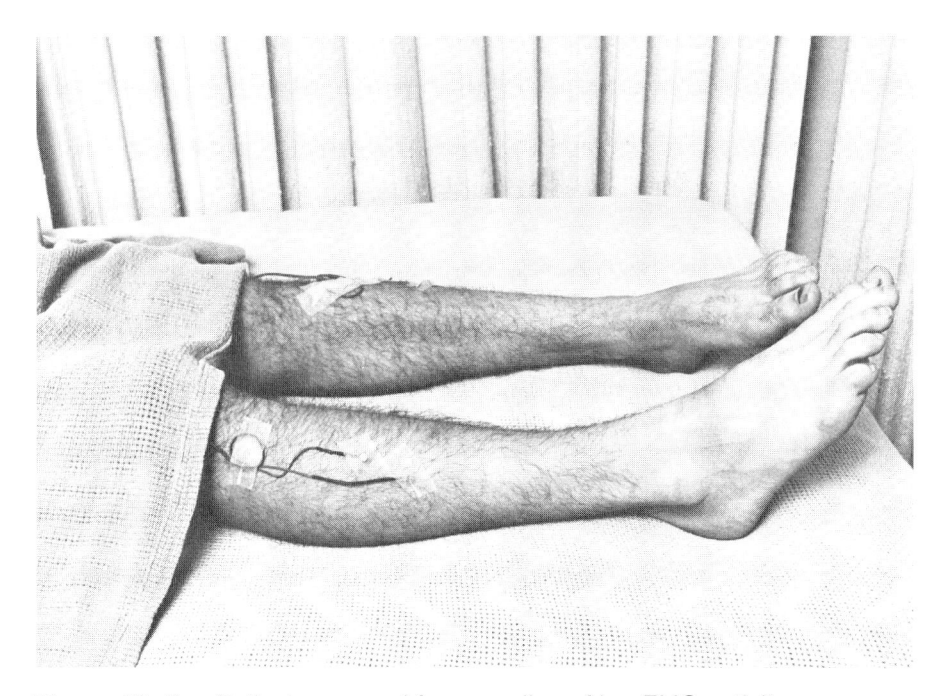

**Figure 12–6.**   Patient prepared for recording of leg-EMG activity.

## Qualitative Analysis of EMG Activity

### Definition of Terms

1. *Body movements, movement time, and movement arousal* refer to extensive EMG activity and/or artifact occurring in recording channels with a duration of at least 10 seconds *(72)*. The waveform is nonspecific. These movements may be followed by long awakenings, are not confined to the leg, and do not have a 20- to 40-second periodicity.
2. *Nonspecific leg movements* are leg movements that appear in isolation. They are not repetitive (periodic) or stereotypic. However, their duration and waveform may be similar to PMS.
3. *Hypnic myoclonus (sleep starts or jerks)* may be either brief (20–100 msec in duration) associated with upper and/or lower extremity movement or longer discharges ($\geq$ 1 second in duration) involving other muscle groups. These jerks occur during the transition from wakefulness to sleep and are not periodic *(7,8)*.
4. *REM extremity movements* are brief movements of the upper and lower extremities that are associated with REM sleep and may be correlated with

dream content *(73)*. The EMG pattern is not periodic or stereotypic. The duration of the movements shows more variability than PMS. These movements are a normal phenomenon occurring in virtually all REM periods. In contrast, PMS is usually inhibited during REM sleep, a stage of sleep where spinal reflexes are diminished *(2)*.

5. *Restless legs syndrome* is primarily a subjective complaint, and polygraphic studies have found that many, but not all, such patients have PMS during sleep. Regardless of the presence of PMS, restless legs patients do show a characteristic leg-EMG pattern during wakefulness and the transition to sleep (stage 1): The leg-EMG channels show excessive activity, a mixture of high background electrical tonic activity with superimposed movements. In some cases, periodic leg movements occur during wakefulness and stage 1 (with an inter-event interval slightly less than seen in PMS during NREM stages) (Figure 12–7). However, in most RLS cases, if PMS develops, it is not evident until the tonic EMG activity subsides and stage 2 sleep begins.

6. *Phasic EMG activity* may occur in the anterior tibialis, even though there is an absence of tonic EMG activity in relaxed nonmimetic skeletal muscles during relaxed wakefulness and sleep *(53)*. During sleep, many patients with PMS have periodic phasic EMG discharges from the anterior tibialis, even when PMS subsides. This activity is characterized by brief (100–500 msec), low-amplitude discharges. They are not accompanied by observable leg movements, but they may precede and indicate the emergence of PMS.

7. *Periodic movements in sleep* are a series of at least four consecutive leg movements, each separated by 4–90 seconds, but usually with an inter-event interval of 20–40 seconds. The duration of a single movement is 0.5–5.0 seconds, and movements typically have a stereotyped EMG waveform on the polysomnogram.

## Quantitative Analysis of PMS

The following parameters can be scored and analyzed:

1. *Total number of movements.* Isolated leg movements (i.e., nonsuccessive) are not counted. Movements occurring synchronously in both legs (within 4 seconds) are counted as one movement.
2. *Total number of epochs.* An epoch is 10 or more minutes of consecutive leg movements. Epochs separated by less than 15 minutes are considered to be the same epoch.
3. *Total number of movements associated with arousal* (K complex, alpha, movement artifact, < 15-sec awakenings) *and awakenings* (i.e., ≥ 15 sec).
4. *Movement index or myoclonus index* is the number of movements per hour of total sleep time (TST). An index for the number of movements per hour of NREM sleep is also helpful because PMS is usually inhibited during REM sleep.

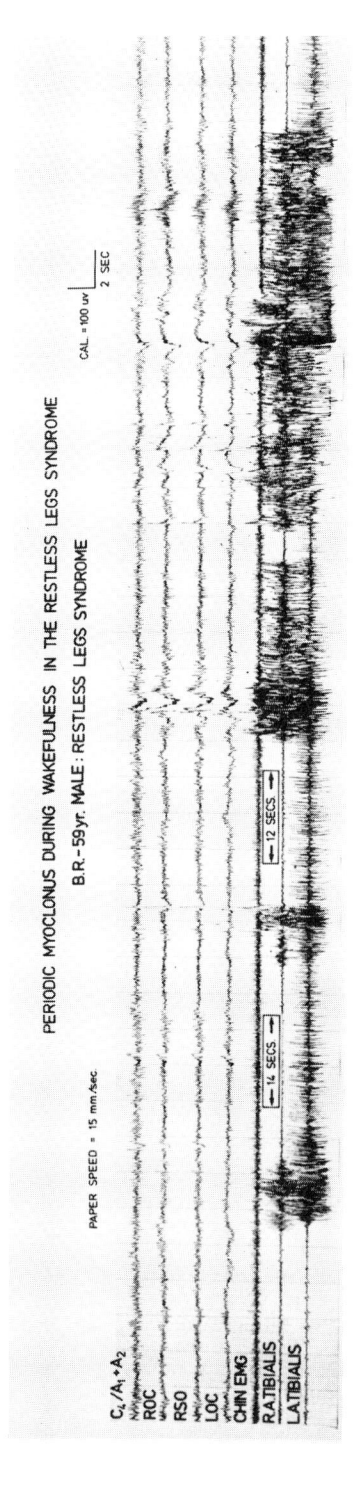

**Figure 12-7.** PMS in restless legs syndrome. Against a background of tonic EMG activity, periodic movements with a 12–14 second interval are present during wakefulness. This inter-event interval will become longer if the patient develops PMS during sleep. Patients complain of motor restlessness during wakefulness, just prior to sleep onset. This is the only known condition where periodic leg movements may occur during wakefulness. Because of the continuous EMG activity, it is difficult to distinguish involuntary periodic leg movements from voluntary movements.

*Sleeping and waking disorders: indications and techniques*

$$\text{Movement Index} = \frac{\text{\# of Movements}}{\text{Total Sleep Time in Minutes}} \times 60$$

5. *Inter-movement event interval* (IMEI) is the interval in seconds between the onsets of two consecutive movement events. This measure indicates the periodicity of the movements.
6. *The average inter-movement event interval* is calculated with the following formula:

$$\frac{\text{Sum of IMEIs}}{\text{\# of Movements}}$$

7. *Histogram of the inter-event interval* (Figure 12–8).
8. *Temporal progression of IMEI through the night* (Figure 12–9).
9. *Histogram of duration of individual movements* (Figure 12–10).

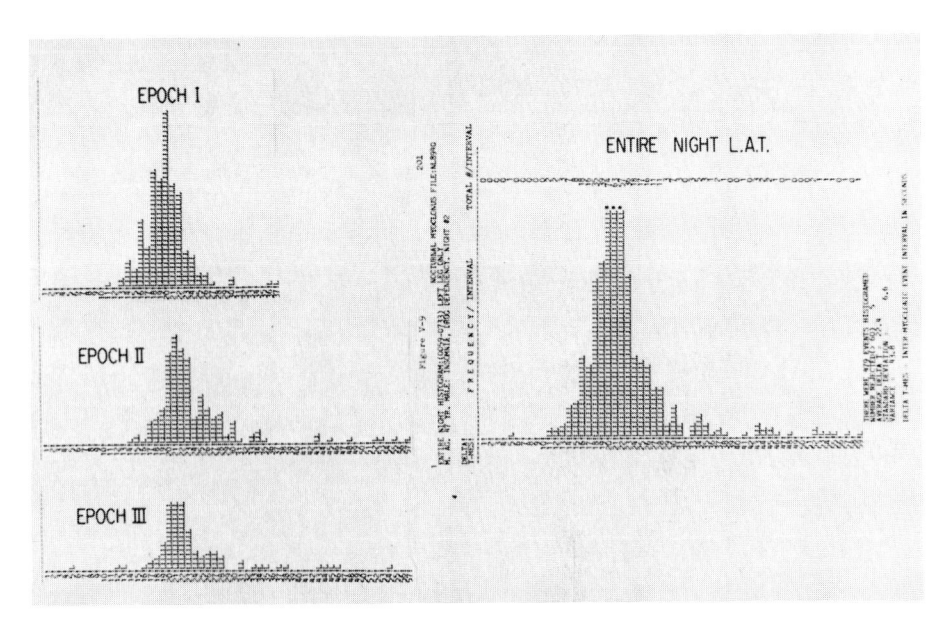

**Figure 12–8.** Histogram of inter-event interval (period length). The intervals between each consecutive leg movement are plotted. The mean period for the entire night was 22.4 ± 6.6 seconds. The histogram shows that the period is similar in each myoclonic epoch.

284

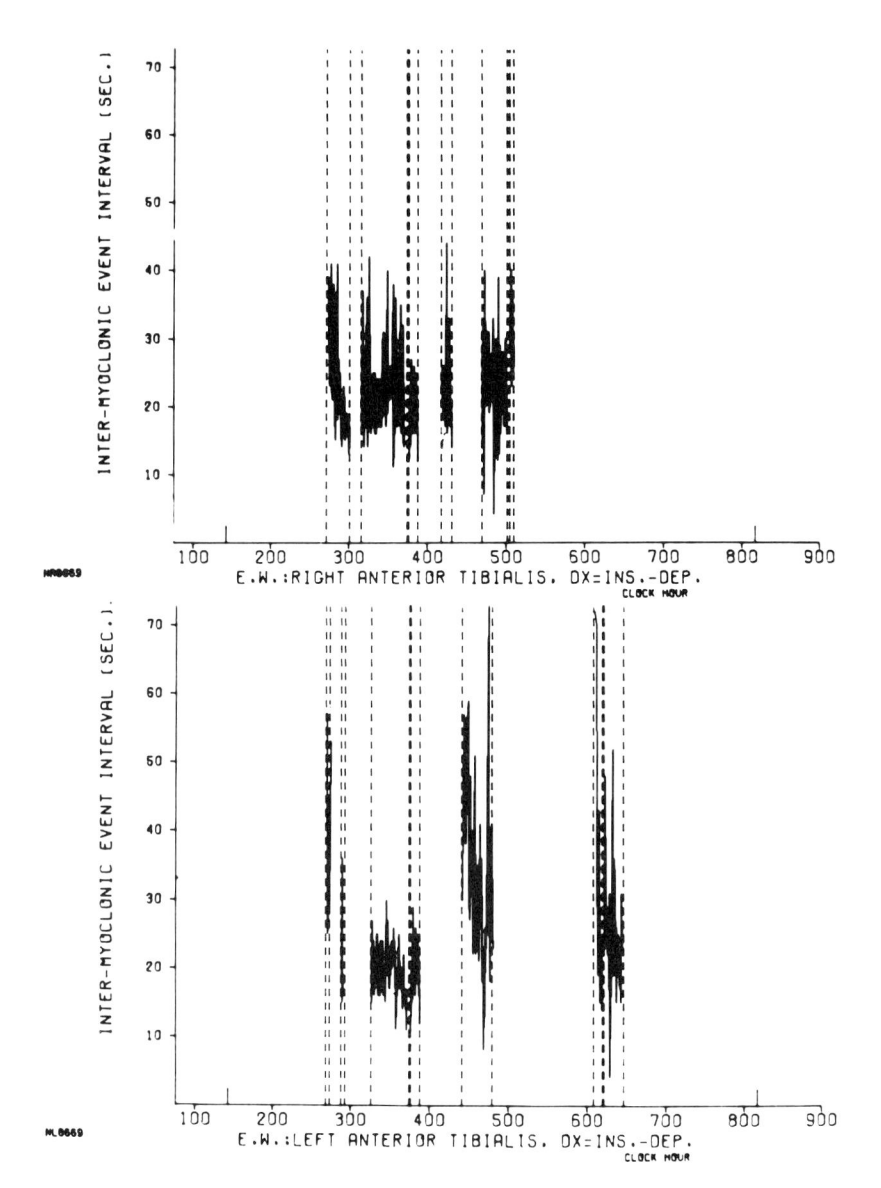

*Periodic movements in sleep (nocturnal myoclonus) and restless legs syndrome*

**Figure 12–9.** Inter-event interval across the night. Every occurrence of five consecutive leg movements during sleep is represented by a dotted horizontal line. Within these consecutive events, the inter-event interval is plotted. Lights-out was at 0130 hours. The period remains stable in the right leg but changes across the night in the left leg.

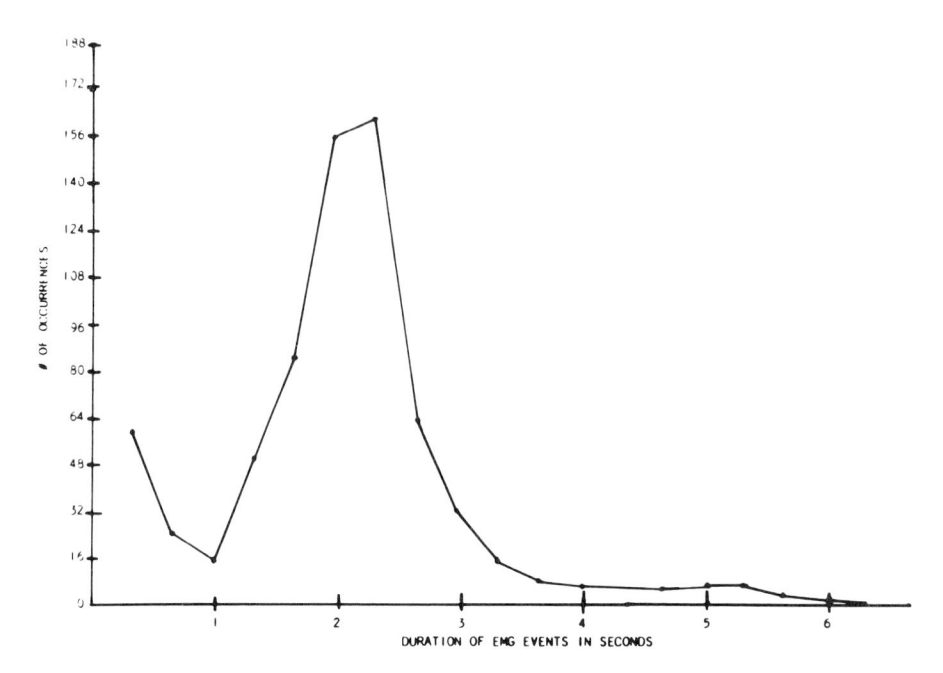

*Sleeping and waking disorders: indications and techniques*

DURATION OF R.A.T. AND L.A.T. EMG EVENTS: T.W., 74M, NIGHT #2
(This plot includes >95% of all EMG events. A few events lasting >6 seconds are not included).

**Figure 12–10.** Duration of OMS. The durations of all leg movements in a nocturnal polysomnogram are plotted (except for those lasting > 6 seconds). In this patient with PMS the modal duration was 2 seconds. This type of histogram is helpful in distinguishing and defining PMS.

## Summary

Most cases of PMS can be easily scored by the suggested methods. However, occasionally cases with variability in periodicity or low-amplitude discharges make it difficult to score PMS. Video monitoring of PMS can be helpful in such cases *(74)*. Another difficulty is whether to score movements with different waveforms that come between two consecutive, well-defined movements. The IMEI (periodicity) analysis is helpful here. Movements occurring within the dominant periodicity should be scored. It is important not to confuse generalized body movements with PMS; however, in a series of periodic leg movements that ends in a body movement, the last movement should be scored.

In patients with periodic sleep apnea, the leg channels may show the characteristic pattern of PMS in association with the end of each apneic episode. These movements should not be scored as PMS unless similar movements also occur in the record in the absence of periodic breathing. PMS will not result in artifact in all recording channels, whereas leg movements associated with sleep apnea arousals usually show movement artifact in all recording channels.

# Ambulatory Home Recording of PMS

There are several methods that can be used for recording PMS on an ambulatory basis. Microprocessors that are utilized for measuring wrist activity to study human circadian rhythms could be placed on the legs at night. Coates et al. *(75)* have reported an ambulatory technique for performing sleep recording at subjects' homes and transmitting information over telephone lines. However, these techniques have not yet been applied to PMS studies.

### Equipment Used

Pollak, Coleman, et al. utilized the Medilog recorder in the only published report to date on ambulatory EMG recordings for PMS *(76)*. Patients are taught to apply surface electrodes to their anterior tibialis muscles. Five electrodes (a pair of recording electrodes from each leg and one ground) are attached in the same manner described for the polysomnographic examination.

The EMG signal is amplified by a miniature amplifier, which is placed near the patient's bed. The amplifiers are constructed with the following characteristics: Frequency response DC-1 kHz, input impedance $< 50$ M$\Omega$, CMMR $> 100$ dB, noise $< 2$ $\mu$V. The EMG signal is recorded on two channels of a miniature magnetic tape recorder, the Medilog, manufactured by Oxford Instrument Company. A standard audio tape cassette is used (Figure 12–11).

The recorder uses batteries, weighs 1 lb, and measures 4 1/2" $\times$ 3 1/2" $\times$ 1 1/2". It is portable and can be placed on a chair at the end of the bed near the patient's legs. With plenty of free wire, the patient has room to move in bed, and electrodes rarely fall off. For example, one patient with PMS and nocturnal seizures was recorded without any missing data.

### Data-Analysis Techniques

There are several ways to analyze the night's data once the cassette tape is returned. To quickly rule out the presence of PMS, the investigator can listen to a replay of the cassette tape on a conventional tape recorder played at fast speed. The presence of PMS is detected by a crackling or popping noise that recurs periodically (every 20–40 seconds in real time). The absence of PMS sounds like a low hum, which reflects background noise. In clinical electromyography, this auditory method is commonly used *(77)*.

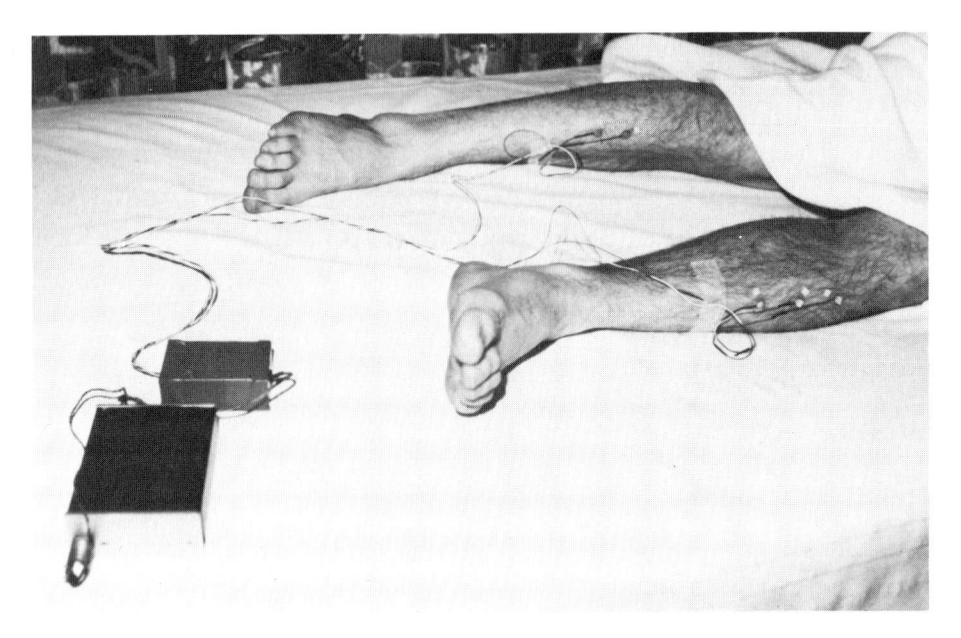

*Sleeping and waking disorders: indications and techniques*

**Figure 12-11.** Ambulatory recording of PMS. Amplifier and Medilog tape recorder are shown on the bed. A fifth (grounding) electrode is also placed on the leg.

In most cases, however, the investigator suspecting the presence of PMS will want a hard copy and detailed analysis of the movements. To obtain this, the cassettes are modulated on a playback unit (Oxford Instrument Company PB-2) at 60 times the original recording speed. Each channel is displayed on an oscilloscope, where PMS is seen as stereotypic, periodic EMG activity against a quiet background. At the same time, each channel is recorded on a slowly moving strip of photosensitive paper (TECA Instagraph). The beam is deflected vertically and modulated in intensity by the EMG signal. The sweep speed of the oscilloscope and paper speed of the Instagraph are selected to match the expected periodicity of the leg movements (usually 20–40 seconds). Figure 12–12 shows an example of PMS recorded with this method.

This ambulatory method allows for quick and efficient retrieval of large quantities of data. For example, at a paper speed of 1 cm/sec an 8-hr all-night recording is replayed in 8 minutes and each leg-EMG pattern appears on a paper strip only 6–8 ft long. The record can then be evaluated for number of movements, periodicity of movements, and distribution of movements throughout the night.

Another ambulatory technique involves gathering information with the Medilog but analyzing data after the EMG-recording information is played back directly onto a polygraph. Utilizing this method, Ancoli-Israel and Kripke (personal communication) analyzed the reliability and validity of 33 simultaneous leg-EMG recordings by the Medilog and standard polysomnogram. Subjects were senior citizens with suspected

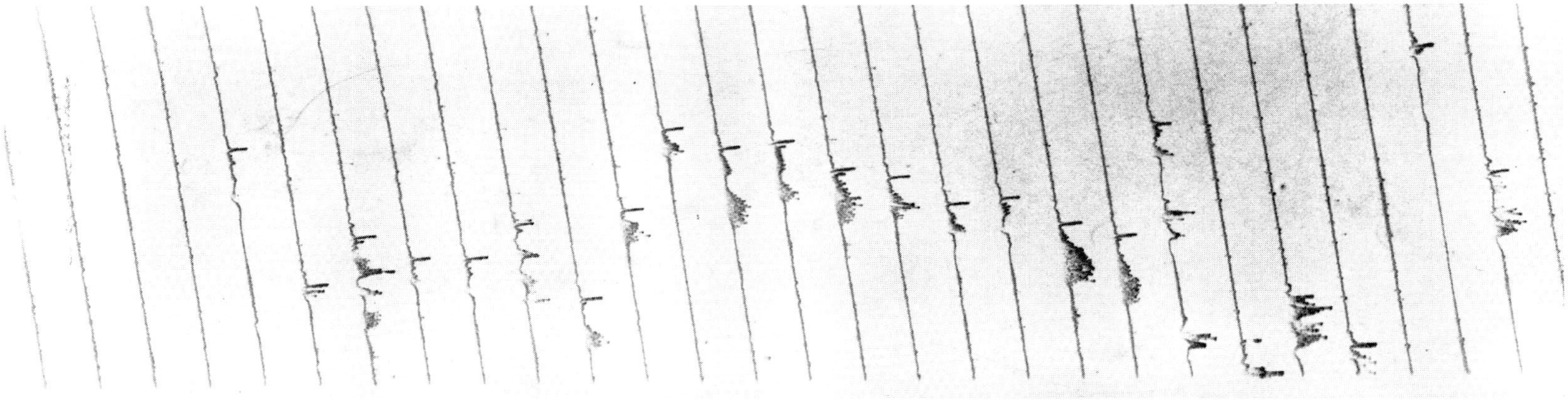

**Figure 12–12.** Results of ambulatory recording of PMS. Periodic movements in sleep are clearly identified in this photographic playback of a Medilog recording. The parallel lines are the background electrical activity, whereas PMS are seen as stereotypic and periodic darkened tracings rising above the baseline. The sweep speed is set so that each horizontal line represents 30 seconds of real recording time. This patient's average period length is approximately 26 seconds.

PMS. The correlation of the myoclonus indexes between the two recording methods was .64 ($p < 0.005$). The correlation between the Medilog on night 1 (recorded simultaneously on the polygraph) and the Medilog used at home on the following night was .43 (not significant). This result probably reflects the night-to-night variability in PMS activity. These data suggest the Medilog is a good screening device for evaluating PMS.

## Problems with Ambulatory Techniques

Problems with the ambulatory techniques are:

1. Data for the entire night can be lost if an electrode falls off, because a technician is not present to replace it.
2. There is currently no way to measure electrode resistance across the night to detect poor recordings.
3. Because the described ambulatory technique does not include EEG, the examiner is unable to determine if leg movements are associated with arousals. However, because the Medilog has four channels, ambulatory EEG could be added. Another technique is to use a wrist activity monitor to measure arousals.
4. More reliability studies (simultaneous recordings of PSG and ambulatory techniques) are needed to distinguish PMS from other movements during sleep.

## Suggested Protocol for Ambulatory Studies of PMS

| Time | | |
|---|---|---|
| 2000 | 1. | Subject is taught how to apply leg electrodes. |
| 2200 | 2. | Subject hooks up his own leg electrodes while technician hooks up remaining electrodes for all-night polysomnogram (PSG). |
| 2300 | 3. | Subject goes to bed with simultaneous PSG and ambulatory recording of leg-EMG activity. |
| 0700 | 4. | Subject awakens, fills out questionnaires, removes and cleans electrodes. |
| 0800 | 5. | Technician and subject listen to Medilog tape and review polygraph record to see if the subject has produced a good recording. |
| Day 1 | 6. | Subject is provided with a home-monitoring kit that includes a Medilog recorder, electrodes, tape cassette, batteries, skin preparation supplies, spare batteries, a sleep log–questionnaire, and instructions. |
| Night 2 | 7. | Subject self-applies two pairs of electrodes to each leg. This allows for a redundant channel of EMG information from each leg, providing the investigator with the opportunity to select the technically superior signal from each leg. The subject will turn on the recorder at lights-off and mark the time on the sleep log. The |

recorder is turned off when the subject gets out of bed in the morning. The time is noted in the sleep log and in a morning-time questionnaire.
8. Subject can mail tapes to the sleep center for analysis.
9. Technically inadequate recordings are discussed with the subject and corrected with additional instructions.

## Summary of State of the Art

Currently, inpatient polysomnographic studies of PMS are routinely performed in sleep disorders centers with few problems. Video and cinematographic techniques are a valuable tool in assessing these movements. Ambulatory recorders will be of critical future importance in providing inexpensive methods for long-term recordings in larger populations. Several important questions have been addressed but not fully answered: *(a)* What are the criteria for reliably diagnosing PMS? *(b)* What is the night-to-night variability in PMS? *(c)* What is the relationship between this variability and subjective sleep-wake complaints? *(d)* Which drugs inhibit PMS? *(e)* What are the differences between patients with insomnia associated with PMS and those with asymptomatic PMS? Answers to these questions will allow a clearer understanding of the relationship of PMS to sleep-wake complaints.

---

This work was supported in part by the National Institute of Mental Health, Grant MH 28461. The author wishes to thank Drs. William Dement, Christian Guilleminault, Charles Pollak, and Elliot Weitzman for their contributions to these studies, the 11 sleep disorders centers that participated in the cooperative case series, Sharon Keenan-Bornstein for her comments on recording techniques, and Liz Davis for her assistance in preparing the manuscript.

# REFERENCES

1. Symonds CP. Nocturnal myoclonus. J Neurol Neurosurg Psychiatry 1953; 16:166–71.
2. Coleman RM, Pollak CP, Weitzman ED. Periodic nocturnal myoclonus occurs in a wide variety of sleep-wake disorders. Trans Am Neurol Assoc 1978; 103:230–5.
3. Willis T. The London practice of physick. 1st ed. London: Bassett and Crooke, 1685:404.

4. Lugaresi E, Tassinari CA, Coccagna G, Ambrosetto C. Particularités cliniques et polygraphiques du syndrome d'impatience des membres inférieurs. Rev Neurol (Paris) 1965; 113:545–55.
5. Lugaresi E, Tassinari CA, Coccagna G, Ambrosetto C. Relievi poligrafici soi fenomeni motori nella syndrome delle Gambe Senze Riposo. Riv Neurol 1965; 35:550–61.
6. Lugaresi E, Coccagna G, Gambi D, Berti-Ceroni G, Poppi M. A propos de quelques manifestations nocturnes myocloniques (Nocturnal Myoclonus de Symonds). Rev Neurol (Paris) 1966; 115:547–55.
7. Oswald I. Sudden bodily jerks on falling asleep. Brain 1959; 82:92–103.
8. Gastaut H, Broughton R. A clinical and polygraphic study of episodic phenomena during sleep. Recent Adv Biol Psychiatry 1965; 7:197–221.
9. Landau WM. Movement disorders. In: Elaisoon S, Prinsky A, Handin W, eds. Neurological pathophysiology. New York: Oxford University Press, 1974:132–40.
10. Lugaresi E, Coccagna G, Montovani M, Berti-Ceroni G, Pazzaglia P, Tassinari CA. The evolution of different types of myoclonus during sleep: a polygraphic study. Eur Neurol 1970; 4:321–31.
11. Lundborg H. Ist univerricht's sogenannte Familiare myoklonie eine Klinische Intitat, Welche in das Nosologie beizechtigt ist? Neurol Centralbl 1904; 23:162.
12. Clark LP. A case of myoclonia occurring only after rest or sleep. J Am Med Soc 1912; 58:1666–8.
13. Symonds C. Myoclonus. Med J Aust 1954; 41:765–8.
14. Ekbom K. Restless legs syndrome. Neurology (NY) 1960; 10:868–73.
15. Dement W, Guilleminault C, Zarcone V. Progress in clinical sleep research. Scientific exhibit presented at the American Medical Association meeting, Atlantic City, New Jersey, June 14–18, 1975.
16. Coccagna G, Lugaresi E, Tassinari CA, Ambrosetto C. La sindrome delle gambe senza riposo. Omni Med Ther 1966; 44:619–67.
17. Coleman RM. Periodic nocturnal myoclonus in disorders of sleep and wakefulness. PhD thesis, Yeshiva University, 1979. Ann Arbor, Michigan: University Microfilms.
18. Ekbom K. Restless legs. Acta Med Scand [Suppl] 1945 158:4–122.
19. Allison FG. Obscure pains in chest, back or limbs. Can Med Assoc J 1943; 48:36–8.
20. Tuvo F. Contributo clinico alla conoscenza della sindrome considetta "irritable legs." Minerva Med 1949; 40:1.
21. Bornstein B. Restless legs. Psychiat Neurol 1961; 141:165–201.
22. Murray T. The restless legs syndrome. Can Med Assoc J 1967; 96:1571–4.
23. Lugaresi E, Coccagna G, Berti-Ceroni G, Ambrosetto C. Restless legs syndrome and nocturnal myoclonus. In: Gastaut H, Lugaresi E, Berti-Ceroni G, Coccagna G, eds. The abnormalities of sleep in man: proceedings

of the 15th European meeting on electroencephalography, Bologna, 1967. Bologna: Aulo Gaggi Editore, 1968:285–94.
24. Ambrosetto C, Lugaresi E, Coccagna G, Tassinari CA. Clinical and polygraphic remarks in the restless legs syndrome. Riv Patol Nerv Ment 1965; 86:244–51.
25. Coccagna G, Lugaresi E. Insomnia in restless legs syndrome. In: Gastaut H, Lugaresi E, Berti-Ceroni G, Coccagna G, eds. The abnormalities of sleep in man: proceedings of the 15th European meeting on electroencephalography, Bologna, 1967. Bologna: Aulo Gaggi Editore, 1968:139–44.
26. Murphy T. The restless legs syndrome. Can Med Assoc J 1959; 17:201.
27. Roth B, Van Thanh L, Vacek J. Syndrom neklidnych nohov, Klinicka a polygraficks studie. Cesk Neurol Neurochir 1974; 37:374–9.
28. Frankel B, Patten B, Gillin C. Restless legs syndrome. JAMA 1974; 230:1302–3.
29. Harriman D, Taverner D, Woolf A. Ekbom's syndrome and burning paraesthesiae. Brain 1970; 93:393–406.
30. Norlander NB. Therapy in restless legs. Acta Med Scand 1953; 145:453.
31. Behrman S. Disturbed relaxation of the limbs. Br Med J 1958; 1:1454.
32. Ekbom K. Restless legs syndrome after partial gastrectomy. Acta Neurol Scand 1966; 2:79–89.
33. Ask-Upmark E, Meurling S. On the presence of a deficiency factor in the pathogenesis of amyotrophic lateral sclerosis. Acta Med Scand 1955; 52:217.
34. Aspenstrom G. Pica och restless legs vid jarnbist. Sv Lakartidn 1964; 61:1174–7.
35. Boghen D, Peyronnard RM. Myoclonus in familial restless legs syndrome. Arch Neurol 1976; 33:368–70.
36. Botez MI, Cadotte M, Beaulieu R, Pichette LP, Pison C. Neurological disorders responsive to folic acid therapy. Med Hypotheses 1976; 2:135–40.
37. Heinze F, Frame B, Fine C. Restless legs and orthostatic hypotension in primary amyloidosis. Arch Neurol 1967; 16:497–500.
38. Ekbom K. Restless legs som tidigsymtom vid cancer. Sv Lakartidn 1955; 52:1875–83.
39. Callaghan N. Restless legs syndrome in uremic neuropathy. Neurology (Minn) 1966; 16:359–61.
40. Tyler HR. Neurological aspects of uremia: an overview. Paper presented at the conference of adequacy of dialysis, Monterey, California, March 20–22, 1974.
41. Keer D. Chronic renal failure. In: Beeson P, McDermott W, eds. Textbook of medicine. Philadelphia: WB Saunders, 1975:1093–1107.
42. Gorman C, Dyck P, Pearson J. Symptoms of restless legs. Arch Intern Med 1965; 115:155–60.
43. Luft R, Muller R. "Crampi" och "restless legs" vid akut poliomyelit. Nord Med 1947; 33:748–50.

44. Billiard M, Besset A, Passouant P. Treatment of chronic insomnia: long-term follow up. Sleep Res 1978; 7:210.
45. Ayres S, Mihan R. Nocturnal leg cramps (systremma): a progress report on response to vitamin E. South Med J 1974; 67:1308–12.
46. Lutz E. Restless legs, anxiety, and caffeinism. J Clin Psychiatry 1978; 39:693–8.
47. Dement WC, Guilleminault C. Sleep disorders: the state of the art. Hosp Pract 1973; 8:57–72.
48. Guilleminault C, Henriksen S, Wilson R, Dement W. Nocturnal myoclonus and phasic events. Sleep Res 1973; 2:151.
49. Guilleminault C, Raynal D, Weitzman ED, Dement WC. Sleep-related periodic myoclonus in patients complaining of insomnia. Trans Am Neurol Assoc 1975; 100:19–21.
50. Coleman RM, Pollak C, Weitzman ED. Periodic movements in sleep (nocturnal myoclonus): relation to sleep-wake disorders. Ann Neurol 1980; 8:416–21.
51. Bixler E, Soldatos R, Scarone S, Martin E, Kales A, Charney D. Similarities of nocturnal myoclonic activity in insomniac patients and normal subjects. Sleep Res 1978; 7:213.
52. Carskadon M, van den Hoed J, Dement W. Sleep and daytime sleepiness in the elderly. J Geriatr Psychiatry, in press.
53. Tauber ES, Coleman RM, Weitzman ED. Absence of tonic electromyographic activity during sleep in normal and spastic non-mimetic skeletal muscles in man. Ann Neurol 1977; 2:66–8.
54. Passouant P, Cadilhac J, Baldy-Moulinier M, Mion C. Etude du sommeil nocturne chez des urémiques chroniques soumis à une épuration extrarénale. Electroencephalogr Clin Neurophysiol 1970; 29:444–7.
55. Cadilhac J, Glaser G, Kuntz D, MacGillivar B. The EEG in renal insufficiency. In: Redmond A, ed. Handbook of electroencephalography and clinical neurophysiology. XV. Amsterdam: Elsevier, 1976:C51–69.
56. Guilleminault C, Raynal D, Takahashi S, Carskadon M, Dement W. Evaluation of short-term and long-term treatment of the narcolepsy syndrome with chlorimipramine hydrochloride. Acta Neurol Scand 1976; 54:71–8.
57. Martinelli P, Pazzaglia P, Montagna P, et al. Stiff-man syndrome associated with nocturnal myoclonus and epilepsy. J Neurol Neurosurg Psychiatry 1978; 41:458–62.
58. van den Hoed J, Kraemer H, Guilleminault C, et al. Disorders of excessive somnolence: polygraphic and clinical data for 100 patients. Sleep Res 1979; 8:212.
59. Lugaresi E, Coccagna G, Montovani M, Lebrun R. Some periodic phenomena arising during drowsiness and sleep in man. Electroencephalogr Clin Neurophysiol 1972; 32:701–5.
60. Zorick F, Roth T, Salis P, Kramer M, Lutz T. Insomnia and daytime excessive sleepiness as presenting symptoms in nocturnal myoclonus. Sleep Res 1978; 7:256.

61. Association of Sleep Disorders Centers. Diagnostic classification of sleep and arousal disorders, 1st ed. Prepared by the Sleep Disorders Classification Committee, HP Roffwarg, chairman. Sleep 1979; 2:1–137.
62. Kales A, Caldwell A, Kales J, Bixler E. Psychological characteristics of insomnia patients and normal subjects with nocturnal myoclonic activity. Sleep Res 1978; 7:190.
63. Coccagna G, Montovani M, Brignani F, Manzini A, Lugaresi E. Arterial pressure changes during spontaneous sleep in man. Electroencephalogr Clin Neurophysiol 1971; 31:277–81.
64. Evans B. Patterns of arousal in comatose states. J Neurol Neurosurg Psychiatry 1976; 39:392–402.
65. Morrison A, Bowker R. A hyperactive startle reflex as one possible cause of hypersomnia or insomnia. Sleep Res 1976; 5:181.
66. Guilleminault C, Raynal D, Phillips R, Dement W. Action of GABA derivative (BA-3467) on sleep patients with nocturnal myoclonus and idiopathic insomnia. Sleep Res 1975; 4:219.
67. Lugaresi E. Some aspects of sleep in man. Proc R Soc Med 1972; 65:173–5.
68. North J, Jennett S. Abnormal breathing patterns associated with acute brain damage. Arch Neurol 1974; 31:338–44.
69. Kjallquist A, Lundberg N, Ponten U. Respiratory and cardiovascular changes during rapid spontaneous variations of ventricular fluid pressure in patients with intracranial hypertension. Acta Neurol Scand 1964; 40:291–317.
70. Oshtory M, Vijayan N. Clonazepam treatment of insomnia due to sleep myoclonus. Arch Neurol 1980; 37:119–20.
71. Basmajian JV. Muscles alive. Baltimore: Williams & Wilkins, 1974.
72. Rechtschaffen A, Kales A, eds. A manual of standardized terminology, techniques, and scoring system for sleep stages of human subjects. Los Angeles: UCLA Brain Information Service/Brain Research Institute, 1968. (Also available as NIH Publ. 204, US Government Printing Office, Washington, DC, 1968.)
73. Wolpert, EA. Studies in psychophysiology of dreams. II: An electromyographic study of dreaming. Arch Gen Psychiatry 1960; 2:231–41.
74. McGregor P, Weitzman E, Pollak C. Polysomnographic recording techniques used for the diagnosis of sleep disorders in a sleep disorders center. Am J EEG Tech 1978; 18:107–32.
75. Coates T, Rosekind M, Thoresen C, Kirmil-Gray K. Sleep recordings in the laboratory and the home: a comparative analysis. Psychophysiology, 1979; 16:345–52.
76. Pollak C, Coleman R, Kokkoris C, Marmarou A, Weitzman E. New techniques for recording and displaying long-term EMG data: application to ambulatory patients with nocturnal myoclonus. Sleep Res 1979; 8:271.
77. Lenman J, Ritchie A. Clinical electromyography. Philadelphia: Lippincott, 1970.

# THIRTEEN
# CHRONOBIOLOGICAL DISORDERS: ANALYTIC AND THERAPEUTIC TECHNIQUES

ELLIOT D. WEITZMAN
CHARLES A. CZEISLER
JANET C. ZIMMERMAN
JOSEPH M. RONDA
RICHARD S. KNAUER

## Introduction to Chronobiology

An important recent development in our understanding of the physiology of human sleep and its disorders has been the recognition of the importance of the laws governing biological rhythm functions in man. Extensive research has taken place in chronobiology since the original report by DeMairan *(1)* of the persistence of 24-hour leaf movements in the absence of a light-dark entraining rhythm. The now well-established biological discipline of chronobiology provides the sleep researcher and sleep disorders clinician with a rich source of biological facts and theories upon which to build a new conceptual understanding of the human circadian time-keeping system *(2)*.

To understand the symptoms and syndromes of circadian rhythm dyssomnias in man, a brief discussion will follow describing important recent findings underlying the present conceptual basis. The recognition that when biological organisms are not entrained by 24-hour "zeitgebers," they develop daily cycles that have periods greater or less than 24 hours has been applied to normal humans in a series of physiologic studies *(2–7)*. All studies carried out for weeks to months in both cave and controlled laboratory conditions have consistently and repeatedly demonstrated that the preferred "free-running" period length of most human subjects is approximately 25 hours. Measurements of body temperature, urinary electrolytes, plasma and urine hormones, psychologic and performance measures, and, recently, sleep duration and sleep-stage organization have been carried out within the structure of time-isolated and nonscheduled human laboratory environments. Many important conclusions have been reached, including the change of phase-angle relationship between temperature and rest time, the ability of different variables to develop independent cycle lengths, the concept of multiple oscillators normally synchronized with each other but which can become desynchronized under free-running conditions *(6)*, and the importance of both "social" contact and the light-dark cycle as entraining signals in man *(8)*. The recent development of methods to obtain very frequent plasma samples (for weeks to months) coupled with detailed and continuous polysmnographic sleep-stage measurements and the application of computer data processing and analysis capability have led to important additional information *(5,7)*. These new insights and methodologic approaches will increasingly form the basis of new concepts toward an understanding of disorders of the sleep-wake cycle in man *(9–16)*.

It has been found that the length of sleep is correlated with the phase of the circadian core-temperature rhythm and not with the duration of prior wakefulness *(17)*. During free-running conditions, prolonged sleep-episode durations of up to 18 hours frequently occurred. We found that sleep length was dependent on when the self-selected bedtimes occurred in relation to the phase of the temperature cycle; long sleep episode durations (12–18 hours) occurred when subjects chose to go to sleep at the peak of the averaged temperature cycle, and shorter sleep-episode durations (6–8 hours), at the nadir *(5,7,17,18)*. There is an associated phase advance of REM sleep relative to sleep onset such that there is a significant shortening of the REM latency, an increase in REM amounts, and often a sleep-onset REM episode during the first third of the circadian sleep episode while the subject is in the free-running condition *(19)*. A phase shift of stages 3–4 sleep, however, does not occur during free-running; the timing and amount of stages 3–4 are linked to the initiation and course of the sleep process and do not appear to be dependent on the total duration of sleep *(19)*. This phase-advance shift of REM sleep, relative to sleep onset, is comparable to a similar phase advance of body temperature relative to sleep onset under free-running conditions. Thus, REM sleep and body temperature remain closely coupled under both conditions *(5,20)*. There are no differences in the REM-NREM cycle length comparing entrained and free-running conditions. In a study, not done in conditions of temporal isolation, but allowing unrestricted sleep in normal subjects who were awake for different intervals prior to bedtime, it was also found that there was a circadian rhythm of sleep-episode duration and a relationship between REM sleep and body temperature similar to that found in subjects with a free-running sleep-wake rhythm under non-scheduled conditions *(21)*.

Measurements of plasma cortisol throughout entrained and free-running conditions demonstrated that one component of the circadian rhythm had a phase advance (six to eight hours) relative to sleep onset, whereas a second component clearly followed sleep onset. The temporal pattern of growth hormone secretion, on the other hand, was directly related to sleep onset. A major episode of hormonal secretion occurred within the first two hours after sleep onset for almost all sleep episodes during both the entrained and free-running conditions *(5,12)*.

Further evidence for the importance of biological rhythm functions in the understanding of sleep disturbances derives from studies of phase shifts of the sleep-wakefulness cycles in either laboratory conditions or after transmeridian rapid flights *(22–24)*. These studies also demonstrate that the daily sleep episode is disturbed after east-west or west-east shifts as well as after 180° acute inversion. Under these conditions, REM sleep also phase advances relative to sleep onset, but the adaptation occurs more rapidly with a phase delay than with a phase advance. These results will be significant in regard to the discussion of the *delayed sleep phase syndrome* and treatment by a chronotherapy regimen *(25–28)*.

The importance of these recent findings and new concepts is illustrated by their direct application to the diagnosis and treatment of affective disorders in man. Wehr et al. *(29)* recently reported that by phase advancing sleep time in several patients with bipolar manic-depressive illness, they repeatedly effected an immediate switch out of depression. Similar results have been obtained by the process of REM deprivation *(30)* and total sleep deprivation *(31)*. On the basis of the REM advance present during sleep in depressive illness, Vogel has postulated a chronobiological explanation for the therapeutic effect of REM deprivation *(32)*.

# Classification of Disorders of Sleep-Wake Cycles

The classification of disorders of the circadian sleep-wake cycle *(33)* has divided the conditions into two major categories: *(a) transient* and *(b) persistent*.

## Transient Disorders

In the *transient* category, the dyssomnia of a rapid time-zone change ("jet-lag") is very similar to that found in an acute "work-shift" change. The sleep disturbance that results is due to both sleep deprivation and the circadian phase-shift change. The symptoms vary considerably from subject to subject but generally consist of an inability to have a sustained sleep episode, with frequent arousals occurring primarily at the end of sleep associated with excessive sleepiness and falling asleep at inappropriate times in relation to social and/or occupational requirements. For varying periods of time (usually from several days to two weeks), the person affected is sleepy, fatigued, and inattentive intermittently during the waking period and has partial insomnia during the sleeping episode. Although this may not very seriously disturb vacationing tourists, it can be a major problem to travelers on important business who must be able to function at high performance levels during their habitual sleep phase. This syndrome is very important in our modern society because it affects people in many critical occupations, e.g., doctors, nurses, airline pilots, air-traffic controllers, police, firemen, military personnel, radar operators, long-distance truck drivers, diplomats, etc.

## Persistent Disorders

The *persistent* category of the sleep-wake cycle disorders is divided into five subcategories: 1. frequently changing sleep-wake schedules, 2. delayed sleep phase syndrome, 3. advanced sleep phase syndrome, 4. non-24-hour sleep-wake syndrome and 5. irregular sleep-wake pattern.

1. **Frequently Changing Sleep-Wake Schedule.** The patient with a frequently changing sleep-wake schedule characteristically has a mixed pattern of excessive sleepiness alternating with periods of arousal, often at inconvenient and inappropriate times during the day. Sleep is usually shortened and disrupted, and waking is associated with decrements in performance and vigilance. The syndrome characteristically disrupts social and family life and often becomes intolerable to the chronic shift worker. However, probably through the process of self-selection, some shift workers prefer (or at least adapt readily to) night work and rotating shift schedules *(34)*.

2. **Delayed Sleep Phase Syndrome.** The delayed sleep phase syndrome (DSPS) has been recently recognized as a chronobiological sleep disorder that can be differentiated from other forms of insomnia *(25,26,28)*. The patient with DSPS reports a chronic inability to fall asleep at a desired clock time to meet required work or study schedules and is typically unable to fall asleep until 0200 to 0600. However, when not required to maintain a struct schedule (e.g., weekends, holidays, and vacation periods), the patient will sleep without difficulty and after a sleep episode of normal length will awaken spontaneously, feeling refreshed. A polysomnogram will demonstrate that the sleep-episode duration and internal organization are normal. However, the patient should be recorded at his usual sleep time (e.g., 0400–1200). If the timing of bedrest onset is attempted at a time considerably earlier for the convenience of the laboratory personnel (e.g., midnight), then there will usually be a long sleep latency, and it will be impossible to make a proper diagnosis. These patients have a long history of many unsuccessful attempts to fall asleep at an earlier time, i.e., phase advance their sleep-onset times. They score high as a "night person" on a standard questionnaire and have been previously considered to have "sleep-onset insomnia." Treatments have included the use of hypnotic drugs, alcohol, behavior modification techniques, sleep hypnosis, psychotherapy, and a variety of home remedies.

    In a series of patients, a successful phase shift of the time of the daily sleep episode has been achieved by a progressive phase delay of the sleep time (chronotherapy) *(27)*. That is, by delaying the time of going to sleep by 3 hours each day (i.e., a 27-hour sleep-wake cycle) the patient's sleep timing can be "reset" to occur at the clock time requested by the patient. Since chronotherapy can clearly be accomplished by a phase delay but not by a phase advance in these patients, we have postulated that differences in the shape of the phase-response curve (PRC) may underlie these patients' chronobiological problems. The phase-advance portion of the curve may be much less prominent than in normal subjects, whereas the phase-delay portion is quite intact. Since the nonentrained biological day length is approximately hours *(2,25,27)*, normal individuals must phase advance the sleep time each day by 1 hour to hold to a 24-hour day. The daily entrainment process requires a well-functioning advance portion of the phase-response curve with a range of entrainment sufficiently broad on both sides of 24 hours to enable normal individuals to adjust to variations in bedtime and time of arising to maintain an appropriate phase sleep time with a period of 24 hours.

3. **Advanced Sleep Phase Syndrome.** There is no clear evidence as yet that there is an advanced sleep phase syndrome. However, it has been suggested that such a category could include individuals who have chronic sleep onset and wake times that are undesirably early but have no disturbance of the sleep process itself. Since the "early to bed–early to rise" concept conforms very well with our socioeconomic and solar day timing system, these individuals probably do not seek medical or psychologic help. However, it has been well documented that the process of aging leads to a characteristic change in the timing of sleep such that the older individual finds himself spontaneously awakening earlier in the morning and becoming sleepy and going to sleep earlier in the evening *(35)*. It is possible that maturational alterations in the shape of the phase-response curve may underlie these aging changes and that many older individuals do in fact have an advanced sleep-phase syndrome. However, it is also clear that other biological rhythm changes of the endogenous circadian and ultradian oscillators occur as a function of aging, including intrusive nocturnal awakenings, fragmentation of the sleep pattern, and repeated daytime brief sleep episodes (i.e., naps) *(36)*.

4. **Non-24-Hour Sleep-Wake Syndrome (Hypernychthemeral Syndrome).** The non-24-hour sleep-wake syndrome has been described recently in several patients and is of considerable interest because of its important relationship to phase-shift disorders and to the free-running sleep-wake pattern of normal humans living in temporal isolation *(37–39)*. Patients with hypernychthemeral syndrome are unable to be entrained to society's 24-hour day and therefore develop a 25- to 27-hour biological day in spite of all attempts to do otherwise. Blindness or a personality disorder may predispose to this condition. No individual living in society has been described thus far who developed a consistent sleep-wake rhythm with a period less than 24 hours. The patient's repeated attempts to hold to a normal 24-hour sleep-wake schedule can lead to cyclic periods of nonsynchronization with society's rhythm as well as to cyclic (three to four weeks) disrupted and delayed sleep with associated daytime sleepiness. Since patients with the delayed sleep-phase syndrome also demonstrate a consistent tendency toward a progressive phase delay, it is postulated that the two syndromes may only differ in degree; the difference being that the patient with the non-24-hour sleep-wake syndrome

has an even further altered phase-response curve with essentially no phase-advance capability.

Support for the concept that there may be large individual differences in phase-advance capability derives from recent studies of phase shift after transmeridian air flight *(23)* and adaptation after phase shifts in the laboratory *(24)*. It was found that an adaptation to eastward flight (phase advance of 6 hours) and a laboratory advance of 8 hours took much longer in some subjects than othes, whereas adaptation to a phase delay (westward flight) occurred more rapidly.

5. **Irregular Sleep-Wake Pattern.** Finally, a syndrome of irregular sleep-wake pattern is described. The pattern is one of considerable irregularity without an identifiable, persistent, circadian sleep-wake rhythm. The condition is presumed to be associated with frequent daytime naps at irregular times in conjunction with a disturbed nocturnal sleep pattern.

# Patient Evaluation

As described elsewhere in this chapter, the evaluation of the endogenous circadian timing system in humans can involve many sophisticated techniques requiring extensively trained personnel and complex equipment. In the description of such techniques, it is possible to obscure the fact that a great deal can be learned without such an elaborate setup.

## Sleep-Wake Diaries

In order to clinically evaluate a patient who may have a disorder of his circadian sleep-wake cycle, it is necessary to inquire into the daily sleep habits in terms of the patient's biological day. It is therefore important to recognize that the patient's functional daily pattern may be quite different from the expected social-clock day. In addition to the detailed clinical history, it is extremely valuable to have the patient keep a detailed daily log of his sleep-wake pattern. In the Montefiore Hospital and Medical Center's Sleep-Wake Disorders Center, we have established a special form for such information (Figure 13–1).

Each log sheet has space for two calendar weeks of information. The patient plots the following information each day:

1. The time the patient started to try to go to sleep.
2. An estimate of the time he thought he fell asleep.
3. The time he woke up and went back to sleep (if sleep was interrupted during the sleep episode).
4. The time of final awakening.

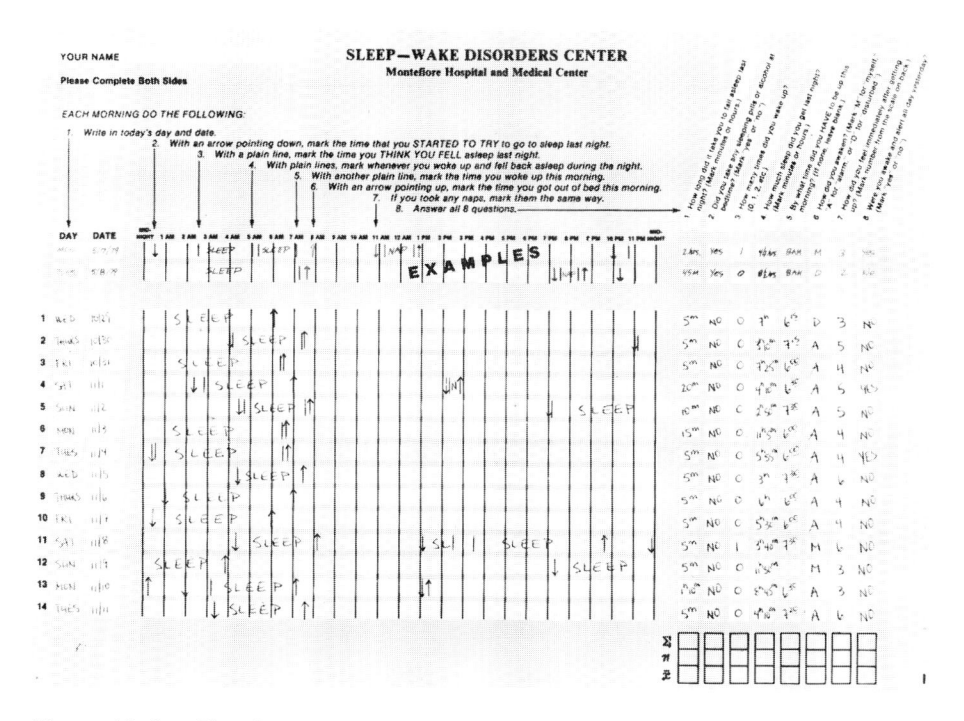

*Chronobiological disorders: analytic and therapeutic techniques*

**Figure 13–1.** The sleep-wake diary form used in the Montefiore Hospital and Medical Center's Sleep-Wake Disorders Center. This particular log was kept by a medical student during a clinical clerkship.

5. The time the patient finally got out of bed for the day.
6. The time of any "nap" periods that occurred outside of the daily sleep episode.

In addition, for each day we ask the following questions:

1. How long did it take you to fall asleep last night? (Mark minutes or hours.)
2. Did you take any sleeping pills or alcohol at bedtime? (Mark "yes" or "no.")
3. How many times did you wake up? (0, 1, 2, etc.)
4. How much sleep did you get last night? (Mark minutes or hours.)
5. By what time did you *have* to be up this morning? (If none, leave blank.)
6. How did you awaken? (Mark "M" for "myself," "A" for "alarm," or "D" for "disturbed.")
7. How did you feel immediately after getting up? (Mark number from the scale on back.)
8. Were you awake and alert all day yesterday? (Mark "yes" or "no.")

From this information, the clinician is at once able to determine several things. First, it is immediately clear if recurrent disruptions of the timing of the sleep-wake

303

cycle, either imposed by work requirements, as in Figure 13–1, or chosen by the patient, are contributing to the patient's sleep-wake complaint. Second, it sometimes reveals patterns of behavior that would be very difficult to determine from the patient's history. An impressive but unusual example of this is illustrated in Figure 13–2. Note how the patient reported sleep episodes occurring later and later each day. Such a pattern revealed that he was unable to entrain his internal circadian pacemaker to the environmental 24-hour day-night cycle. In his case, we were able to correlate his self-reports with simultaneously measured body temperature (recorded using a "Solicorder,"* an ambulatory temperature monitoring device). However, the diagnosis of a hypernychthemeral sleep-wake cycle can be made from such diary data alone *(39)*.

Home sleep-wake diary records can be useful in distinguishing patients with the hypernychthemeral sleep-wake cycle from those who are able to entrain to a 24-hour day but are unable to sleep at a convenient phase of that cycle (Figure 13–3). These are patients with the delayed sleep phase syndrome *(25)*. Finally, a patient's consistent self-report of insomnia can be compared with his self-report during polysomnography to determine the reliability of his diary records. In addition, both ambulatory temperature monitoring and ambulatory wrist activity monitoring can be used in conjunction with those self-reports. We are currently exploring the relationship between those variables and simultaneous polygraphic recording during sleep. This will increase the objectivity of the diary records, especially in patients unable to accurately estimate sleep length.

The sleep-wake diary data, polygraphic recording, and/or long-term ambulatory monitoring data are all instrumental in making a diagnosis of disorders of the sleep-wake schedule *(33)*. Treatment of some disturbances, such as illustrated in Figure 13–1, is as simple as stressing the importance of regulation in the timing of sleep *(20,40–42)*. Often, otherwise sophisticated patients are quite naive in regard to sleep hygiene, thinking that eight hours of sleep is enough, no matter what time of their biological day it is obtained. However, we have shown that both the length and internal organization of sleep are powerfully dependent on its phase within the circadian cycle *(18,19)*. In addition, we have developed a successful nondrug treatment for the delayed sleep phase syndrome based on circadian theory that involves resetting the biological clocks of those patients *(27)*. This technique, which we have called chronotherapy, is most easily performed within a special facility that allows the patient to sleep undisturbed at unusual hours, but it can be done at home under the proper circumstances.

Finally, admission of some patients to the Laboratory of Human Chronophysiology, where they live without time cues, can expose the chronic sleep deprivation and poor sleep hygiene of some patients. For example, Figure 13–4 shows the diary records and the data recorded in the laborabory from a patient with a combined delayed sleep phase syndrome and short sleep time who had convinced himself that he needed very little sleep and therefore held two jobs *(43)*. His complaint of chronic insomnia disappeared once he was returned to a normal sleep-wake schedule in the Laboratory of

---

*Ambulatory Monitoring Corp., Ardsley, New York.

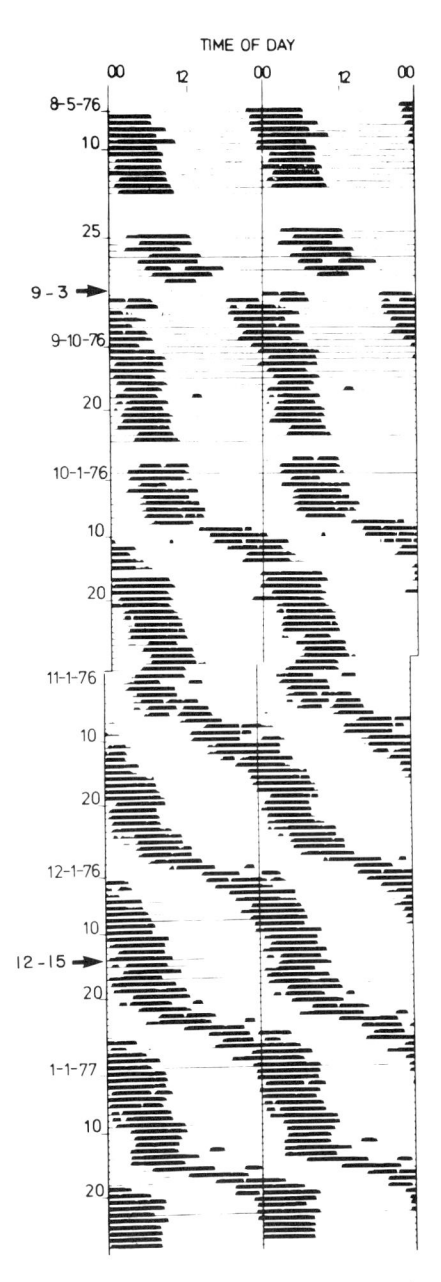

**Figure 13-2.** Double plotting of the lights-off, lights-on, and estimated sleep-onset and awakening times for a period of six months. Black bars represent estimated sleep time and gray bars additional time spent in bed. The arrows indicate the beginning and end of the period during which body temperature was monitored. (From Kokkoris et al. *(37)*).

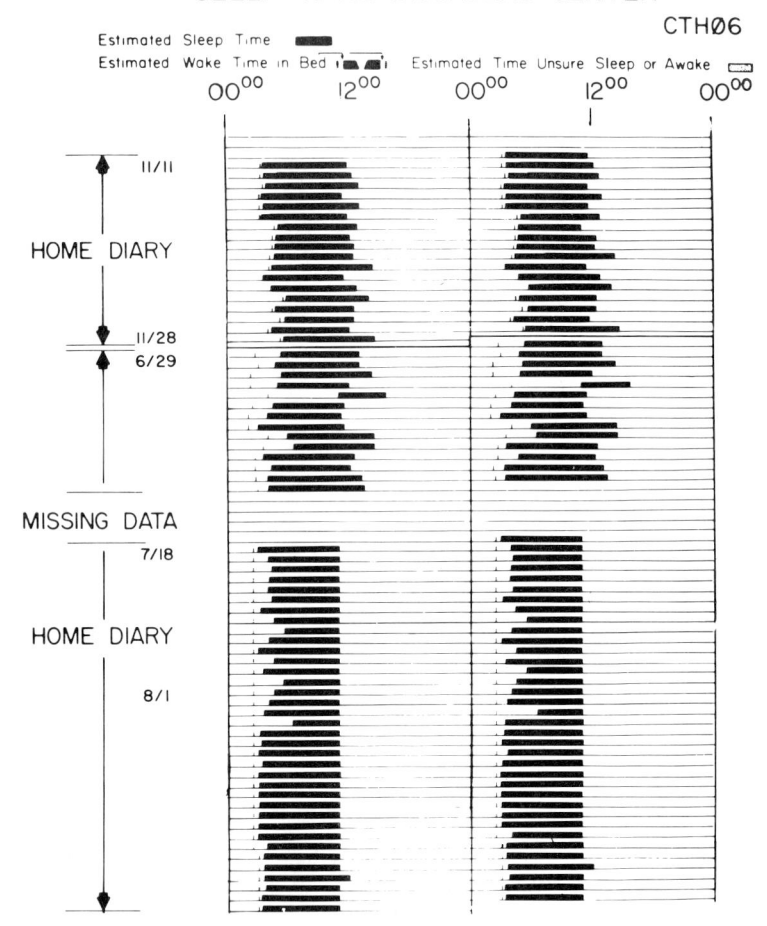

*Sleeping and waking disorders: indications and techniques*

**Figure 13–3.** Double plot of the daily sleep-wake pattern of a patient with a diagnosis of delayed sleep phase syndrome. The dark period is the estimated time asleep. The short vertical lines before and after the lights-out period represent the times of going to bed and arising from bed respectively.

Human Chronophysiology by simply eliminating environmental time cues and allowing him to sleep ad lib.

In summary, we have found that simple techniques of systematically gathering information from patients can be very valuable in the diagnosis of their sleep-wake

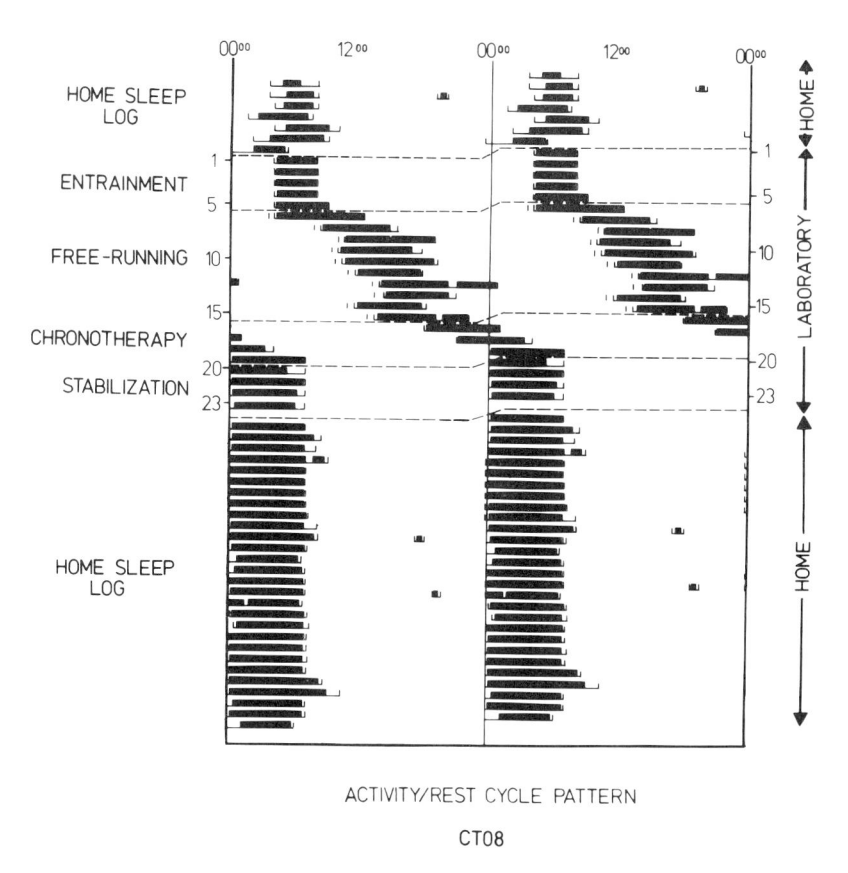

*Chronobiological disorders: analytic and therapeutic techniques*

**Figure 13–4.** Double plot of daily sleep-wake pattern of a patient with combined DSPS and short sleep time recorded before, during, and after chronotherapy. See legend of Figure 13–3 for explanation of symbols. The vertical hatchmark during the free-running section in the laboratory indicates when the patient requested to begin bedtime preparation.

disorders, especially if the basis of the pathology is within the circadian system. We would recommend home sleep-wake diary data recording as a screening device for such disorders in all sleep-disorder patients, as it is a simple, inexpensive, and effective technique. Analysis of such data has already led to the development of a treatment for one type of insomnia. We are confident that the collection and analysis of such data on a large-scale basis will aid in the classification and treatment of an increasing number of sleep disorders as these techniques become more widely utilized.

*Sleeping and waking disorders: indications and techniques*

## Laboratory Monitoring

*Human Chronophysiology Clinical Laboratory*   To study the internal (endogenous) organization of the patient's sleep-wake cycle and related biological rhythmns as well as to provide a suitable milieu for chronotherapy, we have established a special environment (Figure 13–5) free of all time cues for the chronophysiologic study of human beings living in temporal isolation for prolonged periods (5). Two separate apartments were reconstructed to eliminate windows, to sound-attenuate the walls, and to provide a double-door entrance. A background white-noise system further isolates the environment acoustically. A closed-circuit TV system equipped with zoom and infrared features and a voice intercom system allow the staff to monitor and communicate with the subjects. The subjects have direct and frequent contact with the laboratory staff but not with family or friends. Each apartment consists of a bedroom (bed, chest of drawers, exercycle, closet), a study room (desk, typewriter, bookshelves, stereo-phonograph, lounge chair), and a bathroom. Clocks, radios, television, and current newspapers are not permitted.

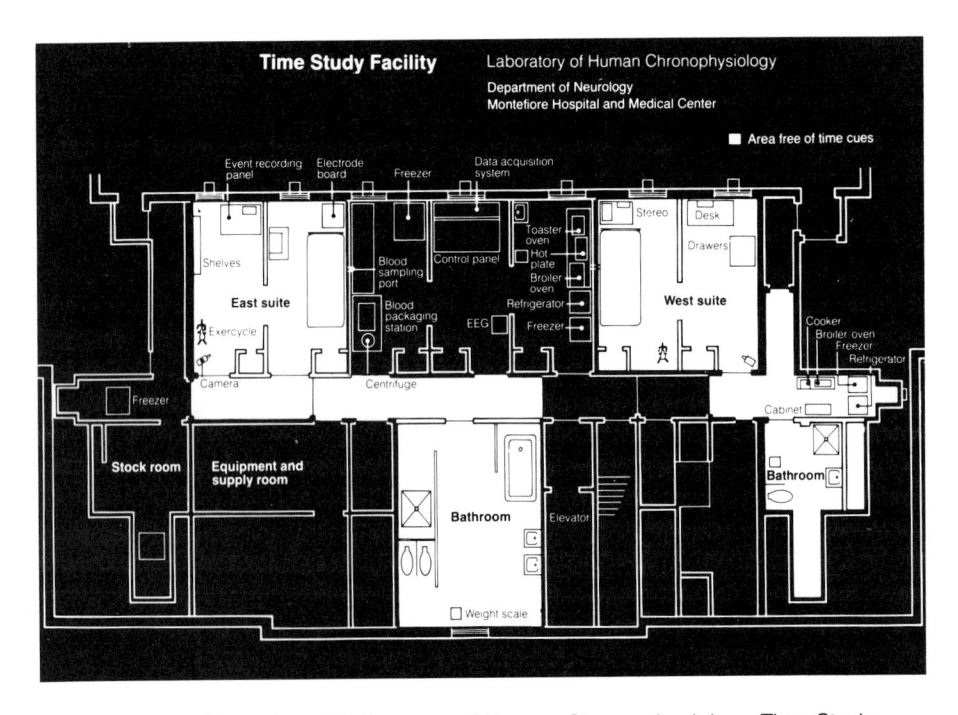

**Figure 13–5.**   Floor plan of Laboratory of Human Chronophysiology Time Study Facility.

The adjacent monitoring and control room is divided into several areas. There is a fully-equipped kitchen for food preparation and storage. In a separate area (equipped with a centrifuge, a packaging station, and freezer-storage space), blood and urine samples are processed and stored. The main data-acquisition area contains a 12-channel polygraph (Grass model 78) for sleep-stage recording and an electronic desk console unit, which houses the equipment used for all electronic monitoring and recording of the subject's physiologic variables. This data-acquisition area is arranged so that the technician can simultaneously watch the subject (via closed circuit TV) and monitor all data recording. To staff a 24-hour, continuously operating chronophysiologic facility, it is necessary to have a well-trained, dedicated, and full staff of technicians.

All staff members are given intensive training in the necessary laboratory techniques, including rapid electrode application, operation of the polysomnograph, the techniques of frequent blood sampling, and maintenance of the electronic data-acquisition system. During interaction with the subject, staff members must avoid communicating time cues. An extensive series of written protocols, checklists, and log books are used to ensure accuracy and uniformity in the execution of standard procedures (e.g., prior to bedrest, at activity onset, etc.) and to provide for staff communication during shift changes. In addition, descriptive narrative information throughout the study and chronotherapy provides important data for evaluation of the patient's status.

Technicians are assigned work shifts by a computer-generated randomized schedule created weekly. The shift lengths vary from 3.5 to 8.5 hours with a half-hour overlap between shifts to assure an orderly transfer of duties.

In addition to the technicians, a highly experienced staff member is always available "on call" for any emergencies (e.g., equipment failure, blood-sampling problems, technician illness). This individual also assists in the preparation for the subject's sleep time. Electrode application for polysomnographic recording is done rapidly (within 15 minutes) to ensure minimal interference with the subject's decision to go to sleep.

*Polysomnography* A 12-channel EEG unit (Grass model 78) is used to polygraphically record sleep stages utilizing a modified electrode array, including frontal EEG, lateral eye movement (EOG), chin EMG, and ECG. Two subjects can be recorded simultaneously. Extension cables with mini–electrode boards connect the polygraph to each subject's bed (Figure 13–6). Bedtime preparation includes a thorough facial scrubbing with a special soap (Clearasil) to remove excess oil and dirt. The technician applies surface electrodes after briskly rubbing the subject's skin with a gauze pad. If the subject's skin resistance is too high ($> 20,000$ ohms), the skin is rubbed with an alcohol pad or with a dab of electrode gel. We avoid the use of acetone and so have been able to use the same skin sites for long periods (up to six months). We use the frontal EEG placements to minimize electrode application time. The polygraphic data are obtained at a paper speed of 10 mm/sec. All polygraphic records are manually scored utilizing standard techniques *(44)* and transferred to a computer-generated time-aligned scoring sheet. These data are then manually entered into the laboratory computer system and checked and edited before analysis.

*Sleeping and waking disorders: indications and techniques*

**LABORATORY OF HUMAN CHRONOPHYSIOLOGY**

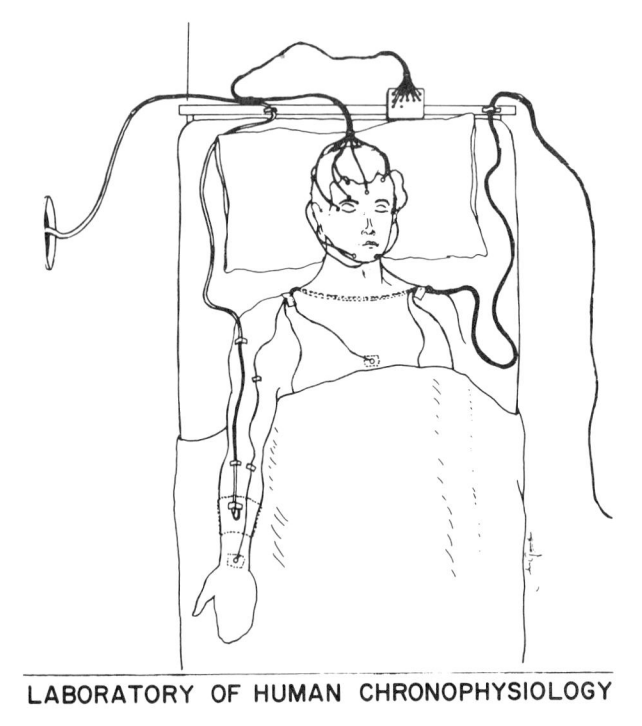

**Figure 13–6.** Diagram of a subject in bed whose sleep is being recorded. Polygraphic electrodes are in place for frontal EEG recording, vertical and horizontal eye movements, and chin electromyogram. For illustrative purposes, the subject's right arm is exposed to reveal the placement of the blood-sampling catheter and the thermistor for recording wrist and skin temperature. (From Czeisler (7)).

*Body-Temperature Recording* Core body temperature (rectal), skin temperature (ankles, wrists, and chest), and room temperature are all recorded automatically every minute by an electronic temperature-acquisition system (Digitec, United Systems Corporation) and transferred to a punch paper tape and paper-strip printout. To minimize loss of data (due to probe malfunction, slippage, etc.), each temperature channel is electronically monitored so that an alarm will sound, alerting the technician, if the temperature reading is beyond an established upper and lower limit. The thermistor skin and rectal probes (Yellow Springs Instrument Company) are placed together into one cable bundle to allow the subject full freedom of movement within the apartment (Figure 13–7). The subject is connected to this cable bundle at all times, although individual probes may be removed for short periods (e.g., rectal for defecation). The punch paper tape and printout with minute-by-minute recording of temperature values and special events (see below) are time-coded with a unique cumulative minute number.

*Chronobiological disorders: analytic and therapeutic techniques*

LABORATORY OF HUMAN CHRONOPHYSIOLOGY

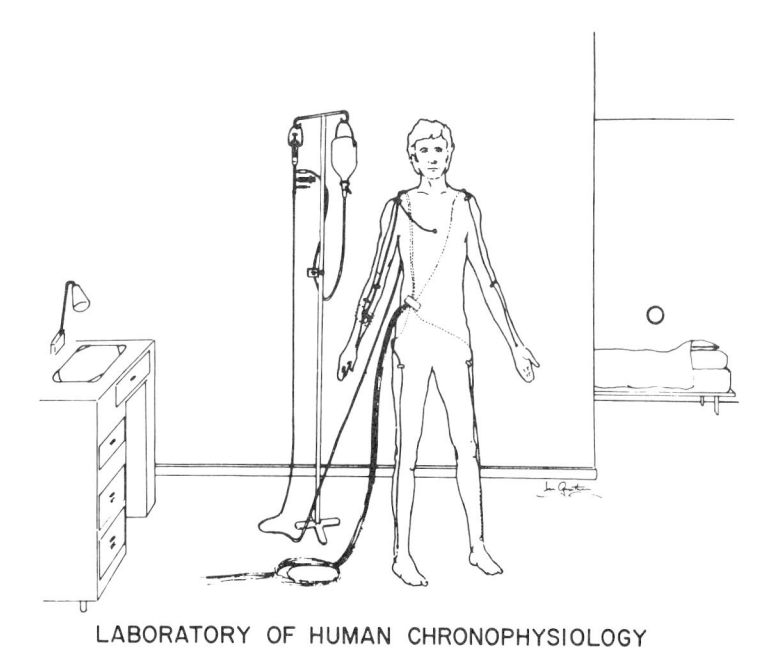

**Figure 13–7.** Diagram of subject living in experimental suite to illustrate placement of skin-temperature thermistors and blood-sampling catheter assembly during "daytime" recording. (From Czeisler *(7)*).

*Special-Event Recording* The timing of certain events occurring during the course of a study (e.g., the time a subject decides to go to sleep or get up, exercise, shower, urinate, etc.) is recorded by an electronic system interfaced with the data-acquisition system to immediately record each event on punch paper tape. This event-recording system consists of a series of button switches located in each of the subject's rooms. The subject presses a button switch that causes the interface device to punch a unique time and event number onto the paper tape. The appropriately coded button switch is lit simultaneously on the subject's button panel and on a master control button panel at the data-acquisition console in the control room. The technician is alerted to the request and responds by pressing the lighted button switch, thereby indicating to the subject that the request or event was recognized.

*Blood-Sample Collection* Multiple frequent blood samples (over 2000 samples per month) are obtained from the subjects for long periods of time (up to 77 days to date). Technicians collect samples according to a computer-generated random schedule with intervals ranging from 16 to 24 minutes *(12)*. Samples are collected through a blood-sampling apparatus (Figure 13–8), including a specially designed polyethylene intra-

*Sleeping and waking disorders: indications and techniques*

**HEPARINIZED SALINE**

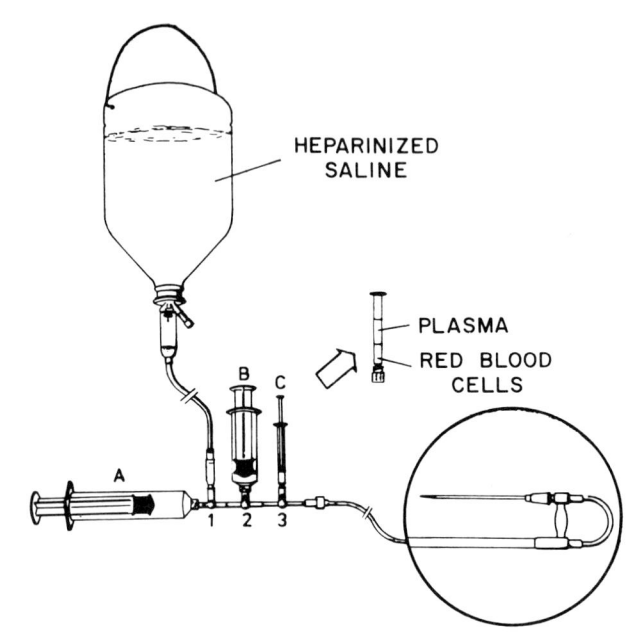

**PLASMA**
**RED BLOOD CELLS**

LABORATORY OF HUMAN CHRONOPHYSIOLOGY
TIME STUDY
BLOOD SAMPLING ASSEMBLY

**Figure 13–8.** Assembly for collection of multiple frequent blood samples. (From Czeisler *(7)*).

venous catheter (18 gauge) with side portholes (Deseret Pharmaceutical Company, Sandy, Utah) located in a suitable forearm vein *(7)*. The side portholes increase the reliability of continued blood collection because the tip of the catheter occasionally becomes occluded by the wall of the vein (especially during sleep).

The intravenous catheter is connected to a series of three-way leur lock stopcocks (Cobe Laboratories, Lakewood, Colorado) and syringes by an IV loop with a 12-foot extension tubing (Deseret Pharmaceutical Company). The narrow-lumen extension tube is protected by an outer tube, which also insulates the subject's skin from temperature changes as blood and saline pass through the inner tubing, allowing undisturbed sleep during blood collection. The series of stopcocks are connected to an IV microdrip, which allows for the controlled infusion of heparinized 0.45% saline (5000 units heparin per liter at 6–12 mL per hour) between blood samples.

During the subject's day, the technician enters the suite to draw blood samples. However, we do not disturb the subject's bedrest. A bedside porthole connects the bedroom and the control room to allow for continued blood sampling. Just prior to the subject's bedrest episode, the intravenous system is disconnected and the tubing is placed through the porthole. After replacing several stopcocks to minimize contamination, the system is reconnected and sampling can continue.

To draw a blood sample, the technician must withdraw the saline in the tubing into syringe B (Figure 13–8). This draws blood out of the subject's arm. After 3 mL of blood have been drawn into syringe B, the sample (0.7 mL) is collected in syringe A. Then, the blood and saline in syringe B are returned to the subject to restrict blood loss to the sample volume. Syringe C is used to flush the line with fresh saline and a drip rate is reestablished. The 1 cc sampling syringe A is preheparinized, dried out, and sterilized before use. After the sample is collected, the syringe tip is fitted with a disposable cap (Becton-Dickinson, Rutherford, New Jersey), and the blood is centrifuged in the syringe. This avoids the loss of blood associated with the transfer of blood to a heparinized test tube (to prevent clot formation) and during the pipetting of the plasma from the separated sample. Plasma is stored in numbered polypropylene microcentrifuge tubes and frozen for susequent radioimmunoassay.

We have been able to maintain a catheter in the same site for periods of up to 25 days before replacement in a vein of the opposite arm. Special care is taken to minimize the chance of infection. Prior to catheterization, a suitable forearm vein is located and the site is prepared by the removal of forearm hair and disinfection with povidone-iodine and alcohol. After the catheter is inserted, the site is cleansed and an antibacterial ointment (Bacitracin) is applied. The catheter is taped down securely (Transpore Surgical Tape, 3M Company). The tape strip (1/2-inch width) is placed with the adhesive side up beneath the catheter stub and is folded to firmly anchor the catheter. Several other strips are used to firmly affix the catheter and the IV loop assembly to the skin up the arm before the sterile gauze dressing is applied. This securing of the intravenous line will minimize to-and-fro motion at the catheter site and will appreciably reduce the risk of bacterial colonization *(45)*. During each of the subject's days, the entire assembly, except for the intravenous catheter, is replaced using sterile technique. During this procedure, the area is cleansed with alcohol and peroxide, and Bacitracin is applied to the venipuncture site. Routine careful inspections are made of the catheter, vein, and surrounding skin for thrombosis, redness, heat, or tenderness; of the IV-bottle solution for clearness and a vacuum seal; and of the subject's core body temperature for fever. Any evidence of infection dictates the immediate removal and culturing of the intravenous catheter, the tubing, and the bottle to determine the precise source of contamination. In the course of our program, we have had to remove a catheter only rarely due to this problem. Normally, we leave catheters in place for the duration of the study or replace catheters that present technical difficulties (e.g., slow or intermittent blood flow due to the catheter position in the vein) if the catheter cannot be adjusted to obtain a better blood flow.

*Subjective Assessment of Alertness*   An important variable in the study of the chronobiology of sleep disorders is a measure of the degree of alertness a patient feels at different times of his biological day. We have instituted a subjective assessment of alertness by recording the degree of alterness at frequent intervals, using a device that has been interfaced with the automatic data-acquisition system. The "alertness scale"

*Sleeping and waking disorders: indications and techniques*

consists of a specially constructed linear potentiometer (8-inch stroke, 100,000 ohms) connected to an adjustable lever. The subject is instructed to move the lever to a position indicating his degree of alertness; the more alert, the higher the lever is placed. The time of the test and the number corresponding to the potentiometer's resistance is recorded on the punch paper tape when the subject presses a push-button switch.

The recorded alertness values are sorted by the computer into a data file and are then converted into a linear scale from 0–10, using the resistance/mm calibration performed at the beginning of each study. Figure 13–9 illustrates by example the relationship between sleep, core body temperature, and the subjective alertness scale during free-running conditions. It is clear that there is a close correlation between rises and falls of temperature and changes in subjective alertness. This close relationship is present at activity onset and prior to bedrest and often during transient daily temperature changes (for example, in Figure 13–9, prior to sleep episode 46, when a drop in core temperature was accompanied by a drop in subjective alertness).

*Performance Tests and Mood Scales*   The performance test, Activation-Deactivation Adjective Checklist, and mood scales are all administered at the same times: before each meal, prior to bedrest, at activity onset, and with each urine collection.

1. **Performance Test.** A card-sorting performance test is administered to subjects before each meal, prior to bedrest, at activity onset, and before each

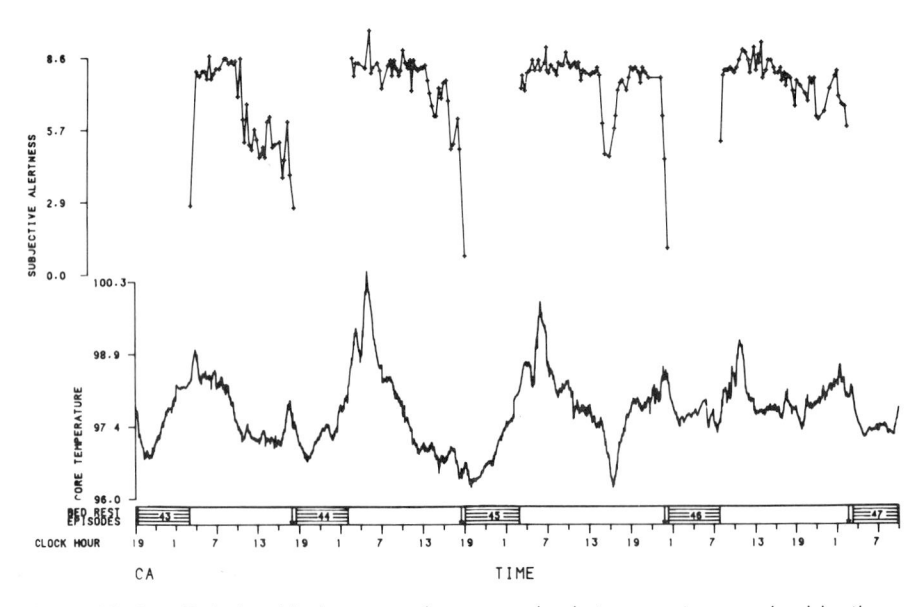

**Figure 13–9.**   Relationship between sleep, core body temperature, and subjective assessments of alertness during free-running conditions in subject CA.

urine collection. The task requires that the subject sort 96 playing cards into red and black groups as rapidly as possible. The time taken and the number of errors are recorded.
2. **Activation-Deactivation Adjective Checklist.** We use the Thayer "Activation-Deactivation Adjective Checklist" (A-DACL) *(46)* to measure fluctuations in "sleepiness" or "wakefulness" throughout the day. The A-DACL, a self-reported test of transitory activation or arousal states, consists of 20 common adjectives. A four-choice scale is used by the subject to rate how closely the adjective describes his feelings at the moment. The A-DACL is administered several times each day.
3. **Mood Scales.** The subject's self-assessed mood ratings are quantified using a series of 100 mm lines. At the beginning and end of each line are mood descriptions representing a continuum, e.g., sad–happy. The subject is instructed to place a mark along the line at a position that reflects his mood at that time. This test takes about one minute to complete and is administered with each performance test. (This test was suggested to us by Dr. Thomas Wehr at the National Institute of Mental Health and is compatible with his assessment forms currently in use with manic-depressive patients.)

*Ambulatory Monitoring* An important new development in the study of biological rhythms in man has been the use of ambulatory monitoring devices. We presently use two such devices, one for core body temperature and one for motor activity.

1. **Ambulatory Temperature Measurements.** Core body temperature is automatically recorded and stored using the Solicorder 16 solid-state recorder module (Ambulatory Monitoring, Inc., Ardsley, New York). The Solicorder 16 is a small (3.8 cm × 7.6 cm × 14 cm, 4 oz) portable, battery-powered, solid-state data logger that can easily be carried by the subject in a pocket or on a belt. It is capable of storing up to 2040 temperatures at 2- or 6-minute preset intervals. In addition, it will store subject identification information consisting of subject code number, start data, and start time. Data from the Solicorder is rapidly transferred to our laboratory computer (HP-MX21), using an electronic interface device, for graphing and statistical analysis.

    The major advantage of the Solicorder ambulatory monitoring unit is that it provides accurate, frequent, or continuous core body temperature readings from subjects or patients who are fully ambulatory and able to perform normal daily activities in regular social and work functions without restrictions. It thus allows accurate documentation of temperature changes during sleep and waking for each circadian cycle.

    Since the subject or patient is responsible for collecting accurate data, he must be instructed on proper instrument care. A special problem is rectal-probe malfunctioning. Subjects are shown how to examine probe connectors for breakage. For this purpose, we have constructed a mini "probe check box" consisting of an ohmmeter attached to a probe connector. This enables the subject to periodically check the probe's resistance and thereby determine whether the probe is functioning. If a probe malfunctions, the subject switches to a spare rectal probe. Battery checks and time markers should also be performed several times daily.

Subjects return to the laboratory to store the Solicorder data in the computer. The frequency of these visits depends on the sampling time interval at which the data are collected.

2. **Ambulatory Activity Monitor.** The activity monitor is a compact, solid-state data logger that is worn on the subject's nondominant wrist at all times, including during sleep. This monitor was developed by Dr. Thomas Wehr and collaborators at the National Institute of Mental Health.

Using an accelerometer and clock, the activity monitor samples activity at 3.5-second intervals and stores the number of active intervals for 15 minutes (maximum = 256 counts). This method of activity sampling provides a continuous distribution of activity at 15-minute intervals. The activity-monitor memory contains 256 locations, thereby providing for 64 continuous hours of data.

The activity monitor has become a valuable tool in the study of sleep disorders because it can document sleep episodes rather closely. Figure 13–10 illustrates a double raster plot (see Data Display section) of activity-rest data from the activity monitor and polygraphic sleep-wake data during entrained and free-running conditions. The top (thin) line represents all activity counts that have a value less than 5, whereas the bottom (thicker) line represents actual sleep time (stages 1–5). It is clear that low activity counts reliably determine the period length of the sleep-wake cycle. The activity monitor is also sensitive to arousals during bedrest and may prove to be a reliable indicator of sleep latency and total sleep time in insomniac patients without the requirement for polysomnographic recording.

## Computer Data Processing for Time-Oriented Data

The study of patients with chronobiological disorders, and the chronophysiology of normal subjects, necessitates accumulating a very large sequential, time-ordered data base. Not only are there thousands of numbers for each physiologic variable, but also it is necessary to determine the relationships among variables. The recent development of inexpensive, large computer memory systems, in association with high-speed random access, has provided the critically necessary capability to process, display, and analyze these extensive data bases. In our Laboratory of Human Chronophysiology, this difficult task has been simplified by the development of a user-oriented system for processing chronophysiologic data.

*Equipment (Hardware)*     Our current computer data-processing configuration consists of a Hewlett-Packard (HP) System 1000 computer, with 384 bytes of main memory, 105 megabytes of on-line disk storage, dual 1600 BPI tape drives, a 36-inch drum

*Chronobiological disorders: analytic and therapeutic techniques*

DC

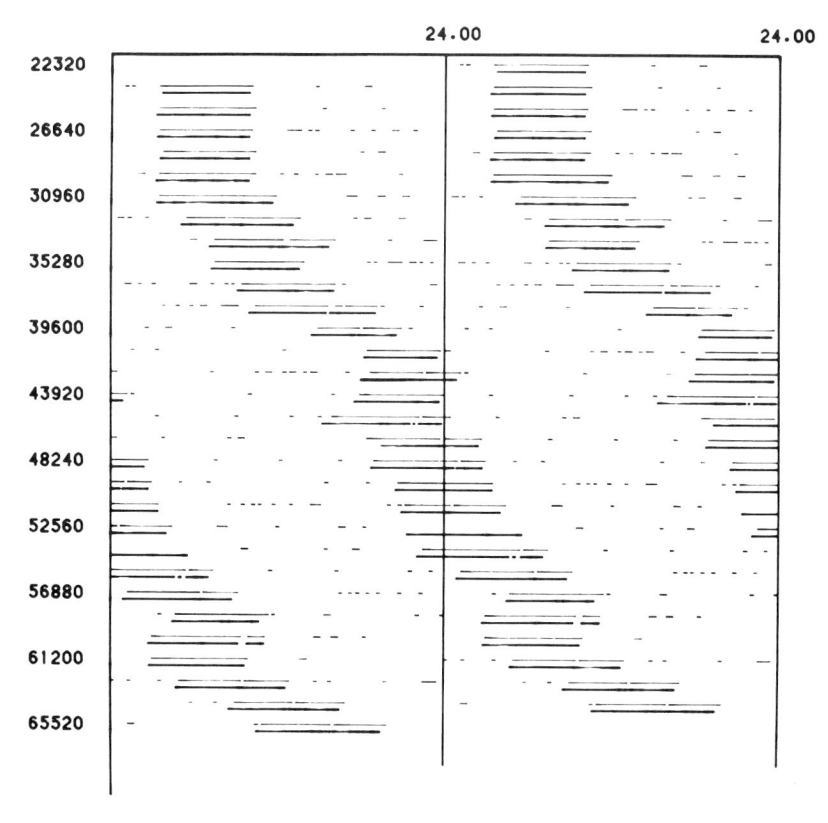

**Figure 13–10.** Double plot of activity-rest and sleep-wake data during entrained and free-running conditions in subject DC. The abscissa spans 48 hours, and each subsequent day is organized in a raster format, with successive 24-hour periods plotted beneath each other. Activity counts from the activity monitor that have a value of less than 5 per 15 minutes are plotted as the top (thin) line. The bottom (thick) line represents actual sleep time (stages 1–5).

Calcomp plotter, and 12 interactive terminals. It is a functionally oriented system, allowing the user to select the proper program for execution based upon an interactive dialogue. For example, if a user wishes to examine a sleep-stage plot, the word "PLOT" would be entered into any terminal, and the dialogue would begin as follows:

Enter In Multi—For A Multi-Variable Plot.
Sleep—For A Sleep-Stage Plot.
Raster—For A Double-Raster Plot.
State—For A Sleep-State Plot.

317

*Sleeping and waking disorders: indications and techniques*

This dialogue continues until all essential information is obtained from the user. This capability allows us to have our technical staff process data in an easy, nonconfusing manner, providing more results in a shorter period of time. Using this system, we are able to derive preliminary results during or shortly after an ongoing patient or subject study.

*Programs (Software)*   Special data-analysis programs have been developed, using Fortran IV programming language. These are described below. Because data storage and retrieval are machine-dependent, these will not be described.

To display an overall picture of the interaction among the variables, we have developed an extensive graphics package that presents the data in several ways. Because flexibility is the key to display processing, our linear-plotting program will display any or all of the data for a given subject on one graph. This general plotting program shows the interrelationships among several variables as well as the time series for a single variable. Figure 13–11 exemplifies such a graph for subject AE. The *x*-axis denotes time of day in both clock hour and elapsed minutes of the experiment. The bedrest episodes are plotted as a rectangle for each episode, and a downward arrow shows the time that the subject requested sleep. The variable lowest on the *y*-axis is growth hormone (GH) concentration in ng/ml. It is clearly seen that individual secretory GH episodes occur during the early part of each sleep episode as well as during the waking

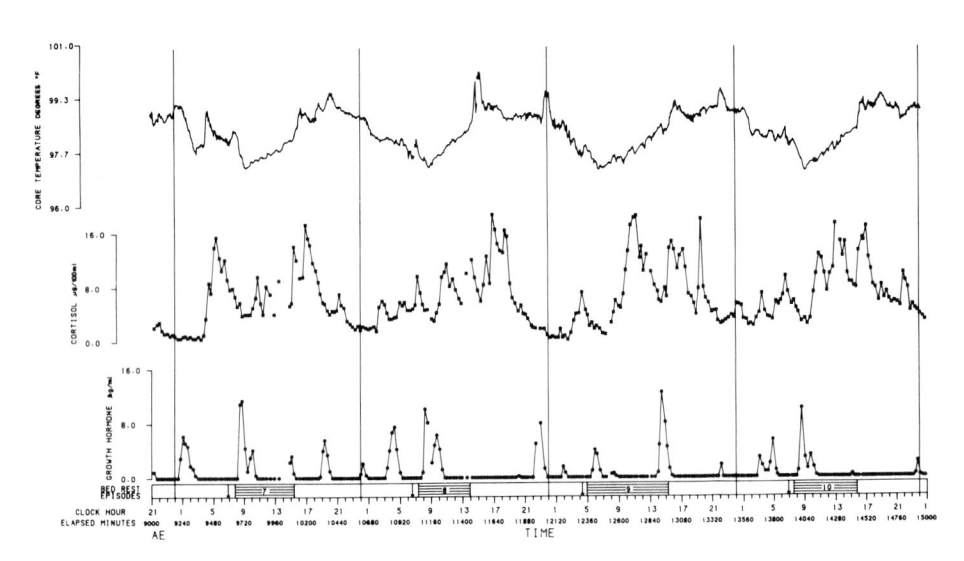

**Figure 13–11.**   Plot of multiple variables recorded under free-running conditions for subject AE. Growth hormone, cortisol, and core temperature are concurrently plotted. Bedrest episodes are indicated by a box for each episode and a downward arrow showing the time that the subject requested sleep.

*Chronobiological disorders: analytic and therapeutic techniques*

day. The next variable is plasma cortisol concentration in mg/100 ml, with a symbol plotted at every data point. It is clear that cortisol and growth hormone do not have episodes occurring at the same time *(47)*. The third variable plotted is core body temperature. In this case, it was chosen to plot the values as a continuous line, an option available to the user.

Because all the biological variables studied are periodic, a useful graphics program is the double-raster plot. This program can display up four variables simultaneously on the same graph. An algorithm filters out a defined range of the periodic function (i.e., any time the function falls within a specified range) and displays the result linearly. Because it is a double plot, on the first line, day 1 is on the left and day 2 on the right. On the next line, day 2 is on the left and day 3 on the right. This process is continued for all the clock days of the study. Figure 13–10 demonstrates an example of activity-rest and sleep-wake data from another subject (DC). The activity data are plotted in counts per 15-minute intervals. In this example, only counts between 0 and 5 are displayed. The sleep-wake data are derived from the scored polysomnographic records. Several plotting routines are used to describe the sleep-stage data. Figure 13–12 is an example of sleep-stage organization for one sleep episode for subject LA. Lights-out and lights-on times are denoted by a down and an up arrow respectively. The graph describes the five stages of sleep, as well as awake, on the y-axis.

As an aid in examining changes that occur in sleep during the course of an experiment, we can graph the total sleep-stage data for the entire study. Figure 13–13 shows a sleep-stage plot of subject AQ for 22 days. In this case, only three states are shown: Awake, REM, and NREM. Awake is the uppermost portion of each small graph, with NREM halfway between Awake and REM. The REM state is denoted by the heavy line drawn below NREM. Each 24-hour clock day is indicated on the y-axis. In this example, it can be seen that REM-onset sleep episodes occurred on clock days 14, 17–20, and 22.

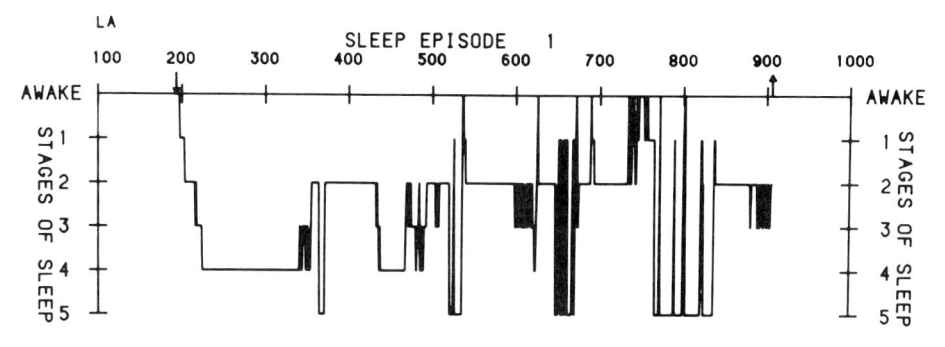

**Figure 13–12.** Sleep-stage organization plot for subject LA. The lights-out and lights-on times are denoted by down and up arrows respectively. The graph shows the five stages of sleep, as well as awake, all on the y-axis.

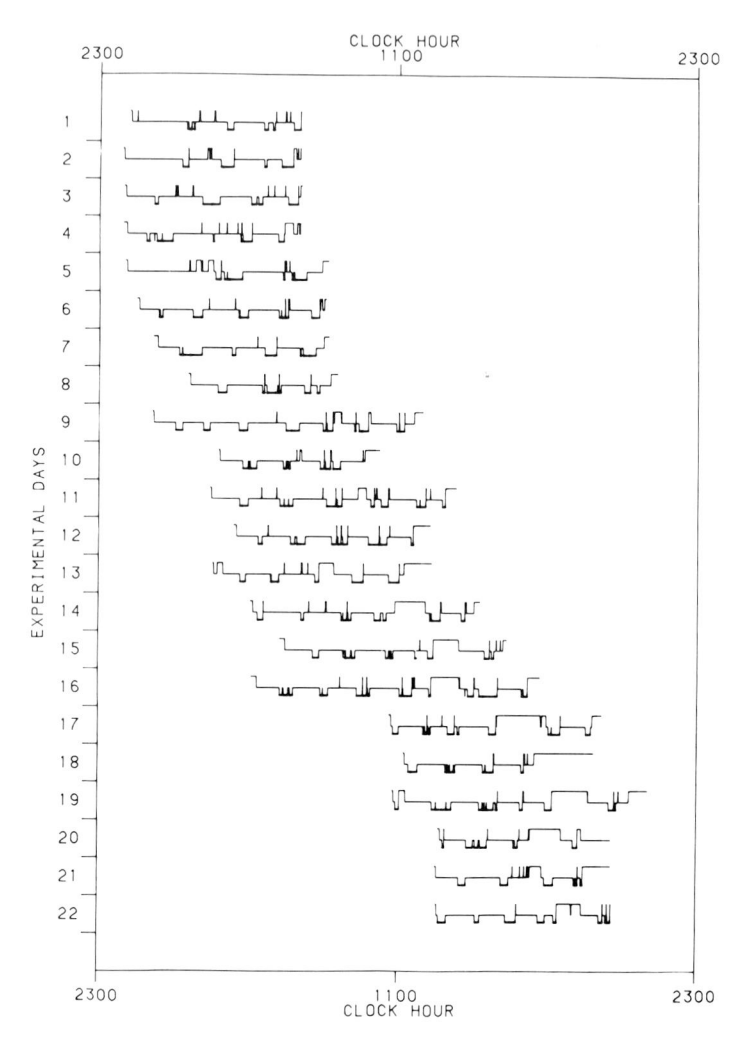

*Sleeping and waking disorders: indications and techniques*

**Figure 13-13.** Sleep-state plot of subject AQ for a 22-day section of his study. There are three states shown here: awake, REM, and NREM. Awake is the uppermost portion of each small graph, with NREM halfway between awake and REM. The REM state is denoted by the heavy line. Each 24-hour day is indicated on the left side of the graph.

A group of individual programs has been developed that generates a series of tables of values. These tables provide quantitative information regarding sleep-stage amounts and percentages, night by night, hour by hour, and across any chosen segments of a study. Some examples are shown in Table 13-1.

*Chronobiological disorders: analytic and therapeutic techniques*

**Table 13–1** Summary Sleep-Stage Statistics Calculated Hour by Hour (A), Night by Night (B) and Averaged Across Nights (C)

A

```
STATS ON F05101 HOUR    1
                #MINUTES  %SLEEP PD TIME  %TOT REC TIME  %TOT SLEEP TIME
------------------------------------------------------------------------
SLEEP PD TIME     60.00       100.00           .00             .00
TOT REC TIME      60.00       100.00         100.00            .00
TOT SLEEP TIME    58.50        97.50          97.50          100.00
WAKE               1.50         2.50           2.50            2.56
STAGE 1            3.00         5.00           5.00            5.13
STAGE 2           18.00        30.00          30.00           30.77
STAGE 3           11.00        18.33          18.33           18.80
STAGE 4           26.50        44.17          44.17           45.30
STAGE 5 REM         .00          .00            .00             .00
MOVEMENT TIME       .00          .00            .00             .00
LOST DATA           .00          .00            .00             .00
SLOW WAVE         37.50        62.50          62.50           64.10
WAKE&MOVEMENT      1.50         2.50           2.50            2.56


STATS ON F05101 HOUR    2
                #MINUTES  %SLEEP PD TIME  %TOT REC TIME  %TOT SLEEP TIME
------------------------------------------------------------------------
SLEEP PD TIME     60.00       100.00           .00             .00
TOT REC TIME      60.00       100.00         100.00            .00
TOT SLEEP TIME    60.00       100.00         100.00          100.00
WAKE                .00          .00            .00             .00
STAGE 1            1.00         1.67           1.67            1.67
STAGE 2           31.00        51.67          51.67           51.67
STAGE 3           14.00        23.33          23.33           23.33
STAGE 4            9.50        15.83          15.83           15.83
STAGE 5 REM        4.50         7.50           7.50            7.50
MOVEMENT TIME       .00          .00            .00             .00
LOST DATA           .00          .00            .00             .00
SLOW WAVE         23.50        39.17          39.17           39.17
WAKE&MOVEMENT       .00          .00            .00             .00
```

B

```
STATS ON F05101
                #MINUTES  %SLEEP PD TIME  %TOT REC TIME  %TOT SLEEP TIME
------------------------------------------------------------------------
SLEEP PD TIME    444.00       100.00           .00             .00
TOT REC TIME     444.00       100.00         100.00            .00
TOT SLEEP TIME   430.00        96.85          96.85          100.00
WAKE              12.00         2.70           2.70            2.79
STAGE 1           20.00         4.50           4.50            4.65
STAGE 2          228.50        51.46          51.46           53.14
STAGE 3           44.50        10.02          10.02           10.35
STAGE 4           51.50        11.60          11.60           11.98
STAGE 5 REM       85.50        19.26          19.26           19.88
MOVEMENT TIME      2.00          .45            .45             .47
LOST DATA           .00          .00            .00             .00
SLOW WAVE         96.00        21.62          21.62           22.33
WAKE&MOVEMENT     14.00         3.15           3.15            3.26
```

C

```
      SL PD  SLEEP  WAKE  STG 1  STG 2  STG 2    3+4   3+4   STG 5  STG 5  MVMT  MVMT
      TIME   TIME   (MIN) (MIN)  (MIN)  %TST    (MIN) %TST   (MIN)  %TST   (MIN) %TST

F05101
      444.0  430.0  12.00 20.00  228.5  53.14   96.00 22.33  85.50  19.88  2.00   .47
F05102
      455.0  442.0   9.00 19.00  170.0  38.46  132.5 29.98  120.5  27.26  4.00   .90
F05103
      449.0  441.5   4.00 49.00  210.5  47.68   75.00 16.99  107.0  24.24  3.50   .79
F05104
      454.0  432.0  17.50 14.00  157.5  36.46  122.5 28.36  138.0  31.94  4.50  1.04

      AVERAGE ACROSS NIGHTS    1 ,   4
      450.5  436.4  10.62 25.50  191.6  43.93  106.5 24.41  112.7  25.83  3.50   .80
      STANDARD DEVIATIONS
        5.07   6.26  5.65 15.89   33.41  7.84   26.04  5.94  22.16   5.08  1.08   .25
      AVERAGES WITH % OF ACTUAL TST
      450.5  436.4  10.62 25.50  191.6  43.91  106.5 24.41  112.7  25.84  3.50   .80
```

*Sleeping and waking disorders: indications and techniques*

To define periodic activity of the data time series, we have developed special mathematical techniques and computer algorithms. One such technique is called the estimate of the *minimum variance (5,7)*. It is based on the intuitive concept that the *variance* of a curve averaged over many periods would be lowest at the "correct" period length. The formula for the estimated mean standard deviation for a specific period length ($\tau$) is:

$$\bar{\sigma}_\tau = \frac{1}{\omega} \sum_{j=1}^{\omega} \sigma_j$$

$\omega$ is the window size (usually set arbitrarily to 1440 data samples).
$\bar{\sigma}_\tau$ is the estimated mean standard deviation at the chosen period length.
$j$ is the displacement within the window.

The following formula is the standard deviation for each point of displacement within the chosen "window."

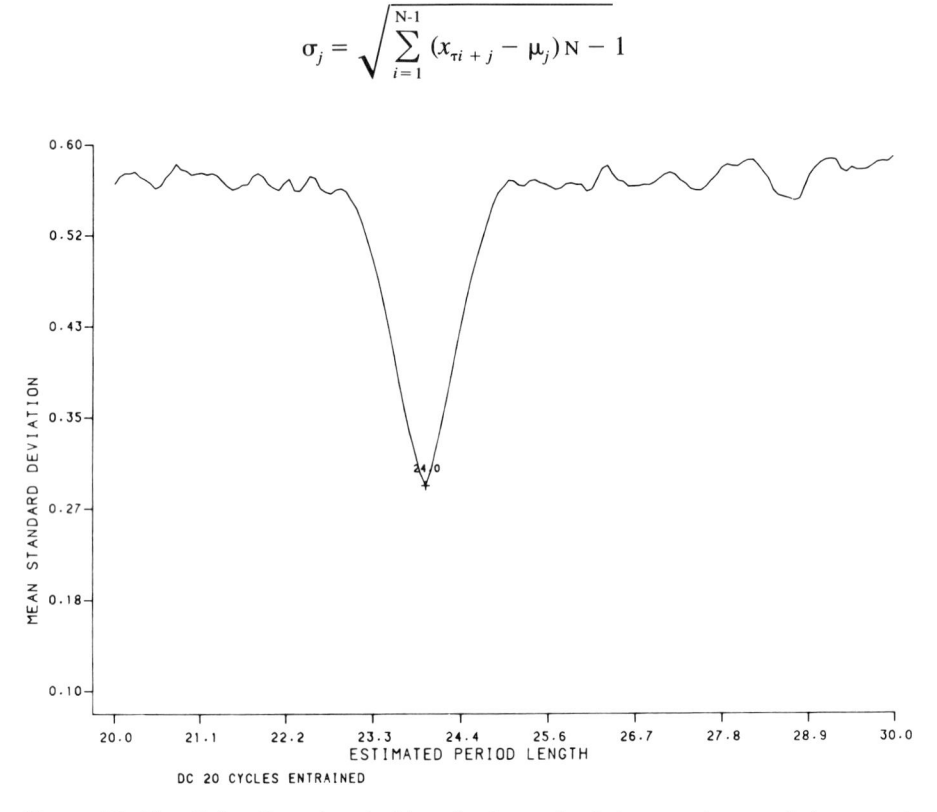

$$\sigma_j = \sqrt{\sum_{i=1}^{N-1} (x_{\tau i + j} - \mu_j) N - 1}$$

**Figure 13–14.** Estimation of period length of core body-temperature cycle by use of minimum-variance technique for subject DC. The x-axis denotes trial period lengths between 20.0 and 30.0 hours. The minimum is seen at 24.0 hours. (see 5,7).

322

*x* is the value of a data point.
N is the number of cycles in the data train.
$\mu_j$ is the mean value of the variable for each point of displacement and is defined as:

$$\mu_j = 1/N \sum_{i=1}^{N-1} x_{\tau i + j}$$

Figure 13–14 demonstrates the graphic result of a minimum-variance analysis on subject DC during days 1–20 for core body temperature. The estimated period lengths tested range between 1200 and 1800 minutes (20.0 and 30.0 hours). A very sharp drop in the mean standard deviation occurs at 1440 minutes (24.0 hours), from a high of 0.55 to a low of 0.29. There are no other large drops during this range. In this case, the subject was entrained to a 24-hour day during this entire experimental period.

Having identified the period length, another special mathematical technique is used to educe the waveform of the data train *(5,7,47)*. This is done by averaging

## TECHNIQUE OF WAVEFORM EDUCTION
PERIOD LENGTH = 26.17 HOURS

AVERAGE S.D. = 0.195 °F

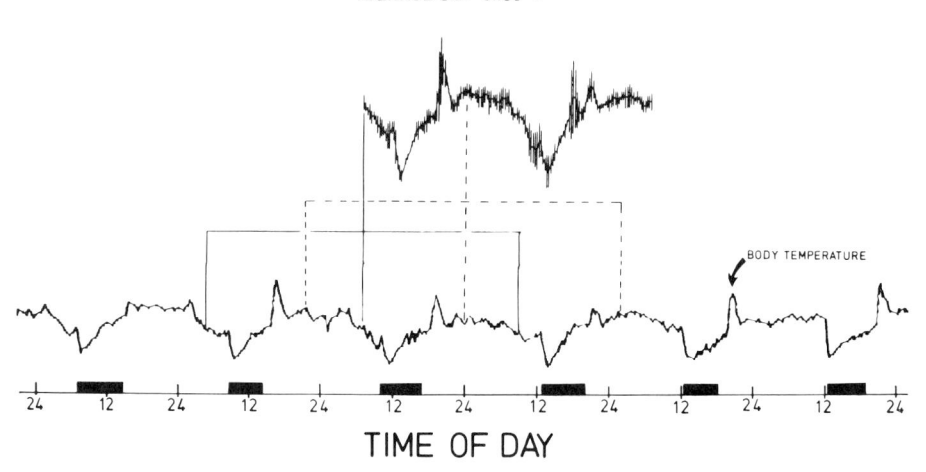

### TIME OF DAY
### LABORATORY OF HUMAN CHRONOPHYSIOLOGY

**Figure 13–15.** Waveform-education technique. The method for determining average waveform is illustrated using the core body temperature for subject AB. The raw data were plotted over time in the lower half of the figure, with sleep episodes indicated by black bars. Temperature values separated by 26.17 hours were averaged together and serially plotted with standard deviation in the upper half of the figure. (From Czeisler *(7)*).

adjacent cycles at the given period length. Every point chosen on the curve of the educed wave has a standard error of the mean associated with it. The formula for the mean value of a given data point for the educed wave is:

$$\bar{x}_j = 1/N \sum_{i=1}^{N-1} x_{\tau i + j}$$

$\tau$ is the period length in minutes.
N is the total number of cycles in the data train.
$j$ is the displacement within the cycle.

Figure 13–15 provides a visual description of the process of obtaining an educed waveform for subject AB, who had a 26.17-hour period length (derived from the minimum-variance algorithm). Figure 13–16 demonstrates an educed waveform of plasma cortisol and the sleep-wake cycle for subject AE during the first four 24-hour entrained days.

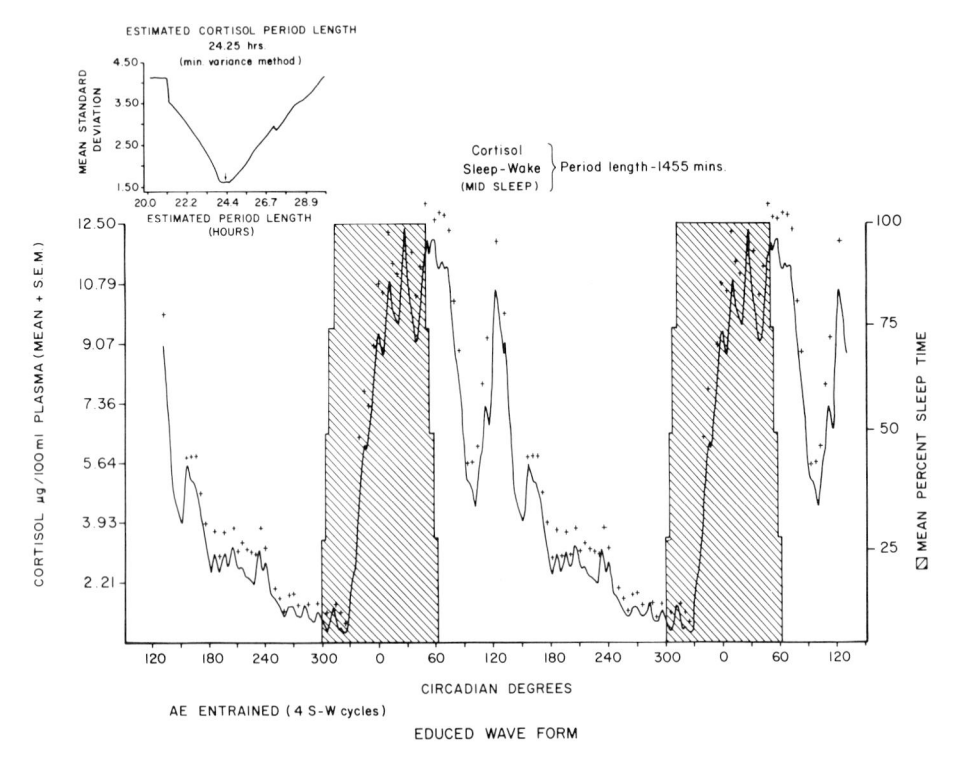

**Figure 13–16.** Educed-waveform and period-length estimate of cortisol level and sleep-wake pattern during entrainment for subject AE. The sleep-pattern-educed waveform was obtained at the same period length as cortisol level and is derived by averaging the percentage of time asleep at each defined data point across the same sequence of circadian cycles.

*Chronobiological disorders: analytic and therapeutic techniques*

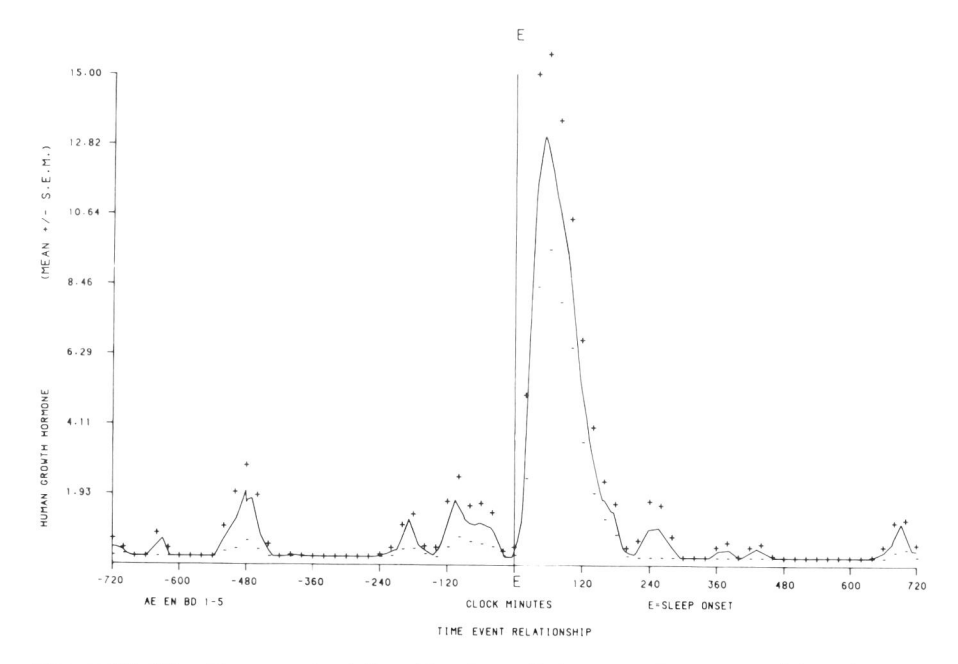

**Figure 13–17.** Time-event relationship of growth hormone (somatotropin) to sleep-episode onset for subject AE during entrained nights 1 to 5. The results are plotted as average growth hormone concentration ± standard error of the mean.

Another technique of analysis (developed here) is the *time-event relationship* (TER). This is used to determine the relationship, if any, of a specific event in time to a particular physiologic variable *(7)*. It is similar in principal to the evoked-response technique used in electrophysiologic studies. Any response of the variable to a defined temporal event will be displayed by averaging values that occur N minutes before and after the event. Figure 13–17 shows a time-event relationship of growth hormone concentration for sleep-onset times for subject AE during 24-hour entrained days 1–5 of the study. There is a large rise in the concentration of the hormone, peaking at approximately 60 minutes after sleep onset. This rise in growth hormone is associated with the occurrence of stages 3–4 sleep.

# Summary

The field of sleep disorders and chronomedicine has now recognized that disorders of the patient's biologic rhythm manifested as a sleep-wake dyssomnia may be a primary cause of specific complaints of insomnia or hypersomnia. In addition, alterations of the daily sleep-wake cycle may be important in a wide variety of other sleep disorders. Emphasis is given in this chapter to methods of assessing abnormalities of these endogenous circadian timing systems. These analytic approaches range from careful clinical methods of history-taking and daily structured sleep-wake logs to sophisticated and elaborate temporal-isolation laboratories and computer-derived statistical data analysis. It is anticipated that recent developments in our understanding of the chronobiology of man's sleep-wake pattern will lead to increasing clinical application in the diagnosis of sleep-wake disorders and new chronotherapeutic regimens.

# REFERENCES

1. DeMairan J. Observation botanique. Paris: Histoire de l'Académie Royale des Sciences. 1729:35.
2. Wever R. The circadian system of man. New York: Springer-Verlag, 1979.
3. Chouvet G, Mouret J, Coindet J, Siffre M, Jouvet M. Périodicité bicircadienne du cycle veille-sommeil dans des conditions hors du temps. Electroencephalogr Clin Neurophysiol 1974; 37:367–80.
4. Aschoff J, Wever R. Human circadian rhythms: a multioscillatory system. Fed Proc 1976; 35:2326–32.
5. Weitzman ED, Czeisler CA, Moore-Ede M. Sleep-wake, neuroendocrine and body temperature circadian rhythms under entrained and non-entrained (free-running) conditions in man. In: Suda M, Hayaishi O, Nakagawa H, eds. Biological rhythms and their central mechanism. New York: Elsevier North-Holland 1979:199–227.
6. Aschoff J. Desynchronization and resynchronization of human circadian rhythms. Aerospace Med 1969; 40:844–9.
7. Czeisler CA. Human circadian physiology: internal organization of temperature, sleep-wake and neuroendocrine function in an environment free of time cues. PhD dissertation, Stanford University, 1978.
8. Czeisler CA, Richardson GS, Zimmerman JC, Moore-Ede MC, Weitzman ED. Entrainment of human circadian rhythms by light-dark cycles: a reassessment. Photochem Photobiol, in press.
9. Weitzman ED, Pollak CP, McGregor P. The polysomnographic evaluation of sleep disorders in man. In: Aminoff MJ, ed. Electrophysiological approaches to neurological diagnosis. New York: Churchill Livingstone, 1980:496–524.
10. Weitzman ED, Czeisler CA, Moore-Ede MC. Sleep-wake, endocrine and temperature rhythms in man during temporal isolation. In: Johnson LC,

Tepas DI, Colquhoun WP, Colligan MJ, eds. Variations in work-sleep schedules: effects on health and performance. Advances in sleep research. Vol 7. New York: Spectrum, in press.

11. Weitzman ED, Kripke DF. Experimental 12-hour shift of the sleep-wake cycle in man: effects on sleep and physiologic rhythms. In: Johnson LC, Tepas DI, Colquhoun WP, Colligan MJ, eds. Variations in work-sleep schedules: effects on health and performance. Advances in sleep research. Vol 7. New York: Spectrum, in press.

12. Weitzman ED, Czeisler CA, Zimmerman JC, Moore-Ede MC. Biological rhythms in man: relationship of sleep-wake, cortisol, growth hormone and temperature during temporal isolation. In: Martin JB, Reichlin S, Bick K, eds. Advances in neurology. New York: Raven Press, in press.

13. Weitzman ED. Sleep and its disorders. Annu Rev Neurosci 1981; 4:381–409.

14. Wagner DR, Weitzman ED. Neuroendocrine secretion and biological rhythms in man. In: Holmes DD, ed. Psychiatric clinics of North America. Vol. 3, No. 2. Philadelphia: WB Saunders, 1980:223–50.

15. Weitzman ED. Neuroendocrine rhythms and the sleep cycle. In: Van Praag HM, ed. Handbook of biological psychiatry. Part III: brain mechanisms and abnormal behavior—genetics and neuroendocrinology. New York: Marcel Dekker, 1980:310–41.

16. Weitzman ED. Disorders of sleep and the sleep-wake cycle. In: Martin JB, ed. Update I: Harrison's principles of internal medicine. New York: McGraw Hill, 1981:245–63.

17. Czeisler CA, Weitzman ED, Moore-Ede MC, Kronauer RE, Zimmerman JC, Campbell C. Human sleep: its duration and structure depend on the interaction of two separate circadian oscillators. Sleep Res, in press (abstract).

18. Czeisler CA, Weitzman ED, Moore-Ede MC, Zimmerman JC, Knauer RS. Human sleep: its duration and organization depend on its circadian phase. Science 1980; 210:1264–67.

19. Weitzman ED, Czeisler CA, Zimmerman JC, Ronda JM. Timing of REM and stages 3+4 sleep during temporal isolation in man. Sleep 1980; 2:391–407.

20. Czeisler CA, Zimmerman JC, Ronda JM, Moore-Ede MC, Weitzman ED. Timing of REM sleep is coupled to the circadian rhythm of body temperature in man. Sleep 1980; 2:329–46.

21. Åkerstedt T, Gillberg M. The circadian pattern of unrestricted sleep and its relation to body temperature, hormones and alertness. Proceedings of the 1979 ONR/NIOSH symposium on variation in work-sleep schedules: effects on health and performance. In: Tepas DI, Johnson LC, eds. Advances in sleep research. Vol 6. New York: Spectrum Publications, in press.

22. Weitzman E, Kripke D, Goldmacher D, McGregor P, Nogeire C. Acute reversal of the sleep-waking cycle in man. Arch Neurol 1970; 22:483–9.

23. Klein KE, Hermann H, Kuklinski P, Wegmann HM, 1977. Circadian per-

formance rhythms: experimental studies in air operation. In: Mackie RR, ed. Vigilance: theory, operational performance and physiological correlates. New York & London: Plenum Press, 1977:117–32.
24. Hume KI. Sleep adaptation after phase shifts of the sleep-wakefulness rhythm in man. Sleep 1980; 2:417–35.
25. Weitzman E, Czeisler C, Coleman R, Dement W, Richardson G, Pollak C. Delayed sleep phase syndrome: a biological rhythm disorder. Sleep Res 1979; 8:221.
26. Weitzman ED, Pollak CP. Disorders of the circadian sleep-wake cycle. Med Times 1979; 107:83–94.
27. Czeisler CA, Richardson GS, Coleman R, et al. Chronotherapy: resetting the circadian clocks of patients with delayed sleep phase insomnia. Sleep 1981; 4:1–21.
28. Weitzman ED, Czeisler CA, Coleman RM, et al. Delayed sleep phase syndrome: a chronobiologic disorder with sleep onset insomnia. Arch Gen Psychiatry, in press.
29. Wehr T, Wirz-Justice A, Goodwin RK, Duncan W, Gillin JC. Phase advance of the circadian sleep-wake cycle as an anti-depressant. Science 1979; 206:710–11.
30. Vogel GW, Thurmond A, Gibbons P, Sloan K, Boyd M, Walker M. REM sleep reduction effects on depression syndromes. Arch Gen Psychiatry 1975; 32:765–77.
31. Rudolf GAE, Schilgen B, Tolle R. Anti-depressive behandlung mittels schlafentzug. Nervenarzt 1977; 48:1–11.
32. Vogel GW, Vogel F, McAbee RS, Thurmond AJ. Improvement of depression by REM sleep deprivation. Arch Gen Psychiatry 1980; 37:247–53.
33. Association of Sleep Disorders Centers. Diagnostic classification of sleep and arousal disorders. 1st ed. Prepared by the Sleep Disorders Classification Committee, HP Roffwarg, chairman. Sleep 1979; 2:1–137.
34. Rentos PG, Shephard RD, eds. Shift work and health: a symposium. Washington, DC: National Institute for Occupational Safety and Health, Office of Extramural Activities, 1976.
35. Weitzman ED. Sleep and aging. In: Katzman R, Terry R, eds. Neurology of aging. Philadelphia: FA Davis, 1981, in press.
36. Lewis SA. Sleep patterns during afternoon naps in the young and elderly. Br J Psychiatry 1969; 115:107–8.
37. Kokkoris CP, Weitzman ED, Pollak CP, Spielman AJ, Czeisler CA, Bradlow H. Long-term ambulatory temperature monitoring in a subject with a hypernychthemeral sleep-wake cycle disturbance. Sleep 1978; 1:177–90.
38. Miles LEM, Raynal DM, Wilson MA. Blind man living in normal society has circadian rhythms of 24.9 hours. Science 1977; 198:421–3.
39. Weber AL, Cary MS, Connor N, Keyes P. Human non-24-hour sleep-wake cycles in an everyday environment. Sleep 1980; 2:347–54.
40. Regestein Q. Treating insomnia: a practical guide for managing chronic sleeplessness, circa 1975. Compr Psychiatry 1976; 17:517–26.

41. Sawyer J. Insomnia: its causes and treatment. 2nd ed. Birmingham: Cornish Bros, 1912:92.
42. Worster-Drought C. The treatment of insomnia: therapeutic measures. Lancet 1927; 213:767–8.
43. Weitzman ED, Czeisler CA, Spielman AJ, Fiss M, Zimmerman JC. Chronotherapy treatment of a patient with a combined chronic short sleep period and delayed sleep phase syndrome. Sleep Res, in press (abstract).
44. Rechtschaffen A, Kales A, eds. A manual of standardized terminology, techniques and scoring system for sleep stages of human subjects. Los Angeles: UCLA Brain Information Service/Brain Research Institute, 1968. (Also available as NIH Publ 204, US government printing office, Washington, DC, 1968.)
45. Reinarz JA. Nosocomial infections. CIBA Clin Symp 1978; 30:2–32.
46. Thayer RE. Measurement of activation through self-report. Psychol Rep 1967; 20:663–78.
47. Weitzman ED, Czeisler CA, Zimmerman JC, Ronda JM. The sleep-wake pattern of cortisol and growth hormone secretion during non-entrained (free-running) conditions in man. In: Nijhoff M, ed. Circadian and ultradian variations of pituitary hormones in man. Brussels, Belgium: in press.

# FOURTEEN
# MEASUREMENT OF GASTROESOPHAGEAL REFLUX DURING SLEEP BY ESOPHAGEAL pH MONITORING

WILLIAM C. ORR
CYNTHIA BOLLINGER
MONTE STAHL

## Introduction

Gastroesophageal reflux (GER) is a common problem associated with considerable morbidity. Recent studies have shown that the highest incidence of esophagitis, as well as the most severe forms (erosion and stricture), are associated with recumbent reflux occurring during sleep, a situation permitting prolonged acid-mucosal contact *(1,2)*. This is presumably due not only to an incompetent lower esophageal sphincter, but also to an inability to effectively clear the refluxed material. It is well known that a variety of physiologic phenomena are substantially altered during sleep, and it is felt that the study of esophageal function during sleep (using appropriate techniques for studying sleep physiology) will significantly improve our understanding of the pathophysiology of esophageal reflux and esophagitis.

Gastroesophageal reflux may be experimentally viewed as consisting of two components: *(a)* the regurgitation of acid gastric juice through the anti-reflux barrier at the esophago-gastric (EG) junction, and *(b)* the return of the acid gastric juice to the stomach (i.e., esophageal acid clearing).

In asymptomatic control volunteers, studies of gastroesophageal reflux using an intraesophageal pH probe have shown that the EG junction is competent to prevent reflux of acid gastric juice while sleeping in a recumbent position. If nocturnal reflux episodes do occur in recumbency, acid gastric juice is rapidly cleared from the esophagus. In contrast, patients with symptomatic reflux have increased acid exposure at night while asleep *(1,2)*. This may result from an increased number of reflux episodes as well as from delayed esophageal acid clearing. When numbers of acid exposures measured while awake in an upright position were compared with those while sleeping recumbent, it was shown that frequent episodes of reflux that cleared rapidly (upright posture) were less caustic to esophageal epithelium than fewer episodes of reflux that were poorly cleared (recumbent posture). Additionally, the highest incidence of esophagitis (all grades), as well as the most severe forms (erosions and strictures), were associated with recumbent reflux occurring during sleep *(2)*. Sleep-associated GER permits prolonged acid-mucosal contact owing to the delayed esophageal clearing of the refluxed acid gastric juice. These studies suggest that the inability of the esophagus to clear refluxed stomach contents while asleep is a major cause of esophagitis.

To date, there has been limited physiologic monitoring of esophageal acid clearing during sleep. Recent studies have shown that the rate of swallowing diminishes from 73 per hour while awake to only 7 per hour while asleep *(3,4)*. Evaluation of esophageal peristalsis or acid clearance was not done in these studies. More recently, a study by Dent et al. *(5)* showed that episodes of reflux during sleep in normals were generally associated with brief arousals from sleep.

The esophageal clearing of 15 mL of 0.1 N HCl (acid clearance test) has been extensively studied. Symptomatic reflux patients required more than ten swallows to clear this bolus of acid from the esophagus, as opposed to asymptomatic control volunteers, who cleared the identical bolus with three to four swallows. However, the acid clearance test has only been performed on individuals while awake. There is a strong suggestion that primary esophageal peristaltic waves are responsible for acid clearing during sleep because the number of swallows to clear a 15 mL bolus of 0.1 N HCl from the esophagus while awake significantly correlates with the mean duration of reflux episodes observed during sleep *(1)*. A recent study in our laboratory has documented prolonged acid clearance times during sleep in both esophagitis patients and asymptomatic controls *(6)*. In addition, the patients showed significantly longer clearance times while awake as well as with arousals (provoked by acid infusion) from sleep. The patients showed shortened arousal latencies subsequent to acid infusion, indicating a more acid-sensitive esophagus.

A significant factor in the morbidity associated with GER is the occurrence of pulmonary aspiration and its complications, e.g., pneumonitis, aspiration pneumonia, and bronchiectasis. Common symptoms associated with this condition are unexplained nocturnal cough, hypoxemia, and awakening with heartburn and a sour taste in the mouth *(7)*.

The documentation of gastroesophageal reflux during sleep, as well as the efficiency of acid clearance, can be a useful diagnostic tool. Although such studies are not indicated frequently, their availability greatly enhances the diagnostic capabilities of both the pulmonary physician and the gastroenterologist.

## Methodology

The esophageal pH is monitored with standard stomach pH probes, which are commercially available from the Beckman Instrument Company or from Microelectrodes, Inc. (see appendixes). The pH probe is swallowed, generally nasally, and the distal tip is placed approximately 5 cm above the lower esophageal sphincter (LES). The sphincter location is determined by performing an esophageal-motility evaluation prior to the overnight study and determining the high-pressure zone that exists between the stomach and esophagus (LES). The pH probe is then placed 5 cm above this high-pressure zone. If the manometry study is not done, the position for the probe during the overnight study should be 32 cm. This measurement can be appropriately altered if the person is over 75 inches in height.

A reference lead is placed on the ventral surface of the forearm (Appendix 14–A). The reference lead and the pH probe are then connected to an electrical isolation box, which is attached to the pH meter.* This measurement is made simultaneously with the standard polygraphic measurements for monitoring sleep, i.e., EEG, EOG, EMG, ECG. A ground electrode is placed on a nonactive site (usually a bony prominence such as the forehead or mastoid).

Two approaches can be taken to the monitoring of esophageal pH. One involves the more prolonged monitoring of esophageal pH to determine the frequency and duration of gastroesophageal reflux. Here it is recommended that recordings last for at least 12 hours, and preferably 24 hours. Complete polygraphic recordings are necessary only during the sleeping interval. We believe that the actual documentation of sleep-related reflux is an important parameter. Reflux is identified by a drop in the pH of the distal esophagus below 4.0. Clearance is arbitrarily defined as a return of the esophageal pH to 5.0 or above. The time between the drop in pH below 4.0 and its return to 5.0 is referred to as the clearing duration, or clearance interval. It is considered clinically significant if the total amount of clearance time occurring in a 24-hour interval exceeds 2%.

In our laboratory, the technique for evaluating esophageal function during sleep has been somewhat different. We have chosen to evaluate the phenomenon of clearance rather than reflux per se. Our protocol consists of infusing 15 mL of 0.1 N HCl during sleep, and evaluating the clearance time (the interval between a drop below 4.0 and return to 5.0). The acid is infused through a small polyethylene tube, which is affixed to the side of the pH probe (Appendix 14–D). After intubation, the patient undergoes two presleep infusions. The first (ad lib infusion) consists of infusing 15 mL of 0.1 N HCl into the distal esophagus over a one-minute time period. Do not let the patient

---

*The pH meter can be purchased from Beckman Instruments Co. or Corning, Inc. (Appendix 14–B), but any commercially available pH meter is suitable.

become aware of the infusion and do not instruct him to swallow. For all infusions, note on the paper record the following:

1. Start of infusion.
2. End of infusion.
3. pH value before and after infusion.
4. Time of infusion.
5. Time pH returns to 5.0 or over.

Record swallowing until after acid is cleared (pH of 5.0 or greater) or until 20 minutes have passed. If the patient has not cleared at this time, infuse 15 mL of sterile water. Wait five minutes before initiating the next infusion.

The second infusion is called the standard acid clearance test. First, tell the patient not to swallow except on command. Infuse 15 mL of 0.1 N HCl. Instruct the patient to swallow once and mark the chart. Request the patient to swallow every 20 seconds until the pH returns to 5.0. If the patient fails to clear within 12–15 swallows, infuse 15 mL of sterile water before beginning the next infusion.

After the patient is asleep, infuse 15 mL of 0.1 N HCl over one minute approximately once per hour during sleep. Do not start another infusion unless *(a)* the pH has gone to 5.0 or above, or *(b)* one hour has passed with the pH below 5.0. Again, if the patient has not cleared within one hour, infuse sterile water before beginning the next infusion. Allow 20 minutes between the time pH returns to 5.0 or above and the next acid infusion. Acid should be infused four to six times during sleep, and each clearance interval assessed. Clearance intervals exceeding 30 minutes are considered abnormal, although there is considerable variability. In general, patients considered at high risk for pulmonary aspiration and/or the development of severe esophagitis have clearing times exceeding 45 minutes to one hour.

## Spontaneous Reflux

Another parameter noted during the night is episodes of spontaneous reflux. This occurs when the pH drops below 4.0 even though no infusion has taken place, because the patient has refluxed acid from the stomach into the esophagus. Again, the number of such episodes and the time to clear to a pH of 5.0 are parameters of interest. In our experience, two or more episodes of spontaneous reflux during an overnight recording are considered abnormal.

There are several methods of quickly determining the occurrence of spontaneous reflux. First, have only the pH recording cabled into a separate recorder operating at a slower paper speed. Second, have the monitor check readings from the pH meter every 15 minutes. If a reflux episode is missed, it will have been less than 15 minutes in duration. Third, have the monitor constantly watch the pH reading and note the spontaneous reflux episodes in the log book. This method is not totally accurate and

*Measurement of gastroesophageal reflex during sleep by esophageal pH monitoring*

should not be the only one relied on because the monitor may miss some of the reflux episodes. We use all of these techniques in our laboratory. The most effective method of identifying reflux episodes is to use a supplemental pH recording at a slow paper speed (approximately 1 cm per minute). This allows a more condensed view of the overnight pH recording. A drop in pH level to below 4.0 that is not associated with acid infusion can be assumed to be caused by an episode of spontaneous reflux. (Transient drops in pH are most often due to movement artifact. Episodes of true GER will generally last at least two to three minutes.)

# APPENDIX 14–A

## Equipment

There are many reliable pH meters that can be purchased for less than $1000. Before purchasing a meter, determine whether it is compatible with electrodes from Microelectrodes, Inc., or with Beckman stomach electrodes. Either type of electrode may be used and there are advantages to each. The Microelectrode electrodes are less expensive as well as smaller and more flexible, which makes them more comfortable for long-term use. However, intubation is slightly easier with Beckman electrodes. Both require a reference electrode attached to the forearm. The Beckman reference electrode is larger and more cumbersome than the Microelectrode reference.

Equipment used in our laboratory:

Beckman pH meter—Electromate model #1009.
Beckman stomach electrode with long lead—item #39042.
Beckman small junction calomel reference electrode with eight-foot lead—item #41239.
Microelectrode stomach electrode with five-foot cable—item #MI500.
Microflexible reference electrode—item #LI402.
Patient isolation box available from either Microelectrodes, Inc., or Beckman Instruments, Inc..
Buffer, available from Beckman or most hospital suppliers (pH of 1.0, 4.01, 7.0).

Equipment settings:

Using a Grass model 78 polygraph, the settings should be as follows:

Signal comes from "Record Out" on back of pH meter to "$J_1$ input $J_2$" on a DC driver amplifier model 7DAC. Amplifier settings are: Polarity "-up use," 1/2 amp high-frequency ".5", driver sensitivity–variable, baseline–variable. Signal now comes out of DC driver amp at $J_6$ and into $J_5$ on an AC amplifier model 7P511. This step is not necessary if you have an oscillograph and pen for this amplifier.

# APPENDIX 14–B

Addresses:   Beckman Instruments, Inc.
Scientific Instruments Division
Campus Drive at Jamboree Boulevard
P. O. Box B-19600
Irvine, California 92713
(714) 833-0751

Microelectrodes, Inc.
Grenier Industrial Village
Londonderry, New Hampshire 03053
(603) 668-0692

Corning, Inc.
63 North Street
Medfield, Massachusetts 02052

# APPENDIX 14–C

## Application of Reference Electrode for Overnight Studies

1. Clean the volar (nonhairy) surface of the arm thoroughly with acetone and gauze.
2. Roll a 4 × 4 gauze pad and place it across the arm perpendicular to the axis of the forearm. Tape this roll of gauze in place.

*Measurement of gastroesophageal reflex during sleep by esophageal pH monitoring*

3. Place the reference electrode perpendicular to the gauze roll so that the tip of the electrode touches the surface of the forearm. The reference electrode should rest at an angle of approximately 30°. Using Micropore (or comparable) tape, secure the top part of the reference electrode to the gauze pad by wrapping the tape completely around the arm.
4. Place a large mound of electrode paste around the tip of the electrode. (We use EEG electrode jelly.) Do not hesitate to place a lot of paste around the electrode.
5. Place another 4 × 4 inch gauze pad lightly over the top of the electrode and paste. Secure the bottom part of the gauze pad to the arm by circling it with tape.
6. Place a piece of plastic (Saran) wrap completely around this preparation.
7. Wrap the preparation completely with a Kling bandage and secure the gauze in place by wrapping tape around the arm and gauze bandage two to three times.
8. Place some tape around the arm at the point where the cable emerges from the wrapping to fix the reference electrode lead to the arm so that it will not put any tension on the electrode.

# APPENDIX 14–D

## Attachment of Infusion Tubing to pH Electrode

1. Cut the end of the polyurethane tubing (5 mm) on a diagonal. This tapers the end close to the probe tip.
2. Measure up 5 cm from the tip of the tubing.
3. Heat an opened paper clip and make a hole through the tubing. The hole should be made in such a manner that when the tubing is glued onto the probe, the hole will be open to allow infusion of liquid (Figures 14–1 and 14–2).
4. This portion of the procedure involves using a syringe and needle. Pour the glue into the syringe, then place the needle in the tapered end of the tubing and fill with glue. This closes the end of the tubing, causing the infused liquid to go out the hole made during step 3. Fill the last one inch of tubing with glue (Figure 14–3).

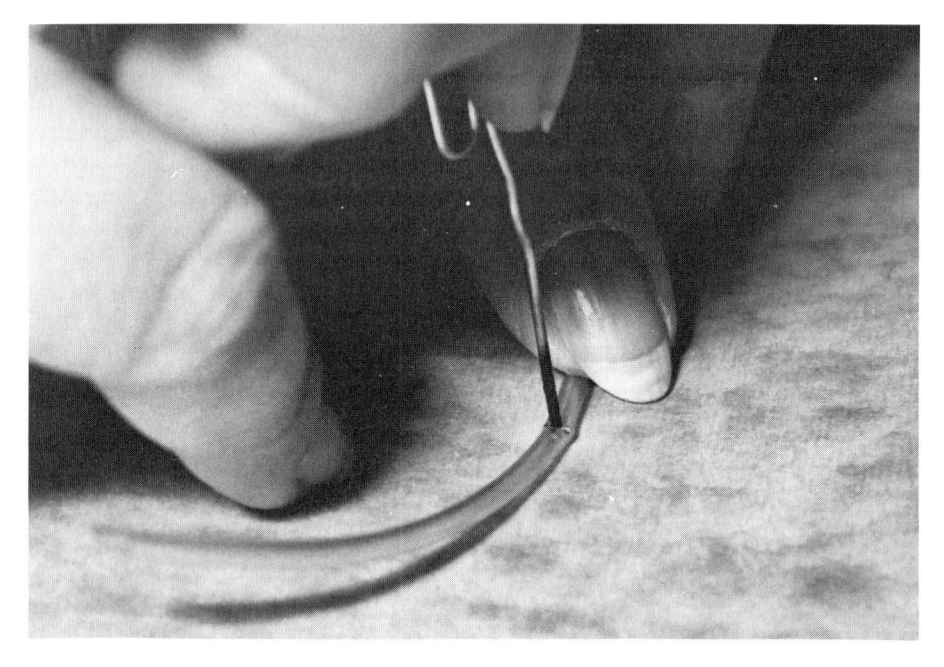

*Sleeping and waking disorders: indications and techniques*

**Figure 14–1.**

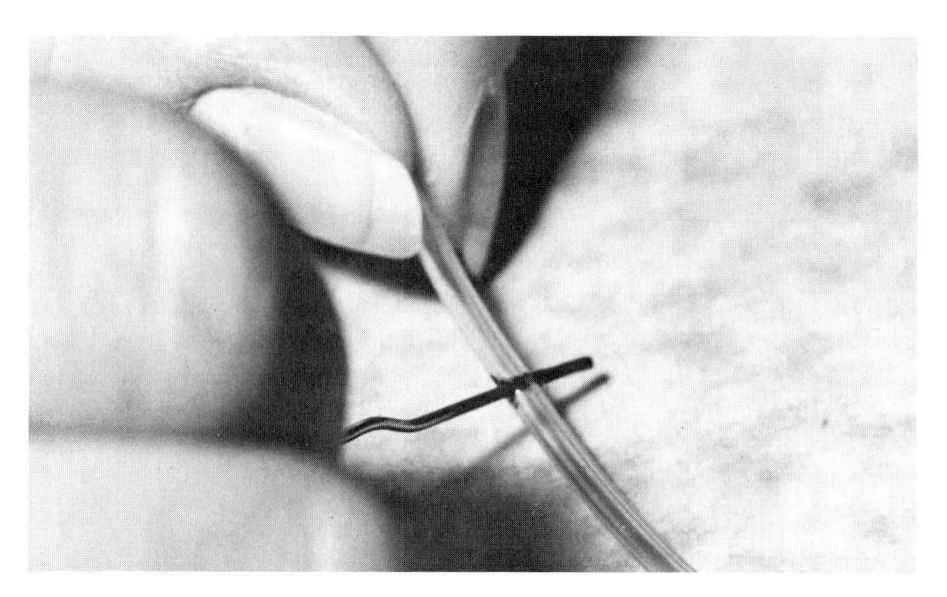

**Figure 14–2.**

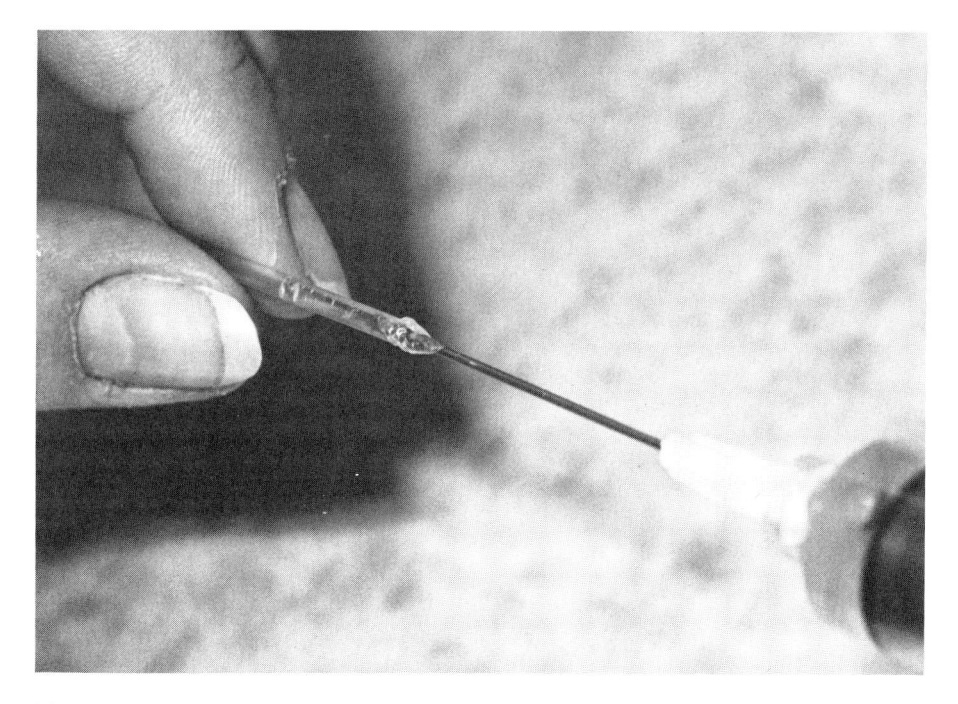

*Measurement of gastroesophageal reflex during sleep by esophageal pH monitoring*

**Figure 14–3.**

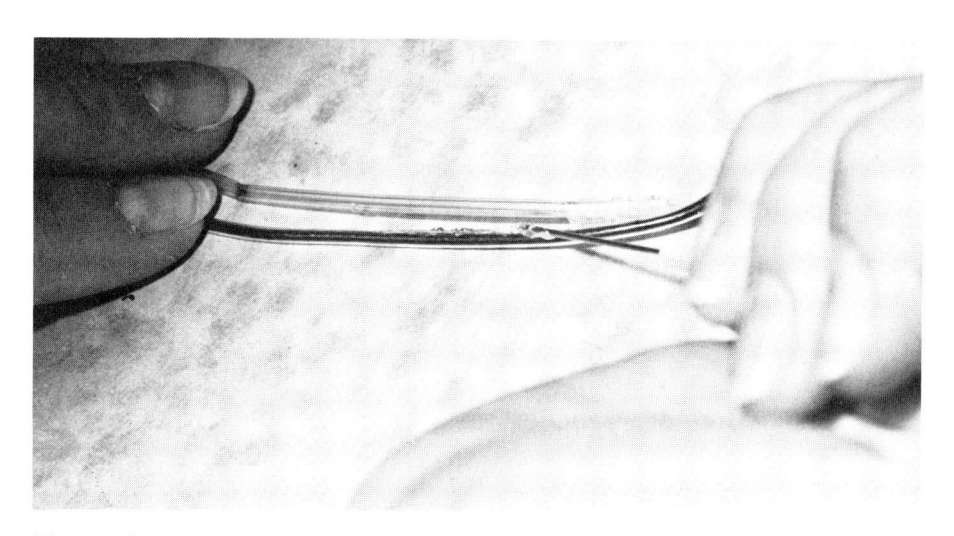

**Figure 14–4.**

*Sleeping and waking disorders: indications and techniques*

5. Allow the glue to dry about ten minutes.
6. Now glue the tubing to the probe, positioning the infusion hole 5–6 cm above the tip of the pH probe. The tip of the tubing and the tip of the probe should be approximately side by side. Place some glue on the tubing to be attached to the probe. Then hold the tubing to the probe with your fingers until it begins to adhere (three to five minutes). Continue this procedure until 26 inches have been attached (Figures 14–4 and 14–5).
7. At this point, lay the probe down and fill in any gaps (Figure 14–6).
8. Allow 24 hours for the glue to dry.
9. Figures 14–7 and 14–8 indicate the appearance of the pH probe before and after the polyurethane tubing has been attached.

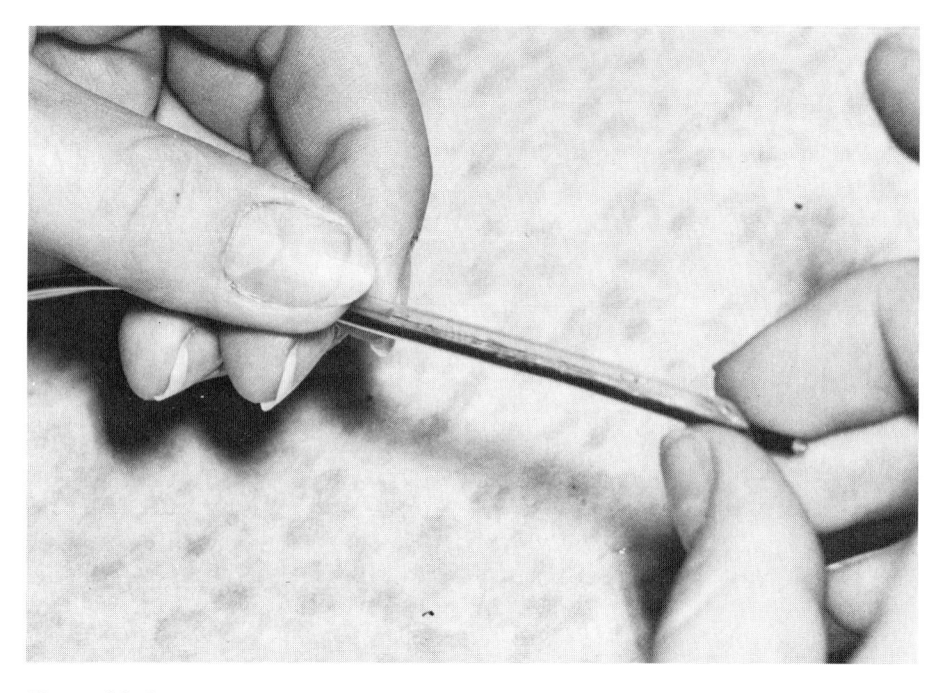

**Figure 14–5.**

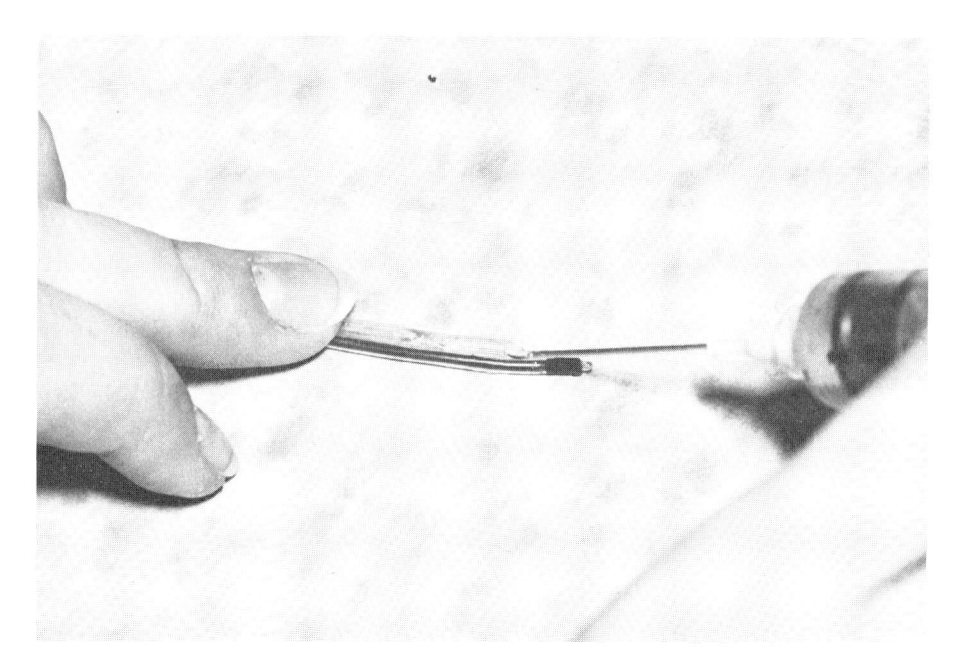

*Measurement of gastroesophageal reflex during sleep by esophageal pH monitoring*

**Figure 14–6.**

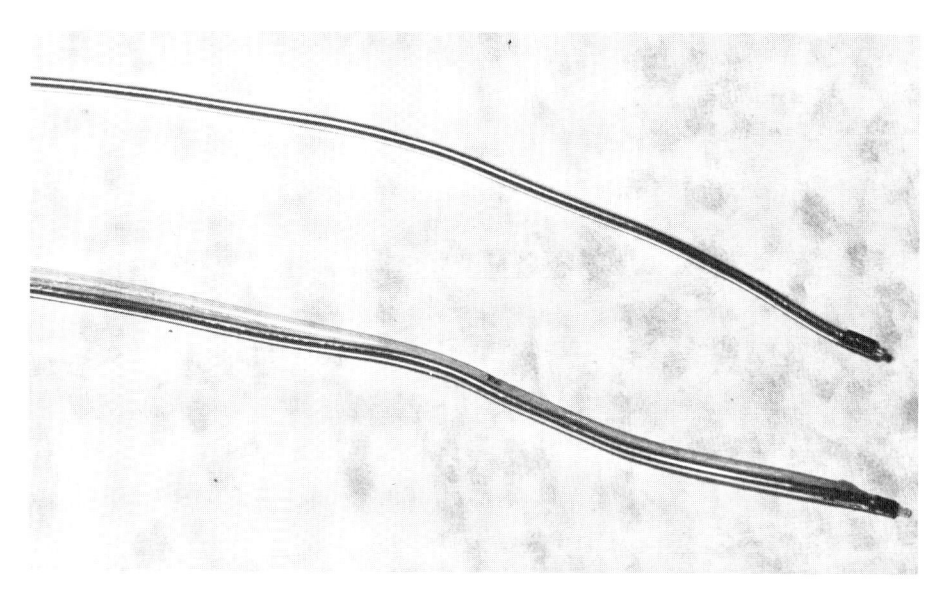

**Figure 14–7.**

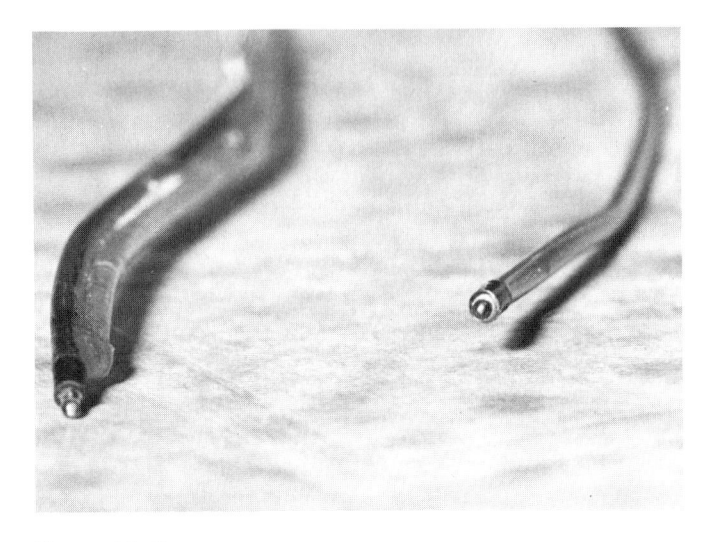

**Figure 14–8.**

# REFERENCES

1. Johnson LF, DeMeester TR. Twenty-four hour pH monitoring of the distal esophagus: a quantitative measure of gastroesophageal reflux. Am J Gastroenterol 1974; 62:325–32.
2. Johnson LF, DeMeester TR, Haggit RC. Esophageal epithelial response to gastroesophageal reflux: a quantitative study. Am J Dig Dis 1978; 23:478–509.
3. Lichter J, Muir RC. The pattern of swallowing during sleep. Electroencephalogr Clin Neurophysiol 1975; 38:427–32.
4. Leon CSC, Flanagan JB Jr, Moorrees CFA. The frequency of deglutition in man. Arch Oral Biol 1965; 10:83–96.
5. Dent J, Dodds WJ, Friedman RH, et al. Mechanism of gastroesophageal reflux in recumbent asymptomatic human subjects. J Clin Invest 1980; 65:256–67.
6. Orr WC, Robinson MG, Johnson LF. Acid clearing during sleep in the pathogenesis of reflux esophagitis. Dig Dis Sci, in press.
7. Bynum LJ, Pierce AK. Pulmonary aspiration of gastric contents. Am Rev Respir Dis 1976; 14:1129–36.

# FIFTEEN
# EVALUATION OF NOCTURNAL PENILE TUMESCENCE AND IMPOTENCE

ISMET KARACAN

## Rationale for the Evaluation

Methods of evaluating, diagnosing, and treating erectile impotence have progressed phenomenally during the past decade. The movement had its genesis in the liberalization of attitudes toward sex that characterized the late 1960s. Many men and women came to believe that it was socially acceptable, if not mandatory, to actively seek qualified help with sexual problems; physicians and scientists discovered that professional interest in sexual matters was no longer as taboo as it had been. Patients' demands for effective treatment spurred improvements in the variety, sophistication, and accessibility of management techniques. By the mid-1970s, for example, treatments for impotence as divergent as behavioral therapy and implantation of a penile prosthesis were widely available. In turn, such advances stimulated a critical examination of the diagnostic process: The existence of a variety of treatments creates a need for careful decisions about which patients receive which treatments; rational decision making is possible only if the diagnostic process equals or exceeds the treatment process in refinement. Many who examined the contemporary procedure for evaluating and diagnosing impotence found it wanting.

The goal of the contemporary procedure was to determine whether a patient's impotence had primarily organic or psychologic origins. To reach this goal, one was typically instructed (1,2) to perform a thorough physical examination to detect relevant physical pathology, and to evaluate the history and characteristics of the complaint to detect presumed symptoms of psychogenic impotence. The symptoms most often listed were the sudden initial onset of impotence, the selective occurrence of impotence, and the persistence of at least occasional spontaneous, masturbatory, or morning erections. Positive physical findings indicated physicogenic impotence, positive psychologic findings indicated psychogenic impotence, and a combination of the two indicated impotence of mixed etiology. In practice, psychogenic impotence was the usual default diagnosis if signs and symptoms were unremarkable.

It is important to note that with this procedure, an accurate differential diagnosis depended directly both on success in identifying relevant physical and psychologic signs and symptoms and on the validity of the assumed relationship between observed signs and symptoms and the nature of the complaint of impotence. Unfortunately, it was a mistake to trust either the sensitivity of the recommended detection methods or the assumption of a link between findings and complaint. Two overriding reasons were the lack of adequate data on the physical and psychologic causes of impotence and, especially in the case of physical causes, the lack of instruments and techniques for locating them. Relying on a routine physical examination to reveal relevant physical pathology was unsatisfactory both because the physical evaluation was too superficial to assure that all relevant physical processes had been examined and because it was impossible to know whether or not positive findings were actually relevant. Relying on the suggested method of assessing psychologic factors introduced greater error. The method was even more superficial than the physical examination, for it included no explicit mention of a thorough evaluation of the patient's psychologic status. Worse, there had been no known study of whether or not the critical symptoms are indeed indicative of psychogenic impotence; it is arguable that they may just as well characterize certain types of physicogenic impotence. But even if a thorough psychologic evaluation were performed, the state of knowledge was such that, as with the physical examination, it was impossible to know whether or not a positive finding truly had etiologic relevance.

Significantly lacking in the recommended procedure was an instruction to verify the patient's complaint of inadequate erection by directly examining his erect penis. Exposing the patient to erotic material or having him masturbate are two methods of stimulating erections for observation. These methods are not free of problems: Even today many men are more uncomfortable than aroused when asked to undergo the procedures. This discomfort may prevent the occurrence of erections representative of the patient's typical function, and negative results will therefore be of little diagnostic use because one cannot determine whether poor or absent erection is due to situational factors or physical pathology. In addition, an important characteristic of erection, duration, is probably not optimally examined with the procedures. Nevertheless, one has the impression that it was often the physician's embarrassment rather than his methodologic concerns that deterred him from arranging to view the patient's erect penis. Yet, direct observation is essential. When it is not made, the physician is forced to rely solely on the patient's report of his erectile function, and there are numerous reasons why a patient might innocently or deliberately misrepresent the facts. In addition, only when the penis is erect can one see certain occult morphologic abnormalities that compromise normal function or determine the degree to which previously detected disease processes, such as Peyronie's plaque, actually interfere with erection. Most important, if the observation is made under conditions that assure that the erection represents the patient's maximal physiologic capacity, it can reveal whether or not the patient has a physical limitation to adequate erection.

Thus, the deficiencies in the contemporary procedure derived from the dependence of the differential diagnosis on insensitive methods of locating deficits that could only be presumed to play a role in the patient's complaint, and from neglect of the basic procedure of directly observing the patient's erection. Admittedly, the state of knowledge and technology was largely responsible for these limitations, but there was a surprising failure of clinicians to recognize that these limitations existed. Generally unacknowledged were the obvious reasons why false-negative physical and false-positive psychologic diagnoses were inherent to the process. As a result, the often-made assertion that up to 90% of impotence has psychologic origins was widely accepted with confidence.

Today, there still exist large areas of ignorance about the types and mechanisms of specific etiologies of impotence, but there have been vast improvements in techniques for evaluating systems known to play a role in erection. Though some progress has been made in psychologic assessment, the greatest advances have involved procedures for locating neural, neuromuscular, vascular, and hormonal deficits. Further, monitoring of nocturnal penile tumescence (NPT) is a reliable method of actually assessing physiologic erectile capacity that is independent of the sensitivity or insensitivity of methods for isolating relevant pathology. As a result of this progress, the modern diagnostic process can be both less circular and more specific than the older procedure, at least with respect to physicogenic impotence.

The major decision facing those who incorporate NPT monitoring into their lists of services is whether they will evaluate impotence or NPT. Choosing to evaluate impotence carries with it the obligation to use all available diagnostic procedures necessary to derive both differential and specific diagnoses. Choosing to restrict service to NPT monitoring alone carries with it the obligation both to recognize and make known to users the precise and limited nature of the results and to assure that users are able to interpret the results properly. The focus of this chapter is use of NPT monitoring and closely related procedures to identify physical impairment. For the benefit of those who elect to evaluate impotence, I will list and briefly describe other techniques that can aid both differential and specific diagnosis.

Since the 1940s, NPT had been known to occur in men *(3–5)*, but the discovery of REM and, later, of the close temporal association between REM and NPT *(6–8)* stimulated active research on the phenomenon. From studies of healthy boys and men aged 3 to 79 years *(9–14)*, we concluded that NPT occurs in all healthy males and undergoes definable age-related changes. The major changes were progressive declines from age 20 years in the frequency and the amount of NPT; also apparent were small but consistent increases with age in the amount of NREM-related NPT. Because all healthy men exhibited NPT and because the nocturnal erections occurred predictably and for extended periods during sleep, when conscious social and psychologic restraints can interfere minimally, the NPT phenomenon seemed to provide an ideal condition for study of the mechanisms of erection. It might also be a useful clinical tool *(15)* for detection of physical impairment if it were demonstrated that characteristics of NPT are reliably related to physiologic erectile capacity in the awake state.

Several kinds of evidence support the assumption that NPT is a reliable index of waking erectile capacity. First, our recordings of over 1000 potent men never revealed impaired or absent NPT. By contrast, high percentages of men with medical conditions likely to impair erectile function—diabetes *(15–19)*, alcoholism *(20)*, end-stage renal disease *(21)*, spinal cord injury *(22,23)*, and Shy-Drager syndrome *(24)*—exhibited significant deficits in NPT. In many of these patients, studies of vascular, neural, and neuromuscular function suggested specific etiologies of impotence. For a number of men with vascular pathology, it was possible to correct the problem surgically. Most of these patients reported a post-surgical improvement in erection, and we observed improvement in NPT, though it was not always sufficient to restore completely normal function. On the other hand, men with major NPT deficits who were referred for behavioral or psychiatric treatment did not show any significant improvement.

In a majority of our medically healthy impotent patients, NPT has been within normal limits, and for many of these men we could identify potentially relevant psychologic problems. Most of these men regained satisfactory erectile function if they conscientiously underwent the behavioral or psychiatric therapy to which they were referred. Although it has been demonstrated *(7,8,25)* that affects such as anxiety, aggression, and rejection in REM dreams are associated with brief, transient reductions in penile circumference (called fluctuations) in accompanying NPT episodes, our clinical experience with some severely neurotic men has provided no evidence that psychologic distress can cause persistent, pervasive decrements in all NPT episodes.

Finally, the temporal association between REM and NPT raises the possibility that NPT deficits may in some cases reflect REM-state disturbances rather than deficits in erectile capacity. Despite their coincidental occurrence, REM and NPT appear to be at least partially independent phenomena. Our studies of age-related changes *(13,14)* showed the peaks of the various measures of REM and NPT to occur at different ages and the patterns of age-related changes to be different. Moreover, both early pilot studies *(7,25)* and our own recent work indicated that when REM is experimentally suppressed, NPT tends to cycle in the normal manner. Likewise, one might argue that characteristics of NPT are dependent on the recency or amount of sexual activity and that reduced sexual activity in impotent men, not reduced erectile capacity, determines observed NPT deficits. Although results of earlier work *(6,7,26,27)* on this question were equivocal, our recent studies *(28)* suggest that neither prolonged abstinence from orgasm, orgastic satiation after this abstinence, nor mere sexual arousal without orgasm before sleep significantly alters characteristics of NPT in healthy men.

Our 18-year experience with NPT monitoring and our more recent experience with the comprehensive evaluation of impotence have convinced us that every man who seeks help with impotence should undergo NPT monitoring as part of the differential diagnostic process. No matter how straightforward the clinical picture appears to be, there can be no substitute for the direct evidence the procedure provides on the patient's physiologic erectile capacity. Without this evidence, the diagnostic process reverts to the outmoded one in which the accuracy of differential diagnosis depends on the ability to identify relevant pathology. Methods of making these identifications are better than in the past, but they are still far from being foolproof, especially in the psychologic realm. The human and economic costs of inaccurate diagnosis can be high. For many men, impotence is an extremely stressful condition, affecting as it does one of the behaviors perceived to be essential to male identity and integrity. Large numbers of our patients have reported long, long histories of going from physician to physician in search of a cure for impotence. These searches have usually both augmented patients' frustration and despair and necessitated expenditures of thousands and thousands of dollars. It is ethically indefensible to add to a patient's stress and society's health care costs by submitting the patient to treatments that are clearly inappropriate if an accurate diagnosis is possible. Moreover, errors in diagnosis made when up-to-date diagnostic procedures are not used can legitimately be considered the results of poor clinical practice, and the physician who makes such errors becomes vulnerable to litigation for malpractice, which further increases stress and health care costs.

# Evaluation of NPT

## Evaluation Schedule

Our standard evaluation protocol includes three nights of polygraphic monitoring. EEG-EOG activity and penile-circumference change are monitored on all three nights. On at least one of the nights, the patient is awakened for a photograph of his erect penis, evaluations of degree and adequacy of erection, and assessment of penile rigidity. We schedule the awakening procedure for the first night but also perform it on the third night if first-night data are not adequate, and on the second and/or third night if the patient's fullest erection occurs on those nights and has not yet been examined. There are several reasons for the three-night protocol. Perhaps the most important is our growing evidence that night-to-night variation in duration and circumference change of nocturnal erections is often greater in men whom we evaluate for impotence than in our control groups. Quite possibly, both physical pathology and advancing age play a role in the variation. Whatever the cause, the necessity of acquiring a representative sample of data under conditions of potential variation demands a sample of reasonable size. Three nights of observation seems to be the minimum adequate number: Our recordings over an eight-night period showed that the nights beyond the third yield little if any new information except in some rare patients with spinal cord injuries. The measurements made during the awakening procedure are critical to the evaluation, but their validity depends on their being made at the optimum time (at the time of greatest penile expansion) and on the absence of technical problems. Prudence dictates that the awakening procedure be possible on more than one night, both to ensure representative measurements and to allow for possible technical problems on one of the nights. Although penile-circumference change is measured on all nights, the data collected on a night when the awakening procedure is not performed should be the best estimates of the characteristics of NPT, *if* substantial night-to-night variation does not suggest otherwise. Finally, because NPT usually appears in association with REM, there may be a first-night effect for NPT just as there is for REM sleep. In our experience, this phenomenon does not occur in all patients, and when it does occur, the reduction in NPT is typically not clinically significant. Nevertheless, the possibility of a first-night effect should be kept in mind; if the effect occurs and is significant, it should be taken into consideration when the data are being interpreted.

## Data Collection for Routine Polygraphic Procedures

*Monitoring EEG, EOG, and EMG Activity*   Sleep is a necessary condition for the occurrence of NPT, and relatively undisturbed and normal sleep would seem to be a necessary condition for the occurrence of a patient's normal amount and quality of NPT. EEG, EOG, and chin-EMG channels are monitored because they provide the most accurate information on the quantity and quality of the patient's sleep and therefore on a necessary condition for valid NPT data. In addition, movement artifact visible in the tracings is often the best guide to the occurrence of artifact in circumference-change tracings. For patients who exhibit unusual or abnormal movements in the lower body or limbs, the possibility exists that nocturnal erections are segmental reflex erections rather than typical NPT episodes that are presumably under suprasegmental control. A means of obtaining data to explore this possibility is to monitor, with EMG electrodes, activity in the area that sustains the movement.

Data-collection procedures are the same as for any routine polysomnographic evaluation. All channels necessary for sleep-stage scoring should be used.

*Monitoring Penile-Circumference Change*   Changes in circumference at the base and the tip of the penis define the occurrence of NPT. The tracings yield the basic data on the duration and magnitude of each nocturnal erection. Circumference changes are monitored at both the base and the tip because in some patients the primary sign is an abnormal discrepancy in expansion at the two locations. For our early work on NPT, we used only a tip gauge. About five years ago, recordings from a young man with corpus-cavernosum atresia at the penis base first suggested the need for two gauges. In our experience, base expansion in normal men is on average double that of the tip, though in some men it is as little as 50% greater or as much as four times greater; the size of the difference depends on the shape of the man's penis. In most impotent men with impaired penile circulation, and in some patients with Peyronie's plaque deposits, base expansion may be normal while tip expansion and rigidity would be insufficient for vaginal penetration. In rare cases, tip expansion and rigidity seem normal, but base changes are so small that the rigid penis flops down or to the side and would be difficult to aim in the normal manner.

## Data-Collection Procedures

*Materials*   The essential materials are mercury-filled strain gauges (29), Wheatstone-bridge and amplifier circuits (29), two calibration cylinders of known and different circumferences, surgical gloves, surgical tape, and a Polaroid camera with flash attachment. Gauges 7.0, 7.5, 8.0, 8.5, 9.0, and 9.5 cm in circumference meet most needs; smaller or larger gauges should be constructed as needed. Penile-circumference measurements made during the physical examination usually suggest the proper sizes for the patient. A gauge with circumference 1–5 mm smaller than that of the penis provides the best fit—snug, but not binding, on the flaccid organ. Gauge output directly enters the bridge, and bridge output feeds into the polygraph pen-driver amplifier. We use specially constructed, solid-plastic calibration cylinders 5 cm in length; the circumference of half of a cylinder is 2 cm greater than that of the other half. The 2-cm difference is optimal because in most normal men 2 cm is the average maximal circumference change during NPT, especially at the penis tip. We find it convenient to maintain a supply of cylinders suitable for calibrating gauges of all the standard sizes.

*Precautions* The strain gauge is rather fragile and must be carefully handled, especially when it is being placed on the calibration cylinder or the patient's penis. The electrical circuit breaks if the silastic tubing ruptures, the mercury-to-lead-wire junction is damaged, the lead wires are severed, or air bubbles invade the mercury column. A short circuit occurs if the lead wires touch each other. The linear characteristics of the gauge can be destroyed if the tubing is twisted and the diameter of the mercury column is reduced. Special attention to the construction of the junction reduces its fragility and prevents short circuits. When handling the gauge, support the junction firmly, do not roll or twist the tubing, and do not pull the lead wires. When placing the gauge on the cylinder or the penis, stretch the tubing gently and slowly, and only to the degree necessary. If an air bubble develops, discard the gauge and use another. When the polygraph pen fails to respond to changes in balance control, check the resistance across the gauge with an ohmmeter. Resistance should be 0.5–2.0 ohms. Lesser resistance signals a short circuit; greater resistance indicates some break or distortion in the circuit.

*Prerun Calibration* Details of calibration will vary with the machinery used. The procedure should include these steps: Test and document the maximal pen deflection; establish the baseline; with the gauge on the smaller calibration cylinder mimicking placement on the flaccid penis, set the gauge tracing at baseline; with the gauge on the larger cylinder mimicking placement on the erect penis, adjust the gain; and with the gauge on the smaller cylinder, verify the baseline. With our system, we set the gain so that the 2-cm gauge expansion produces a 1.5-cm pen deflection. Whatever the setting, it should be such that the patient's penile tip and base can expand at least 3 and 4 cm respectively without causing pen saturation; this allowance will accommodate the majority of patients. The circumference of the smaller calibration cylinder should be approximately that of the gauge (i.e., 1–5 mm smaller than penile circumference). When the gauge is placed on the penis, the tracing will rise 1–5 mm above baseline; it should be lowered to baseline before recording begins. If the rise is larger, the gauge is too small for the patient; if there is no rise or a negative deflection, the gauge is larger than the penis. In either case, a properly fitting gauge should be substituted and calibrated.

*Application of Gauges* A trained, competent technician, *not* the patient, applies the gauges: The patient may damage a gauge or cause it to malfunction by not handling or placing it correctly. Wearing surgical gloves, the technician expands the gauge just enough to pass it around the penis without its rolling or twisting, and turns it so that the junction will rest at the midline of the dorsal surface of the penis and the lead wires

*Sleeping and waking disorders: indications and techniques*

will point toward the penis base. The patient then guides his penis through the gauge. The technician positions the base gauge first, as far down the penile shaft as possible. He then applies the tip gauge, just behind the corona in circumcised men and about 1 cm beyond the corona in uncircumcised men (a gauge placed just behind the corona of uncircumcised men frequently rolls off during the night). The technician checks to be sure the gauges are not twisted and that the junctions and lead wires are in the proper position. He applies small pieces of surgical tape just beyond the junctions of both gauges to fix the lead wires to the penile skin, being sure to tape the tip wires especially well in uncircumcised men. He gathers the wires together and leads them across the patient's pubic area, around his trunk, up his back, and into the set of other lead wires. He applies surgical tape at regular intervals along this path to secure the wires to the patient's body. He takes special care to leave slack in the wires between the penis and the first piece of body tape sufficient to allow the penis to move freely in all directions without expansion of the gauges. As a final step, the technician photographs the dorsal aspect of the patient's penis in such a way that the gauges and proximal parts of the lead wires are clearly visible.

*Recording of Data*  The night monitor's primary technical tasks while recording proceeds are to watch for evidence of, and find solutions for, displaced or broken gauges, baseline shift, and other technical problems; to keep track of the maximum circumference changes during each NPT episode, especially on nights when the awakening procedure is performed; and to perform the awakening procedure.

*Removal of Gauges*  At completion of recording, the technician, wearing surgical gloves, removes the gauges. He first examines the gauges for any changes in position or damage and makes appropriate notes. He then removes the surgical tape, being careful not to cause the patient undue pain when lifting the tape from hairy areas. He removes the gauges in the same manner and with the same care, but in the reverse sequence, as when he applied them. He leaves the gauges in the bedroom until he can perform the postrun checking procedures.

*Postrun Checking*  Prior to turning off the polygraph, the technician tests whether calibration has been maintained throughout the night. First he measures the amplitude difference between smaller-cylinder and larger-cylinder tracings. He then raises the baseline by the amount it was lowered after the gauge was initially placed on the penis for prerun calibration and measures the amplitude from baseline of the larger-cylinder tracing.

## Data Collection for Routine Awakening Procedures

*General Procedures*  The scheduled awakening of the patient provides an opportunity to obtain information on the patient's nocturnal erection that cannot be obtained when he is asleep. It is mandatory that the procedure be performed during at least one erection when the patient's penis expands to its fullest degree so that the assessments will describe the patient's maximal erectile capacity. It is also necessary that the procedure be conducted with the greatest possible speed. Speed is critical because some patients rapidly lose their erections when they are awakened. An experienced technician should be able to collect all the needed data in 15 seconds or less. The manner in which the procedure is performed is very important, for any behavior or event that makes the patient anxious when he is awakened could affect his degree of erection. The technician must be efficient and entirely professional in his approach, and the patient must be carefully instructed beforehand about the purposes and methods of each of the procedures. All steps necessary must be taken to assure that the patient does not develop any undue sexual fantasies or fears.

Given the necessity to perform the awakening procedure during an episode representative of the patient's maximal function, flexibility must characterize the process of deciding whether or not to awaken a patient during a given episode. If data collected on the first evaluation night are representative and complete, there is no need to awaken the patient on later nights. If, however, the first-night data are not representative or complete, the procedure should be conducted on at least one of the later nights.

The onset of REM sleep is generally the best signal to the technician that he must soon decide whether and, if so, when to awaken the patient, although it should be remembered that a certain small proportion of NPT episodes occur during NREM sleep. The procedure is actually begun when the circumference-change tracings indicate that the penis has attained a stable, maximally erect state. After he enters the patient's bedroom, the technician takes the photograph and then measures the buckle force. As he performs these tasks, he has the patient provide the subjective evaluations. After he leaves the patient's room, he notes on a data form all pertinent information.

*Photographing Erect Penis*   The photograph documents the appearance of the patient's maximally erect penis and aids interpretation of the numerical data on circumference change and rigidity. It is particularly useful when it reveals or confirms that a structural anomaly or disease process, such as Peyronie's deposits, plays a role in erectile inadequacy. At times, a urologic surgeon may use the photograph to visualize a structural defect scheduled for surgical correction or to determine the size of penile prosthesis to implant.

The data-collection procedures are as follows: The technician uses a Polaroid camera with flash attachment to take the picture. Standing at the bedside, he aims the camera from above the patient's genital area and composes the image so that the patient's body is in the horizontal plane. Later, he writes the necessary identification information on the picture and labels the directions of the patient's head and feet.

*Evaluating Degree and Adequacy of Erection*   Obtaining the patient's subjective evaluations of the degree and adequacy of his erection is a means of testing the accuracy of the patient's perception of his erection. Some of our preliminary analyses suggest that impotent men with normal NPT may underestimate degree of erection more often than impotent men with deficits in NPT. If more systematic research confirms this suggestion, it will then be necessary to explore the mechanisms of the phenomenon (e.g., true perceptual failure, self-image problems, deliberate misestimation, deficit in subtle internal cues, etc.). A by-product of the estimation procedure is that the patient is able to view his penis when it has attained its presumed maximal physiologic expansion. Depending on his fears and expectations, the patient may be either reassured or disappointed by the view. If handled with care, however, the experience can often be used to help the patient accept the evaluation results and positively approach whatever treatment is ultimately recommended.

The data-collection procedures are as follows: Before the patient goes to bed, the technician carefully explains to him that after he is awakened he will be asked to estimate his degree of erection as a percentage of his best erection ever and to state whether the erection would or would not be sufficient for vaginal penetration. When he has awakened the patient and is in the process of photographing the penis, the technician elicits the patient's judgments.

*Assessing Penile Rigidity* A patient's success in effecting normal vaginal penetration with his penis is directly dependent on the rigidity of the organ. The changes in penile circumference and length that accompany erection are simply results of the process that produces a rigid penis. A direct measure of penile rigidity is necessary both because good clinical practice demands that the basic complaint—inadequate penile rigidity during erection—be explored directly and because of the possibility in pathologic conditions of a breakdown in the normally close relationship between penile expansion and rigidification. Progress in measurement techniques has been slow but consistent. The procedure we used for several years provided a means of measuring the force that caused the penis to buckle, but it suffered from the fact that it involved the technician's subjective evaluation of when penile buckling occurred. We now use more sophisticated devices that allow automatic detection of penile bending; we are still exploring the more esoteric aspects of the procedure. Still to be fully developed is the ideal system—a method of measuring rigidity by remote control, on command, and without having to awaken the patient.

*Data-Collection Procedures*

1. **Materials.** Two types of equipment are required: a device for applying force to the penile tip and measuring the force that causes the penis to buckle, and a sensor and related circuitry that indicate when the penis buckles. Our force-application device is shown in Figure 15–1; it contains a pressure transducer that responds in a linear fashion to pressures between 1 gm and 1000 gm. The transducer's signal is amplified and metered in an associated piece of machinery, from which the output feeds into a polygraph pen-driver amplifier. The buckle detector is the constantin-foil, precision strain gauge (weight less than 1 gm) shown in Figure 15–2; gauge output enters a Wheatstone-bridge and amplifier circuit, and from there the signal feeds into a

*Evaluation of nocturnal penile tumescence and impotence*

polygraph pen-driver amplifier. Gauges are available in various lengths. The gauges chosen for a particular patient should be shorter than the distance between the corona and the base of the patient's flaccid penis. The user can select either AC or DC gauge output; an AC signal is adequate for routine clinical recordings.

2. **Precautions.** The force-application and -measuring device should be checked periodically for accuracy in measuring the full range of pressures between 1 gm and 1000 gm. To prevent damage to the buckle detector, we seal each gauge in a small plastic envelope with smooth edges.
3. **Prerun Calibration.** For the pressure system, the calibration procedure consists of adjusting the gain on the polygraph according to the selected

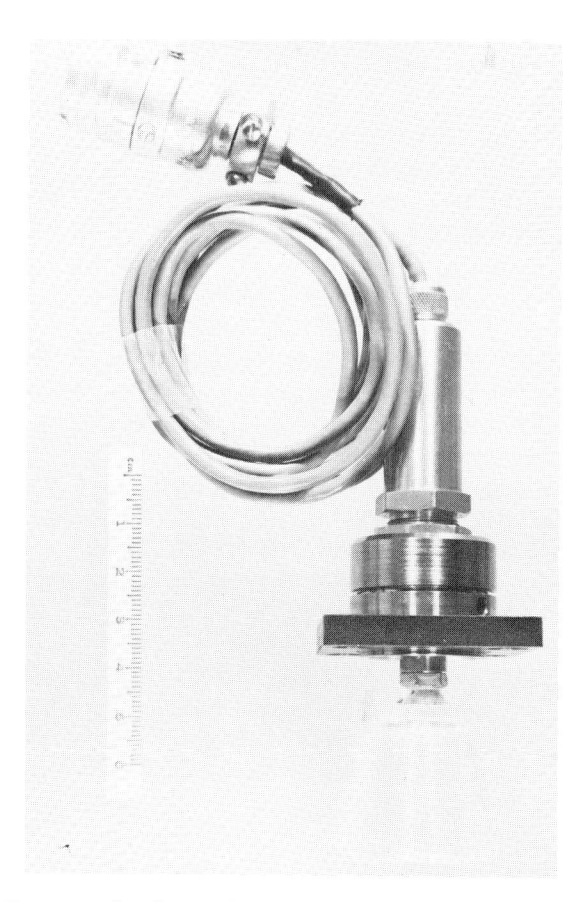

**Figure 15–1.** Force-application and -measurement device, containing a pressure transducer.

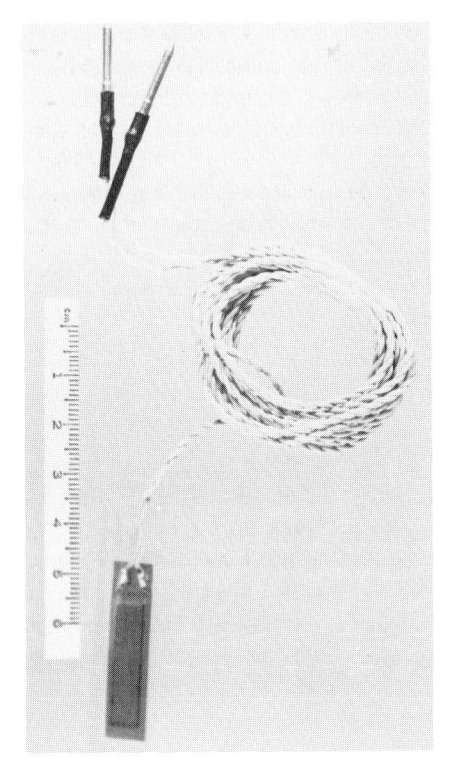

*Sleeping and waking disorders: indications and techniques*

**Figure 15–2.** Constantin-foil, precision strain gauge for detection of penile bending.

calibration ratio. With our system, we set the gain so that 1000 gm in pressure causes a 3-cm pen deflection. For the buckle sensor, no on-line calibration is required when an AC-spike signal is generated. The signal threshold of the gauge can be adjusted electronically to any desired setting. We have found that an experienced observer cannot accurately or reliably detect penile bending of less than 15°, so we have chosen to set the signal threshold at 15° for routine clinical use.

4. **Application of Gauge.** The technician positions the gauge at the same time he applies the other transducers. He places one gauge along the midline of the ventral or dorsal surface of the penis, with the lead wires directed toward the base, and fixes the plastic cover securely to the penile skin with surgical tape. If it seems appropriate, a second gauge can be positioned on one of the lateral surfaces of the penis. The technician joins the gauge lead wires to the others that pass up the patient's body from the genital area.

*Evaluation of nocturnal penile tumescence and impotence*

5. **Measuring Buckle Force.** The technician measures the buckle force immediately after he has taken the photograph. He places the cap of the pressure device over the tip of the glans and presses toward the penis base until the penis visibly bends (about 45°) or the force reaches 1000 gm, whichever occurs first. A force greater than 1000 gm may give the patient discomfort. We have found that a force of 450 gm causes buckling in a penis that is just rigid enough to be functional, so the 1000-gm upper limit is entirely adequate for evaluation purposes.
6. **Removal of Gauge.** The technician removes the gauge in the morning when he removes the other transducers.

## Data Scoring for Routine Procedures

*EEG, EOG, and EMG Activity*   Sleep stages are scored according to standard procedures *(30,31)*, and values for the descriptors of interest are derived. The most important descriptors are those related to the induction, maintenance, and amount of sleep (e.g., sleep latency, number of awakenings, number of stage shifts, total sleep time, sleep efficiency), and to the amount and distribution of each stage (especially REM sleep). Special EMG tracings of abnormal movements, when made, are examined when penile-circumference-change tracings are scored.

*NPT Episodes*

1. **Penile Rigidity.** Scoring consists of identifying the time when the penis bends and measuring the force being applied at that time (the *buckle force*). When AC output is selected, the buckle detector generates a discrete spike (Figure 15–3) at the moment the penis bends beyond the threshold value.

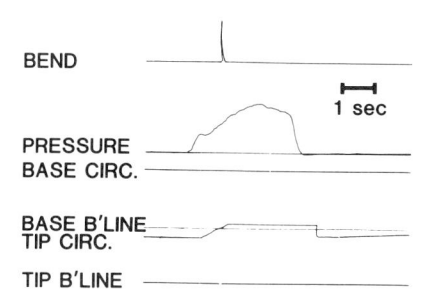

**Figure 15–3.** Sample polygraph tracing showing signals from the constantin-foil gauge, the pressure transducer, and the base and tip mercury gauges during measurement of buckle force.

The sudden appearance of artifact in circumference-change tracings also signals penile bending. To obtain the buckle force, measure the amplitude from baseline of the force signal at the time the spike appears in the buckle-detector tracing. Using the appropriate formula, convert the amplitude value to a force value. For example, with our 1000-gm:3-cm calibration ratio, a 1.5-mm amplitude would represent a 500-gm buckle force.

2. **Penile-Circumference Change**
   a. Score the tracings without knowledge of the patient's history, medical status, or psychologic status.
   b. Score base and tip tracings separately.
   c. Use a scoring epoch of at most 20 seconds (significant events may be missed if longer epochs are used).
   d. Inspect the tracings made during the prerun calibration and the postrun checking procedures. The data are invalid if initial calibration was not properly performed and questionable if calibration was not maintained.
   e. Identify all *episodes*. An episode is a complete, discrete nocturnal erection in which the flaccid penis swells to a partially or fully erect state and then returns to a completely flaccid state. It is signalled by a non-artifactual pen excursion that lasts at least 20 seconds and is at least 1 mm above baseline (adjusted for upward baseline shift, if it has occurred), and that is separated from preceding and succeeding episodes by at least one minute of baseline recording.
   f. For each episode, identify in base and tip tracings any of the following events and take the suggested actions:

   1) **Artifact.** Artifact is a transient pen excursion caused by some event (usually body movement) other than penile-circumference change. It appears in the tracing as either a brief, abrupt change that may or may not be accompanied by movement artifact in EEG, EOG, and EMG tracings (abrupt changes are not characteristic of the physiologic signal), or a long, gradual slope that indicates stretching of the gauge. Ignore episodes that appear to be artifactual.
   2) **Baseline Shift.** Baseline shift is a change from the originally calibrated baseline caused by electrical problems that produce DC drift (proper amplifiers eliminate this problem), by a gauge that does not fit properly, or by tension in the lead wires. The shift appears as a discrepancy between the calibrated baseline and pre- or post-episode gauge tracings. If the baseline has shifted upward, take this fact into consideration when scoring the data. If it has shifted downward, the data are invalid.
   3) **Pen Saturation.** Pen saturation is deflection of the recording pen to its maximal level. It appears as a tracing at the known maximum pen-excursion level. Saturation may occur when the penis expands

beyond the calibrated limits, when artifact-producing conditions (e.g., lead wires get pulled) expand the gauge beyond the limits, or when the gauge breaks. Determine the cause and note it for future reference.
g. For each episode, inspect the base and tip tracings for evidence of unusual divergence between circumference increases at the base and the tip (i.e., erect base but flaccid tip, or vice versa).
h. In patients with spastic disorders, inspect special EMG tracings and determine whether NPT episodes are predominantly or exclusively related to abnormal movements rather than to REM sleep.
i. For each episode, write down the maximum pen deflection after measuring the amplitude of the tracing from baseline at the point of greatest pen excursion. Take account of upward baseline shift if it has occurred. If pen saturation has occurred, note this fact. Using the appropriate formula, convert the maximum pen-deflection value to the *maximum circumference-increase* value. For example, if a ratio of 1.5 cm on tracing:2.0 cm on penis is used, a maximum pen deflection of 1.0 cm represents a maximum circumference increase of 1.3 cm.
j. For each episode, write down the *phase-onset times* (Figure 15-4), which are the points during an episode that signal distinct phases of the episode and of the overall degree of penile expansion.

   1) **T-Up.** The time when the tracing first rises visibly above baseline.
   2) **T-Max or T-Semi.** The time when pen excursion attains the maximum level for the episode; T-Max occurs in full episodes and T-Semi occurs in partial episodes. (Full and partial episodes are defined below.)
   3) **T-Down.** The time when pen excursion first begins a more or less continuous decline to baseline. (See item l below for procedures to distinguish the T-Down phase from a fluctuation.)
   4) **T-Zero.** The time at the end of the T-Down phase when the pen first reaches baseline. (See item k below for procedures for cut episodes.)

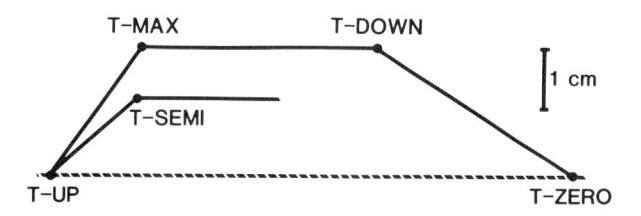

**Figure 15-4.** Schematic representation of phase onsets in an NPT episode.

*Sleeping and waking disorders: indications and techniques*

    k. Score the last episode of the night as a *cut episode* if it is interrupted by the final morning awakening. The onset time of the awakening is the *cut time*. The cut time is treated as the end of the episode. To distinguish a cut in the T-Max or the T-Semi phase from one in the T-Down phase, determine whether or not penile circumference at the time of the cut has dropped at least 2 mm below the maximum circumference-increase value for the episode. If it has not, the cut has occurred in the T-Max or the T-Semi phase; if it has, the cut has occurred in the T-Down phase. A cut episode and the phase during which the cut occurs are considered to be artificially terminated, and they are excluded when average lengths of episodes or of the phase in question are calculated.

    l. For each episode, write down the total number of fluctuations (Figure 15–5a). A fluctuation is a transient reduction in penile circumference and pen excursion during the course of an episode; it typically occurs during the T-Max phase or the T-Semi phase. For an event to be scored as a fluctuation:

      1) It must contain no artifact.

      2) The trough must represent a penile circumference that is at least 2 mm below the maximum circumference-increase value for the episode. (If this criterion is not met, the event is ignored.)

      3) A period of complete return to baseline must last no longer than 59 seconds. (If the pen remains at baseline for one minute or longer, the episode has ended and the event is part of the T-Down phase.)

      4) The event must end with a return of penile circumference to a level that is at least 80% of the maximum circumference-increase value for the episode. (If this criterion is not met, the episode is ending, and the event is part of the T-Down phase.)

    m. For each episode, write down the total number of *pulsations* (Figure 15–5b). A pulsation is a brief increase in penile circumference that lasts about 1 second and is at least 1 mm in amplitude. Be sure that artifact is not erroneously called a pulsation; when pen excursion is greater after the event than before, a true pulsation has occurred.

    n. Note any relevant or unusual features of the tracing or recording. For example, indicate periods when the patient arose to urinate or was awakened for the awakening procedure.

3. **Summary Values**

    a. After all records for a patient have been scored, classify each episode in each record as a full or a partial episode. A *full episode* is one in which the penis becomes at least 80% fully rigid; a *partial episode* is one in which the penis becomes at most 79% fully rigid.

      1) Identify the episode with the largest maximum circumference-increase value (the *criterion episode*) and note the buckle-force value for the episode.

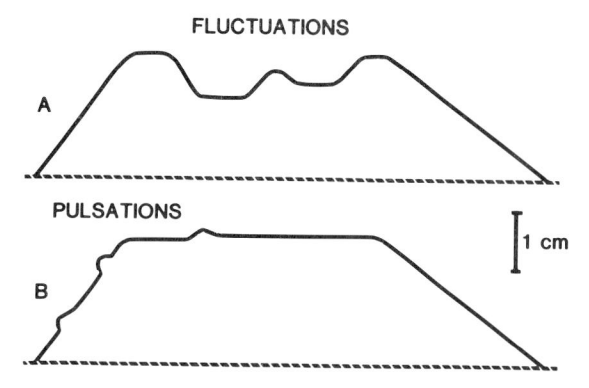

*Evaluation of nocturnal penile tumescence and impotence*

**Figure 15–5.** Schematic representation of fluctuations *(A)* and pulsations *(B)* in an NPT episode.

2) Categorize the criterion episode. If the buckle-force value is 450 gm or greater, the episode is a full episode. If the buckle-force value is less than 450 gm, the episode is a partial episode.
3) If the criterion episode is a full episode, categorize all other episodes individually. Episodes with maximum circumference-increase values greater than or equal to 80% of the maximum circumference-increase value for the criterion episode are full episodes. Episodes with values less than 80% of that for the criterion episode are partial episodes.
4) If the criterion episode is a partial episode, categorize all other episodes as partial episodes.

b. For each record, calculate and tabulate the number of full episodes, the number of partial episodes, the average durations of the T-Up, T-Max, and T-Down phases, and the ranges of those durations. Exclude from the calculations of durations episodes during which the awakening procedure was performed and phases that were interrupted by the final morning awakening.

## Data Interpretation

The general goal of data interpretation is to determine whether a patient's NPT is or is not within normal limits. If it is below the normal range, the implication is that there is a physical component to the impotence. If it is in the normal range, the implication is that there is *probably* no physical component. (See the section on differential diagnosis for the exceptions.) The interpretation process includes several steps: assessing the validity of the data, assessing the amount and quality of NPT, and assessing information that can contribute to refining conclusions or to understanding certain etiologic factors.

Determining the validity of the data involves examining the sleep data and unusual aspects of the scoring of circumference-change data. The descriptors derived from sleep-stage scoring indicate the overall quantity and quality of the patient's sleep. If amount of sleep or of REM is low, or if sleep is unusually fragmented, consider the possibility that NPT may be abnormal because of the patient's disturbed sleep. The accuracy and persistence of prerun calibration for circumference-change tracings should have been checked when the tracings were scored. If the scored data look suspicious, the photographs of the patient's penis may suggest the reason. Any or all of the pictures may reveal that the gauges were applied improperly; the photograph made during the awakening procedure may show that the gauges had shifted, twisted, or rolled off at some point. If there is a suspicious discrepancy between the circumference-change reading at the time of the awakening and the appearance of the erect penis in the picture, explore the possibility of some technical problem.

Once there is assurance that the NPT data are valid, assess the NPT descriptors. Determine whether the patient's values differ substantially from normal. For a patient with one or more abnormal values, assess the meaning of the abnormalities. For example, a reduced number of full episodes and an increased number of partial episodes suggest that there is no problem with initiation of erection but that the processes that carry erection to the functional level are defective. A reduced duration of the T-Max or the T-Semi phase suggests defects in the processes that maintain erection. Prolonged T-Up phases may indicate penile arterial disturbance, whereas abrupt or brief T-Down phases may signal venous disturbance. Large variability in measures suggests some less-than-normal stability in the system.

The conclusion about NPT should be weighted by several other factors. An abnormal discrepancy between penile expansion at the base and the tip may have been suggested by the circumference-change tracings. Further evidence may come from the technician's observation and the photograph made during the awakening procedure.

The relationship of NPT episodes to REM and to abnormal movements must also be considered. The usual temporal association of NPT and REM suggests that under normal conditions there is close interplay between the neural mechanisms of the two phenomena. If most of a patient's NPT episodes are not related to REM, there is suggestive evidence of a central neural deficit during sleep; the possibility that the deficit may also impair erection during the awake state should be entertained. Similarly, when most NPT episodes are related to spasms in a patient with spinal cord injury, the probability is high that the patient can have only reflex erections in the awake state, not erections controlled by higher neural mechanisms.

A large discrepancy between the various direct measures and the patient's estimates of the degree and adequacy of his erection may need further exploration. At times it is helpful to show the patient the photograph of his erect penis and to determine whether he verifies the original estimate; it may also be useful to have the patient describe in detail how he arrived at his estimate. In any case, one should use whatever information is available to formulate an explanation for the discrepancy.

The report of conclusions should include a description of both the NPT findings and any other relevant observations that may aid the referring physician to identify the etiology of the patient's impotence. I generally state first that a patient's NPT is or is not within normal limits (on occasion, a conclusion of low normal or borderline normal seems most accurate). I then describe any unusual features of the episode frequencies; the phase durations; the patterns of NPT, REM, and spasms (where appropriate); and the patient's subjective evaluations. Finally, I offer my interpretations of the unusual features and suggest to the physician any additional evaluations that I believe might be indicated.

## Miscellaneous Matters

A few final comments and suggestions of a general nature deserve mention. The first concern the kinds of knowledge and experience one should acquire before inaugurating routine patient evaluation. Needless to say, basic knowledge and understanding of both the mechanisms of erection and the causes of impotence are prerequisites for competent evaluation. Unfortunately, there is no single adequate source of this information, but studying several different publications *(32–39)* can provide a good beginning. On a less theoretic level, it is highly advisable, once all equipment appears to be operational, to perform both the polygraphic and the awakening procedures in a series of healthy men of various ages. The aims of the process should be to debug the equipment and procedural systems, to acquire knowledge of the normal range of data, and to explore systematically the recording results of various artifact-producing conditions. No amount of reading will substitute for this first-hand experience. Finally, the threshold values (i.e., an 80% value separates a full from a partial erection, a 450-gm buckle force reflects the 80% value) are derived from our own experience. In the initial period of patient evaluation, special effort should be made to develop a feel for how these guidelines can be most realistically used.

I cannot emphasize enough the necessity of creating and maintaining the proper atmosphere for the evaluation. A sexual complaint is *not* like other medical complaints; it can carry with it any number of special sensitivities and concerns. Every possible effort must be made to assure that the evaluation does not induce or aggravate negative feelings in the patient. Scrupulously professional behavior must be demanded of every person who interacts with the patient. Careful selection of technicians is of primary importance. Well-trained and competent technicians, wearing white coats at all times, can contribute significantly to the patient's confidence and ease because the technicians are typically the ones who perform the most intimate procedures. Likewise, thorough orientation of the patient beforehand about the purposes and methodology of the evaluation will minimize the chance that he will feel threatened during his stay in the laboratory. This orientation should be conducted by a professional staff member. It may be convenient to develop a videotape or sound-and-slide show for this purpose.

Several aspects of data collection require comment. We ask patients to refrain from taking naps, excessive caffeine, and alcohol during the evaluation period so that these potential contaminants will not affect the physiologic data. For the same reason, we typically ask the patient to refrain from taking drugs (especially psychoactive agents) that he normally consumes only occasionally. On the other hand, we usually have him continue taking any drugs that he normally consumes daily because these drugs could well contribute to his erectile problem, and we wish to study him under representative conditions. If we find in the initial evaluation that NPT is impaired, we typically try to reevaluate the patient after he has discontinued the drugs so that we can directly determine the role of the drugs in his impotence.

As stated earlier, we strongly recommend that circumference be routinely recorded from both the base and the tip of the penis. Our normative data were collected before we discovered the importance of the dual recordings. Only a tip gauge was used for those studies. If it is impossible to use two gauges, the location of choice is the penis tip. The location of the gauge should be described in both clinical and research reports. Some existing published work on NPT is difficult to evaluate because this information is missing.

Ideally, the circumference-change recordings should be made on a polygraph, not with one of the portable NPT monitors that are now on the market. Paper speed on the portable devices is too slow to allow detection of brief artifact, and the separate chart prevents detailed assessment of the relationship between NPT and REM and between NPT and gross or abnormal movements. The portable devices are suitable only for NPT screening. In a laboratory that monitors more than one or two patients per night, it may be useful to install on the polygraph an alarm that sounds when penile-circumference change reaches a certain level (say 10 mm). This alarm may minimize failures to perform the awakening procedure at the appropriate time.

We have for years scored the circumference-change tracings manually, but recently we have implemented a microprocessor on-line scoring system. We will share the system software with any who are interested in it. Use of an automated scoring system should be considered in any laboratory where NPT evaluations are performed frequently. Also in progress is research on the DC recordings of buckle force, and we invite others to join in that endeavor. Needed first are studies of the relationships between amount of applied force and amount of penile bending. The relationship is almost certainly not linear. After these data are available, it will then be necessary to determine whether DC readings have any clinical usefulness.

Last, but most important, I caution that under no circumstances should the responsibilities for NPT data collection and data interpretation be delegated entirely to the technical staff. A professional staff member must always oversee data collection and be closely involved in the scoring and interpretation of data. For virtually every case, the professional's knowledge, experience, and common sense are necessary in order to conduct a proper evaluation.

# Evaluation of Impotence

## Differential Diagnosis

The goal in differential diagnosis is to determine whether the patient's complaint has physical and/or psychologic components. The first step in the evaluation is, of course, to learn the nature and history of the patient's chief complaint and to obtain a detailed sexual and marital history. Published interview guides *(34,40)* can aid this process. The next step is to separately assess physical and psychologic involvement. NPT monitoring is the method we recommend for identifying physical involvement. As noted earlier, methods of assessing a patient's physiologic erectile capacity with sexual arousal are useful only if the patient manages to attain a representative degree and duration of erection, but there may be cases in which these procedures are indicated in addition to NPT monitoring. There are two general conditions—penile sensory deficit and penile pain—that we know can yield false-positive NPT results (i.e., NPT is normal, but there is a relevant physical problem). NPT occurs in the absence of external stimulation of the penis, but such stimulation has a prominent role in sexual erection. Thus, in a patient with a sensory deficit, NPT may be normal, but during intercourse the deficit compromises the initiation and/or maintenance of adequate erection. On the other hand, in some patients, pain with erection interferes with initiation or maintenance during intercourse. This pain may also be present during NPT, but because the patient is asleep it may not affect erection to the same degree, if at all. In some rare patients, however, penile pain is perceived during sleep, and awakening with painful erection is one of the patient's chief complaints. Because of these exceptions to the basic assumption about NPT, the final step in assessing physical involvement must be evaluation of penile sensory function and penile pain. In the sensory evaluation, vibrotactile *(41)* and pain thresholds should be tested.

Assessment of psychologic involvement is the least satisfactory part of the diagnostic process. Despite recent research *(42–45)* in which attempts have been made to describe the psychologic profiles of men presumed to have psychogenic impotence and to use these profiles for differential diagnosis, there is still great ignorance about the psychologic manifestations and causes of impotence. Moreover, there exists no equivalent to the NPT procedure in the psychologic realm—that is, a method of determining psychologic involvement that is independent of identification of relevant psychologic pathology. In a sense, a diagnosis of psychogenic impotence remains essentially a default diagnosis. The best one can now do is to derive an informed clinical impression from the available information. A comprehensive assessment of the patient's intrapsychic and interpersonal status is mandatory. In addition to a standard psychiatric interview, we also administer a battery of tests that includes the Shipley Institute of Living Scale *(46)*, the Minnesota Multiphasic Personality Inventory *(47)*, the Loevinger Sentence-Completion Test for Men *(48)*, the Profile of Mood States *(49)*, the State-Trait Anxiety Inventory *(50)*, the Derogatis Sexual Functioning Inventory *(44)*, the Locke-Wallace Marital Adjustment Scale *(51)*, and a special Reactions-to-Situations

Scale *(52)* that attempts to assess performance anxiety in sexual and other situations. Because of our suggestive evidence that men with psychogenic impotence tend to underestimate their degree of erection, we evaluate the patient's estimate when formulating a conclusion about psychologic involvement.

Evidence of physical involvement indicates a diagnosis of physicogenic impotence. Evidence of psychologic involvement indicates a diagnosis of psychogenic impotence. Positive findings in both realms indicate impotence of mixed etiology. A diagnosis of physicogenic impotence should be followed by a workup to explore the specific physical causes (see below). In the absence of positive physical or psychologic findings, the diagnosis must perforce be impotence of unknown nature and etiology—undetected, intermittent, or transient physical or psychologic pathology.

## Diagnosis of Physical Etiology

The goal in the workup for physical etiology is to identify the structural, neural, neuromuscular, vascular, endocrine, and/or drug conditions that appear to be at least the proximal causes of physicogenic impotence. To be noted immediately is that we still lack solid demonstrations of cause-effect relationships between many pathophysiologic processes and erectile inadequacy, and we have virtually no information on the role of the various neurotransmitters in erection and erectile failure. Nevertheless, even with the present limited knowledgte, somewhat stronger causal statements are possible with respect to physical pathologies than with respect to psychologic factors.

Table 15–1 lists the evaluation procedures that are presently available. The ideal workup would include every procedure, for multiple deficits may determine physicogenic impotence. In reality, clinical intuition is typically used to guide the selection of the subset of evaluations appropriate for a given patient. The routine medical history and review of systems, the physical examination (including examination of the genitals), and the routine laboratory tests (especially for diabetes and kidney dysfunction) should be performed on every patient. Though these procedures cannot be considered sufficient for the workup, the results often suggest what should be done next. Evaluation of the morphologic system includes aspects of the physical examination and of the NPT monitoring procedures. In some cases cavernography *(53)* may also be indicated.

A variety of tests are available for assessment of neural and neuromuscular function. Tests of penile sensory thresholds performed as part of the differential-diagnosis procedure yield information on sensory neuropathy. Comparison of results from measurement of response latencies for the coronal *(54)* and the urethral *(55)* bulbocavernosus reflexes may differentiate local somatic from autonomic dysfunction because the coronal reflex involves the somatic system, whereas the urethral reflex is believed to involve the autonomic system. The characteristics of the response may help differentiate neuropathy from myopathy. Examination of orthostatic blood pressure, heart rate variation, and pupil responses are established ways *(56)* of detecting autonomic dysfunction. We have found *(57)* that the pattern of penile electrodermal activity during sleep (normally, low or absent activity during REM and the T-Max phase) is disrupted in some men with abnormal NPT, suggesting that an imbalance between sympathetic and parasympathetic activity may contribute to erectile inadequacy. It needs to be established whether this imbalance is also present in the awake state. A combination of tests can be used to explore the contributions of central and peripheral neural deficits. A dissociation between NPT and REM suggests a central deficit. Although earlier investigators of the bulbocavernosus muscle in man *(32,58)* concluded that it played no role in erection, we have discovered *(59)* that spontaneous bursts of bulbocavernosus muscle activity precede slightly and accompany pulsations during NPT episodes. This finding suggests that the muscle may function to pump blood into the penis during erection. Assuming that the activity is initiated in the higher central nervous system, a comparison of results from the monitoring of NPT-related bulbocavernosus muscle activity and from testing of coronal and urethral bulbocavernosus reflexes may aid differentiation of central and peripheral neural deficits.

Assessment of the penile arterial system can also include several procedures. Methods of measuring penile blood pressure are now widely available *(18,60)*. We are exploring the usefulness of data on penile pulse volume, which is collected during NPT monitoring *(59)*, and on urethral temperature. Finally, arteriography *(61)* can be performed when noninvasive tests so indicate. Cavernography *(62)* is a means of exploring penile venous pathology.

The last steps are to examine the patient's endocrine status and drug status. Although the relationship in intact men between low testosterone levels and erectile inadequacy is still not fully understood *(63–65)*, it appears that measures of free testosterone may be more informative than measures of bound testosterone. Prolactin should be studied because of evidence *(66,67)* that hyperprolactinemia may be associated with impotence. Information on luteinizing hormone and follicle-stimulating hormone contributes to a comprehensive assessment of endocrine status. Finally, many and varied drugs have been reported *(68)*, usually anecdotally, to induce impotence. Given present ignorance about the mechanisms of action for most drugs and about the involvement of various neurotransmitters in erection, conclusions about drug-induced impotence can only be hypotheses. Nevertheless, suspicious drugs (especially antihypertensive and psychoactive agents) should be reported as possible contributors to physicogenic impotence.

In most cases, once the workup is completed, there will be positive findings that point to the pathophysiologic process or processes responsible for the patient's impotence. The positive findings are named as the probable etiology of the complaint. However, in a certain number of cases (at least 10% in our experience), there are no positive physical findings after a complete workup of a patient with abnormal NPT. In such cases, the diagnosis of unknown etiology must be invoked, though it may be possible to offer hypotheses about possible contributors.

---

Some of the work reported herein was supported by the Houston Veterans Administration Medical Center.

**Table 15–1** Evaluations for Diagnosis of Physical Etiology

| System | Item | Pathology Identified | Follow-Up Item |
|---|---|---|---|
| Physical | Medical history & review of systems<br>Physical examination results<br>Laboratory test results | Relevant disease states | |
| Morphologic | Appearance & feeling of flaccid penis<br>Penile circumferences during NPT: base vs. tip<br>Appearance of erect penis in photograph<br>Cavernogram | Structural | |
| Neural and Neuromuscular | Penile sensory thresholds | Sensory neuropathy | |
| | Bulbocavernosus reflex response latencies: coronal vs. urethral | Somatic vs. autonomic | Response characteristics: neuropathy vs. myopathy |
| | Heart rate variation<br>Orthostatic blood pressure | Autonomic | |

|  |  |  |
|---|---|---|
|  | Pupil responses |  |
|  | Electrodermal activity during sleep |  |
|  | NPT-REM relationship | Central |
|  | Bulbocavernosus function: NPT-related activity vs. coronal & urethral reflex-response latencies | Central vs. peripheral |
| Vascular | Blood pressures in flaccid penis | Arterial |
|  | Urethral temperature in flaccid penis |  |
|  | Penile pulse volume during NPT |  |
|  | Arteriogram |  |
|  | Cavernogram | Venous |
| Endocrine | Testosterone & prolactin levels | Endocrine |
|  | Luteinizing & follicle-stimulating hormone levels | Central vs. end-organ deficit |
| Various | Drug history | Relevant drug states |
|  | Drug levels in urine |  |

# REFERENCES

1. Keshin JG, Pinck BD. Impotentia. NY State J Med 1949; 49:269–72.
2. Compere JS. Office recognition and management of sexual dysfunction. Am Fam Physician 1978; 17:186–90.
3. Halverson HM. Genital and sphincter behavior of the male infant. J Genet Psychol 1940; 56:95–136.
4. Ohlmeyer P, Brilmayer H, Hüllstrung H. Periodische Vorgänge im Schlaf. Pfluegers Arch 1944; 248:559–60.
5. Ohlmeyer P, Brilmayer H. Periodische Vorgänge im Schlaf. II. Mitteilung. Pfluegers Arch 1947; 249:50–5.
6. Fisher C, Gross J, Zuch J. Cycle of penile erection synchronous with dreaming (REM) sleep: preliminary report. Arch Gen Psychiatry 1965; 12:29–45.
7. Karacan I. The effect of exciting presleep events on dream reporting and penile erections during sleep. Brooklyn: State University of New York, Downstate Medical Center, 1965. (Doctoral dissertation.)
8. Karacan I, Goodenough DR, Shapiro A, Starker S. Erection cycle during sleep in relation to dream anxiety. Arch Gen Psychiatry 1966; 15:183–9.
9. Hursch CJ, Karacan I, Williams RL. Some characteristics of nocturnal penile tumescence in early middle-aged males. Compr Psychiatry 1972; 13:539–48.
10. Karacan I, Hursch CJ, Williams RL, Littell RC. Some characteristics of nocturnal penile tumescence during puberty. Pediatr Res 1972; 6:529–37.
11. Karacan I, Hursch CJ, Williams RL, Thornby JI. Some characteristics of nocturnal penile tumescence in young adults. Arch Gen Psychiatry 1972; 26:351–6.
12. Karacan I, Hursch CJ, Williams RL. Some characteristics of nocturnal penile tumescence in elderly males. J Gerontol 1972; 27:39–45.
13. Karacan I, Williams RL, Thornby JI, Salis PJ. Sleep-related penile tumescence as a function of age. Am J Psychiatry 1975; 132:932–7.
14. Karacan I, Salis PJ, Thornby JI, Williams RL. The ontogeny of nocturnal penile tumescence. Waking Sleeping 1976; 1:27–44.
15. Karacan I. Clinical value of nocturnal erection in the prognosis and diagnosis of impotence. Med Aspects Hum Sex 1970; 4:27–34.
16. Karacan I, Scott FB, Salis PJ, et al. Nocturnal erections, differential diagnosis of impotence, and diabetes. Biol Psychiatry 1977; 12:373–80.
17. Karacan I, Salis PJ, Ware JC, et al. Nocturnal penile tumescence and diagnosis in diabetic impotence. Am J Psychiatry 1978; 135:191–7.
18. Karacan I, Ware JC, Dervent B, et al. Impotence and blood pressure in the flaccid penis: relationship to nocturnal penile tumescence. Sleep 1978; 1:125–32.

19. Karacan I. Diagnosis of erectile impotence in diabetes mellitus: an objective and specific method. Ann Intern Med 1980; 92:334–7.
20. Karacan I, Snyder S, Salis PJ, Williams RL, Derman S. Sexual dysfunction in male alcoholics and its objective evaluation. In: Fann WE, Karacan I, Pokorny AD, Williams RL, eds. Phenomenology and treatment of alcoholism. New York: Spectrum, 1980:259–66.
21. Karacan I, Dervent A, Cunningham G, et al. Assessment of nocturnal penile tumescence as an objective method for evaluating sexual functioning in ESRD patients. Dialysis Transplant 1978; 7:872–6, 890.
22. Karacan I, Dimitrijevic M, Lauber A, et al. Nocturnal penile tumescence (NPT) and sleep stages in patients with spinal cord injuries. Sleep Res 1977; 6:52.
23. Karacan I, Dervent A, Salis PJ, et al. Spinal cord injuries and NPT. Sleep Res 1978; 7:261.
24. Moore C, Karacan I, Taylor A. Erectile dysfunction in Shy-Drager syndrome. Sleep Res 1979; 8:240.
25. Fisher C. Dreaming and sexuality. In: Loewenstein RM, Newman LM, Schur M, Solnit AJ, eds. Psychoanalysis—a general psychology. New York: International Universities, 1966:537–69.
26. Kahn E. The sleep and other characteristics of the aged. New York: Yeshiva University, 1968. (Doctoral dissertation.)
27. Karacan I, Williams RL, Salis PJ. The effect of sexual intercourse on sleep patterns and nocturnal penile erections. Psychophysiology 1970; 7:338–9.
28. Karacan I, Ware JC, Salis PJ, Williams RL, Goze N. Sexual arousal and activity: effect on subsequent nocturnal penile tumescence patterns. Sleep Res 1979; 8:61.
29. Karacan I. A simple and inexpensive transducer for quantitative measurements of penile erection during sleep. Behav Res Meth Instr 1969; 1:251–2.
30. Rechtschaffen A, Kales A, eds. A manual of standardized terminology, techniques and scoring system for sleep stages of human subjects. NIH Publication No. 204. Washington, DC: US Government Printing Office, 1968.
31. Williams RL, Karacan I, Hursch CJ. Electroencephalography (EEG) of human sleep: clinical applications. New York: John Wiley & Sons, 1974.
32. Bors E, Comarr AE. Neurological disturbances of sexual function with special reference to 529 patients with spinal cord injury. Urol Surv 1960; 10:191–222.
33. Cooper AL. Factors in male sexual inadequacy: a review. J Nerv Ment Dis 1969; 149:337–59.
34. Masters WH, Johnson VE. Human sexual inadequacy. Boston: Little, Brown, 1970.
35. Weiss HD. The physiology of human penile erection. Ann Intern Med 1972; 76:793–9.

36. Kaplan HS. The new sex therapy: active treatment of sexual dysfunctions. New York: Brunner/Mazel, 1974.
37. Levine SB. Marital sexual dysfunction: erectile dysfunction. Ann Intern Med 1976; 85:342–50.
38. Money J, Musaph H, eds. Handbook of sexology. New York: Excerpta Medica, 1977.
39. LoPiccolo J, LoPiccolo L, eds. Handbook of sex therapy. New York: Plenum, 1978.
40. Committee on Medical Education. Assessment of sexual function: a guide to interviewing. GAP Report No. 88. Group Adv Psychiatry (Rep) 1973; 8:755–850.
41. Edwards AE, Husted JR. Penile sensitivity, age, and sexual behavior. J Clin Psychol 1976; 32:697–700.
42. Beutler LE, Karacan I, Anch AM, Salis PJ, Scott FB, Williams RL. MMPI and MIT discriminators of biogenic and psychogenic impotence. J Consult Clin Psychol 1975; 43:899–903.
43. Beutler LE, Scott FB, Karacan I. Psychological screening of impotent men. J Urol 1976; 116:193–7.
44. Derogatis LR. Psychological assessment of sexual disorders. In: Meyer JK, ed. Clinical management of sexual disorders. Baltimore: Williams and Wilkins, 1976:35–73.
45. Derogatis LR, Melisaratos N. The DSFI: a multidimensional measure of sexual functioning. J Sex Marital Ther 1979; 5:244–81.
46. Shipley WC. A self-administering scale for measuring intellectual impairment and deterioration. J Psychol 1940; 9:371–7.
47. Dahlstrom WG, Welsh GS, Dahlstrom LE. An MMPI handbook. Vol. I. Clinical interpretation. Minneapolis: University of Minnesota, 1972.
48. Loevinger J, Wessler R. Measuring ego development. Vol. I. Construction and use of a sentence completion test. San Francisco: Jossey-Bass, 1978.
49. McNair DM, Lorr M, Droppleman LF. Manual for the profile of mood states. San Diego: Educational and Industrial Testing Service, 1971.
50. Spielberger CD, Gorsuch RL, Lushene RE. STAI manual: for the state-trait anxiety inventory ("self-evaluation questionnaire"). Palo Alto: Consulting Psychologists Press, 1970.
51. Locke HJ, Wallace KM. Short marital-adjustment and prediction tests: their reliability and validity. Marr Fam Living 1959; 21:251–5.
52. Schalling D. The trait-situation interaction and the physiological correlates of behavior. In: Magnusson D, Endler NS, eds. Personality at the crossroads: current issues in interactional psychology. Hillsdale, New Jersey: Lawrence Erlbaum, 1977:129–41.
53. Ginestié J-F. Cavernography. In: Zorgniotti AW, Rossi G, eds. Vasculogenic impotence. Springfield, Illinois: Charles C Thomas, 1980:185–90.
54. Ertekin C, Reel F. Bulbocavernosus reflex in normal men and in patients with neurogenic bladder and/or impotence. J Neurol Sci 1976; 28:1–15.

55. Dick HC, Bradley WE, Scott FB, Timm GW. Pudendal sexual reflexes: electrophysiologic investigations. Urology 1974; 3:376–9.
56. Clarke BF, Ewing DJ, Campbell IW. Diabetic autonomic neuropathy. Diabetologia 1979; 17:1–18.
57. Ware JC, Karacan I, Salis PJ, Hirshkowitz M, Thornby JI. Patterning of electrodermal activity during sleep: relation to impotence. Sleep Res, in press.
58. Kollberg S, Petersén I, Stener I. Preliminary results of an electromyographic study of ejaculation. Acta Chir Scand 1962; 123:478–83.
59. Karacan I, Salis PJ, Williams RL. The role of the sleep laboratory in diagnosis and treatment of impotence. In: Williams RL, Karacan I, eds. Sleep disorders: diagnosis and treatment. New York: John Wiley & Sons, 1978:353–82.
60. Abelson D. Diagnostic value of the penile pulse and blood pressure: a Doppler study of impotence in diabetics. J Urol 1975; 113:636–9.
61. Michal V, Pospíchal J, Blažková J. Arteriography of the internal pudendal arteries and passive erection. In: Zorgniotti AW, Rossi G, eds. Vasculogenic impotence. Springfield, Illinois: Charles C Thomas, 1980:169–79.
62. Fitzpatrick T. The venous drainage of the corpus cavernosum and spongiosum. In: Zorgniotti AW, Rossi G, eds. Vasculogenic impotence. Springfield, Illinois: Charles C Thomas, 1980:181–4.
63. Rennie TAC, Vest SA Jr, Howard JE. The use of testosterone propionate in impotence: clinical studies with male sex hormones (III). South Med J 1939; 32:1004–7.
64. Raboch J, Stárka L. Reported coital activity of men and levels of plasma testosterone. Arch Sex Behav 1973; 2:309–15.
65. Lawrence DM, Swyer GIM. Plasma testosterone and testosterone binding affinities in men with impotence, oligospermia, azoospermia, and hypogonadism. Br Med J 1974; 1:349–51.
66. Thorner MO, Besser GM. Hyperprolactinaemia and gonadal function: results of bromocriptine treatment. In: Crosignani PG, Robyn C, eds. Prolactin and human reproduction. New York: Academic Press, 1977:285–301.
67. Carter JN, Tyson JE, Tolis G, Van Vliet S, Faiman C, Friesen HG. Prolactin-secreting tumors and hypogonadism in 22 men. N Engl J Med 1978; 299:847–52.
68. Story NL. Sexual dysfunction resulting from drug side effects. J Sex Res 1974; 10:132–49.

# SIXTEEN
# EPILEPSY AND SLEEP

BARRY R. THARP

## Introduction

The relationship between sleep and epilepsy has been known since antiquity *(1,2)*. Early investigators were concerned primarily with the time of occurrence of seizures. They noted that many epileptic patients had seizures during sleep and in some instances seizures occurred only during sleep (nocturnal epilepsy). It has been reported that 0.5% to 24% of epileptics have seizures exclusively during sleep *(3,4,5)*. Janz *(6)* studied 2110 patients with generalized convulsive seizures and reported that 45% had seizures predominantly during sleep.

Since the introduction of electroencephalography (EEG), a more detailed analysis of nocturnal seizures has been possible. It was soon found that not only did clinical seizures occur more frequently during sleep in some patients, but also that abnormal electrical discharges (spikes, sharp waves, and a variety of generalized spike and wave activity) were often more abundant in EEGs recorded when the patient fell asleep during a routine clinical EEG recording. This latter finding was noted in patients with diurnal as well as nocturnal seizures and occasionally in asymptomatic individuals. White et al. *(7)* found that patients whose seizures were predominantly nocturnal showed more EEG abnormalities during sleep than patients with primarily diurnal or mixed diurnal and nocturnal epilepsies.

The relationship between the frequency of potentially epileptogenic discharges and the stage of sleep has been extensively studied. There is a tendency for generalized discharges (usually generalized spike and slow-wave activity) to occur more frequently in NREM sleep, particularly in stages 1 and 2 *(8)*. Focal activity (usually spikes and sharp waves) is also increased during NREM sleep but, in contrast to generalized discharges, may also be activated during REM sleep. In some cases of childhood epilepsy, there may be a dramatic increase in epileptogenic activity with sleep that has been referred to as subclinical "electrical status epilepticus" *(9)*.

Sleep deprivation has been recognized as a precipitant of seizures *(10)*. It is well known that lack of sleep will lead to an increase in seizure frequency in some epileptics

*(11,12)*. Sleep deprivation has also precipitated seizures in healthy individuals without a prior history of epilepsy and who subsequently remain free of seizures if significant sleep deprivation is avoided.

# EEG Evaluation of Patients with Epilepsy

In most patients, the clinical history is sufficient to make a diagnosis of epilepsy. The routine clinical EEG, particularly if it includes a waking and sleep recording, often provides data that are consistent with the diagnosis of epilepsy and also allows the physician to classify the type of epilepsy more accurately. This in turn may result in a more rational selection of anticonvulsant drugs. In addition, a more accurate localization of the epileptogenic area may be possible if one is dealing with a partial epilepsy. Unfortunately, a significant number of epileptic patients have negative EEGs. Ajmone-Marsan and Zivin *(13)* studied 308 patients with epilepsy who had had at least three EEGs. Only 55.5% of these patients had an initially "positive" EEG as defined by the presence of distinct "epileptiform activity."

If the patient's attacks are typically epileptic in nature, a positive EEG is more likely to be recorded if the tracing is obtained within several days of a seizure, if the duration of the diurnal recording is extended beyond the usual 1/2- to 1-hour recording time, and if the patient is deprived of sleep for 24 hours or is withdrawn from some or all of the anticonvulsant drugs he is ingesting. If all these maneuvers fail to uncover potentially epileptic discharges on the EEG, therapy for epilepsy can be started or continued if the description of the patient's attacks is otherwise typical for epileptic seizures. If the episodes are atypical, further EEG recording and observation is required to establish a definitive diagnosis.

Included in this latter group are individuals with abnormal episodic nocturnal behavior that cannot be readily classified by history alone. In some cases, a more detailed description of the episodes by witnesses will provide sufficient information to allow the nocturnal events to be identified as pavor nocturnus, sleepwalking, or epileptic seizures. In the absence of sufficient historical data, some patients are considered epileptic on the basis of abnormal interictal EEGs or by a satisfactory response to anticonvulsant drugs, as was the case, for example, with the patients described by Pedley and Guilleminault *(14)* with episodic nocturnal wanderings.

It should be pointed out, however, that the presence of potentially epileptogenic activity on an EEG does not "confirm" the diagnosis of epilepsy. A small percentage of normal individuals have abnormal EEGs. An even greater percentage of healthy individuals with epileptic siblings have abnormal discharges on routine clinical EEGs.

The response to medications is also nonspecific. Many drugs that are effective in the treatment of epilepsy may also control nonepileptic disorders.

It should be added that patients with epilepsy may also have nonepileptic nocturnal disorders of behavior. Tassinari et al. *(15)* have described epileptic patients with pavor nocturnus, and Saint-Laurent et al. *(16)* have shown that nocturnal enuresis in some epileptics is idiopathic and not the result of nocturnal seizures.

## Indications for All-Night EEG Recording

Long-term EEG monitoring may be necessary in the evaluation of patients with a variety of episodic disorders of behavior. The following types of patients should be considered for prolonged EEG recording:

1. Patients with episodic diurnal attacks that cannot be definitely classified as epileptic. These might include individuals with suspected hysterical ("pseudo") seizures, syncopal-like episodes, dissociative states, unexplained confusional states, and episodes of altered behavior.

    In the majority of such patients, prolonged daytime recording will yield sufficient information to establish the etiology of the patient's episodes, particularly if one of the episodes occurs during the recording session. In some instances, telemetric equipment or a portable, miniaturized magnetic-tape unit should be employed. A discussion of these daytime recording techniques is outside the scope of this chapter.
2. Patients with nocturnal disturbances of behavior that are not typically epileptic, or those in whom there is a suspicion that nocturnal seizures may not be primarily epileptic, e.g., the individual with sleep apnea whose nocturnal tonic seizures are being precipitated by profound hypoxemia.
3. Patients with documented epilepsy who have, in addition to typical seizures, nocturnal events that may or may not be related to brief or subclinical seizures, e.g., the child with frequent diurnal seizures and enuresis.
4. Patients with epilepsy and excessive daytime sleepiness (EDS). In most cases, the sleepiness can be explained on the basis of anticonvulsant drugs; however, in rare instances, frequent minor or subclinical seizures may sufficiently disrupt nocturnal sleep to produce EDS. A nocturnal sleep recording will provide information about the presence of seizures and allow quantification of sleep stages.

## Technical Considerations for Performing All-Night EEG and Polygraphic Recordings on Patients with Possible Nocturnal Epilepsy

All patients considered for this type of extended recording should have a complete neurologic evaluation. If the physician in charge of the polysomnography laboratory is not a neurologist or is not knowledgeable about the field of epilepsy, a neurologic consultant or an experienced electroencephalographer should collaborate with laboratory personnel.

The technologist should be familiar with the clinical manifestations of the various seizure types to provide accurate notations of the patient's behavior during the recording. (See reference list for several excellent clinical references.) He should also be familiar with the large variety of potentially epileptogenic patterns that occur in the EEG and should ideally have training in clinical electroencephalography.

Every patient should have a clinical EEG performed prior to the all-night recording. This tracing should be recorded by a trained, preferably board-certified, EEG technologist during wakefulness and natural sleep following a 24-hour period of sleep deprivation. Nasopharyngeal leads should be used routinely. Optionally, sphenoidal electrodes can be used. The guidelines published by the American EEG Society for performing clinical EEGs should be followed.*

The purpose of this clinical recording is to determine the presence of potentially epileptogenic discharges and their location as well as to characterize their morphology to allow easier recognition during the all-night tracing. If these potentials are of sufficient abundance, portions of the routine clinical EEG should be recorded at the same paper speeds to be employed during the all-night polysomnographic recording.

## Polygraphic Recording

A 16- to 18-channel EEG machine should be used for the all-night recording. The following utilization of channels is suggested:

1. Sixteen-channel machine
   a. Ten channels of EEG.
   b. Two channels for EEG sleep scoring.
   c. One channel for submental muscle activity.
   d. One channel for ECG.
   e. One channel for electro-oculogram (EOG).
   f. One channel for thoraco-abdominal respirations.
   g. Optionally, two channels for anterior tibialis muscle recordings may replace two EEG channels.
2. Eighteen-channel machine—same as above but 12 channels of EEG.

It is recommended, but not essential, that portions of the polygraphic data be recorded on 14-channel magnetic tape. A time-code generator should be used to record the date and time in hours, minutes, and seconds on the video and magnetic tape. These tapes can be reviewed after the recording is completed to compare the patient's behavior with electrophysiologic activity.

---

*Guidelines in EEG—1980* may be purchased from the Executive Secretary of the American EEG Society, 2163 Northlake Parkway, Suite 105, Tucker (Atlanta), Georgia 30084.

Additionally, some type of event-marker apparatus should be included. This is activated by the patient and/or the technologist or other witnesses at the time of the patient's attack. The marker placed on the magnetic tape or the EEG paper can be searched for during the off-line review of the data and allows for more rapid identification of the critical portions of the record.

The magnetic tape recorder and the EEG machine should be connected in such a way as to allow flexibility in channel selection. A switching system should be available for selecting the channels to be recorded on magnetic tape. The technologist should have the option of recording variable combinations of electrode pairs during the all-night recording session in the event that abnormal patterns appear that are not maximally expressed in the initial montage selected for storage on magnetic tape.

## Electroencephalogram

Ten or 12 channels of EEG should be recorded according to the recommended guidelines of the American EEG Society. The 10–20 system should be used for determining placement of the scalp electrodes *(17)*. The montage chosen should include coverage of all scalp areas. If an abnormality is found on the routine clinical EEG, the electrode(s) at which it was maximally expressed should be included in the montage for the all-night recording. Two additional channels are used for sleep scoring ($C_4$ and $O_2$ referred to linked ear or mastoid electrodes $A_1$ and $A_2$).

Two basic methods of electrode application are acceptable:

1. Disk electrodes applied with electrode paste and covered with adhesive tape and a protective cap.
2. Cup electrodes applied with collodion. This type of attachment is preferable to paste. Collodian electrodes are more stable and are essential in patients whose nocturnal behavior is characterized by vigorous motor activity.

Needle electrodes should never be employed.

Immediately following electrode application, and at intervals during the recording session, electrode *impedance* (rather than resistance) should be measured. Interelectrode impedance should not exceed 5000 ohms or be less than 100 ohms.

If potentially epileptogenic abnormalities are present in the nasopharyngeal electrode(s) during the routine clinical EEG, $T_1$ and $T_2$ electrodes should be applied for the all-night recording. Preferably bilateral sphenoidal electrodes can be inserted in lieu of the anterior temporal electrodes for recordings during sleep.

*$T_1$ and $T_2$ Electrodes*   These scalp electrodes are located 1 cm above the point one-third of the way forward on a line from the external meatus of the ear to the lateral canthus of the eye. The electrodes overlie the tip of the temporal lobes and are thought to provide a more accurate recording of the activity from the anterior temporal regions (a common site of focal epileptogenic abnormalities) than the $F_7$ and $F_8$ electrode sites of the 10–20 system.

*Nasopharyngeal Electrodes*   Nasopharyngeal electrodes (NP leads) consist of long, roughly S-shaped metal rods that are insulated except at the tip. They are coated with a topical anesthetic ointment, and one is inserted through each naris of the nose. Each electrode comes to rest, after rotation, in the superolateral aspect of the nasopharynx. They are secured below each naris with tape. They record the cerebral activity from the inferomesial portion of the temporal lobe. *They should never be used for all-night recordings;* $T_1$ and $T_2$ or sphenoidal electrodes are preferred.

*Sphenoidal Needle Electrodes*   Sphenoidal needle electrodes consist of fine silver or stainless-steel wires, insulated except for the tip, that are introduced under sterile conditions by the use of a hypodermic needle or other comparable cannula. The electrode is inserted perpendicular to the surface, at a point approximately 2.5 cm anterior to the incisura intertragica of the ear, passes below the zygomatic arch and through the mandibular notch until it contacts the bone in the region of the foramen ovale at a depth of approximately 5 cm. The needle is removed and the wire is left in place, covered by sterile gauze, and attached to the skin by tape or collodion to prevent dislodging of the wire.

*Filter, Sensitivity, and Paper Speed*   The electroencephalogram should be recorded with the following filter, sensitivity, and paper-speed settings:

>Sensitivity 5–10 μV/mm (may be reduced to 15 μV/mm if high-voltage background is present, e.g., in infants and children).
>Time constant should be 0.10–0.12 sec (0.25 sec and 0.60 sec for newborns and young infants respectively).
>High-frequency filter should be such that 70-Hz activity is not attenuated by more than 30% of the activity in the alpha range.
>Paper speed should be 10 or 15 mm/sec. This can be increased to 30 mm/sec (standard EEG recording speed) if abnormal patterns or activity appear during the recording. The faster paper speed may allow a more detailed visual analysis of abnormal rhythms or paroxysmal patterns and facilitates comparison with abnormal activity in the routine clinical EEG.

*Montage*   The proper montage selection is dependent on the particular clinical situation and the findings on the routine waking and sleep EEG obtained following a 24-hour sleep deprivation. If abnormalities are present in this tracing, the electrode site(s) in which they occurred should be included in the montage used for the all-night recording. The principles governing the selection of montages are discussed in a guideline published by the American EEG Society.*

---

*\*A Proposal for Standard Montages to be Used in Clinical Electroencephalography,* which can be obtained from the Executive Secretary of the American EEG Society.

*Epilepsy and sleep*

The following montages are suggested for all-night monitoring of patients with epilepsy or nocturnal behavioral or motor disturbances that may be epileptic. One montage can be used for the entire recording.

16-channel machine

| | | | |
|---|---|---|---|
| 1. | $T_1$ (or sphenoidal $T_3$) | 1. | Left Sph $T_1$ |
| 2. | $T_3 T_5$ | 2. | $T_1 T_3$ |
| 3. | $T_2$ (Sph) $T_4$ | 3. | $T_3 T_5$ |
| 4. | $T_4 T_6$ | 4. | $T_5 O_1$ |
| 5. | $F_3 C_3$ | 5. | Right Sph $T_2$ |
| 6. | $C_3 P_3$ | 6. | $T_2 T_4$ |
| 7. | $P_3 O_1$ | 7. | $T_4 T_6$ |
| 8. | $F_4 C_4$ | 8. | $T_6 O_1$ |
| 9. | $C_4 P_4$ | 9. | $F_3 P_3$ |
| 10. | $P_4 O_2$ | 10. | $F_4 P_4$ |

The remainder of the channels are used for EEG, electro-oculogram (EOG), recording of submental EMG activity, thoraco-abdominal respiration, and, optionally, leg movements for nocturnal myoclonus. The recording parameters for these channels are discussed in the chapter on routine polysomnography (Chapter 1).

If the polygraphic data are being stored on magnetic tape, selected channels from the above montages should be included with the non-EEG data. These channels can be selected arbitrarily but should include a similar number of electrode pairs on homologous scalp regions of each hemisphere. Electrode pairs that contain abnormal activity on the clinical EEG and/or those that contain abnormal patterns during the all-night recording should also be recorded on magnetic tape. The technologist should be sufficiently trained in EEG interpretation so that the channels selected for magnetic-tape storage can be changed during the all-night recording.

## Video Monitoring

It is strongly recommended that simultaneous video monitoring and recording of the patient's activity accompany the EEG. In many instances, the direct observation of the behavioral manifestations of the seizure pattern is diagnostic. One or two cameras equipped with a lens capable of recording in infrared light can be positioned about the patient. If one camera is used, a full-length view of the patient should be recorded. Optionally, this camera can be equipped with a pan tilt mechanism and a zoom lens to allow close-up views of portions of the patient's body, e.g., the face or an extremity in a patient with partial seizures or other localized abnormal motor activity. If two cameras are available, one can be used for close-up views and the other for a full-length view of the patient.

Time-lapse videotape recording is preferable. An all-night recording can be placed on a single tape, which obviates the need for frequent replacement of video cassettes when real-time recording is used. A switch can be activated by the technologist to convert the video recording to real time during periods of abnormal behavior or if he wants to record the patient's behavior during periods when abnormal EEG patterns are appearng on the EEG.

### Responsibilities of the Technologist

The technologist should observe the patient during the entire recording session either directly or by video monitoring. The patient's behavior should be frequently noted on the EEG paper, particularly if video recording is not done. It should be written directly adjacent to the pens and be accompanied by the time in hours and minutes if a time-code generator is not available. The technologist should have sufficient training to run the EEG, magnetic-tape, and video-recording equipment. The mode of video recording (time-lapse or real-time) should be determined by the technologist. If the patient has several episodes during the night, the technologist should attempt to record at least one with real-time video recording. In some cases, a characteristic alteration of the EEG may precede the actual clinical attack and provide enough time for the change from time-lapse to real-time. Electrode impedance should be checked frequently during the recording session. Electrodes with excessively high impedance should be reapplied or, if the patient cannot be disturbed, disconnected from the recording circuit.

---

This chapter was prepared by the EEG and Sleep Committee of the American EEG Society, B. Tharp, Chairman.
Other committee members are: R. Broughton, C. Guilleminault, H. Lemmi, and E. Weitzman.

# REFERENCES

1. Daly D. Circadian cycles and seizures. In: Brazier M, ed. Epilepsy, its phenomena in man. New York: Academic Press, 1973:215–33.
2. Pompeiano O. Sleep mechanisms. In: Jasper H, Ward A, Pope A, eds. Basic mechanisms of the epilepsies. Boston: Little, Brown, 1969:453–73.
3. Gibbard F, Bateson M. Sleep epilepsy: its patterns and prognosis. Br Med J 1974; 2:403–5.
4. Langdon-Down M, Brain W. Time of day in relation to convulsions in epilepsy. Lancet 1929; 2:1029–32.
5. Patry F. The relation of time of day, sleep and other factors to the incidence of epileptic seizures. Am J Psychiatry 1931; 87:789–813.

6. Janz D. The grand mal epilepsies and the sleeping-waking cycle. Epilepsia 1962; 3:69–109.
7. White P, Dyken M, Grant P, Jackson L. Electroencephalographic abnormalities during sleep as related to the temporal distribution of seizures. Epilepsia 1962; 3:167–74.
8. Gastaut M, Batini C, Fressy J, Broughton R, Tassinari C, Vittini F. Le sommeil de nuit normal et pathologique. Études électroencéphalographiques. Electroencéphalographie et neurophysiologie clinique (Nouvelle Serie) In: Fischgold H, ed. Sommeil de nuit normal et pathologique. Vol. 2. Paris: Masson, 1965:239–54.
9. Patry G, Lyagoubi S, Tassinari C. Subclinical "electrical status epilepticus" induced by sleep in children. Arch Neurol 1971; 24:242–52.
10. Janz D. Conditions and causes of status epilepticus. Epilepsia 1960; 23:170–7.
11. Scollo-Lavizzari G, Pralle W, Radue E. Comparative study of efficacy of waking and sleep recordings following sleep deprivation as an activation method in the diagnosis of epilepsy. Eur Neurol 1977; 15:121–3.
12. Kajtor F. The influence of sleep and the waking state on the epileptic activity of different structures. Epilepsia 1962; 3:274–80.
13. Ajmone-Marsan C, Zivin L. Factors related to the occurrence of typical paroxysmal abnormalities in the EEG records of epileptic patients. Epilepsia 1970; 11:361–81.
14. Pedley T, Guilleminault C. Episodic nocturnal wanderings responsive to anticonvulsant drug therapy. Ann Neurol 1977; 2:30–5.
15. Tassinari C, Mancia D, Della Bernardina B, Gastaut H. Pavor nocturnus of non-epileptic nature in epileptic children. Electroencephalogr Clin Neurophysiol 1968; 24:391.
16. Saint-Laurent J, Batini C, Broughton R, Gastaut H. A polygraphic study of nocturnal enuresis in the epileptic child. Electroencephalogr Clin Neurophysiol 1963; 15:904.
17. Jasper H. The ten-twenty electrode system of the International Federation. Electroencephalogr Clin Neurophysiol 1968; 10:371–3.

# General References on Epilepsy

1. Gastaut H. Clinical and electroencephalographical classification of epileptic seizures. Epilepsia 1970; 11:102–13.
2. Tassinari C, et al. Epileptic seizures during sleep in children. In: Penry JK, ed. Epilepsy, the eighth international symposium. New York: Raven Press, 1977:345–54.
3. Schmidt R, Wilder B. Epilepsy. New York: Raven Press, 1968.
4. Aminoff M. Electrodiagnosis in clinical neurology. New York: Churchill Livingstone, 1980.

# APPENDIX I

## LAUGHTON MILES

The following is an example of a sleep questionnaire, reproduced with permission (copyright, Laughton Miles, M.D., Ph.D.). This questionnaire, filled in by patients before they are seen in the sleep clinic, has proven to be helpful in investigating sleep-wake disorders.

*Appendix I*

PATIENT'S NAME _____

AGE _____

TODAY'S DATE _____

TOR NUMBER _____

<u>SLEEP QUESTIONNAIRE AND ASSESSMENT OF WAKEFULNESS</u> (SQAW)

(copyright 1979)
Rev. 18 Oct. 1979

Stanford Sleep Disorders Clinic

and

Stanford Sleep Research Center

Stanford Sleep Disorders and Sleep Research Program
Stanford University Medical Center
Stanford, California  94305

*Appendix I*

KEEP THIS SHEET ALONG SIDE YOU
AS YOU ANSWER THE QUESTIONS

PROCEDURE FOR ANSWERING DIFFERENT TYPES OF QUESTIONS

1. DEGREE TYPE

        ①  ②  ③  ④  ⑤

none (not at all)  slight  moderate  considerable  very great (a lot)

  EXAMPLE: HOW GREAT a problem do you have with paying your bills? . . 1  2  3  ④  5

2. FREQUENCY TYPE

        ①  ②  ③  ④  ⑤

never  just a few times  sometimes  quite often  usually (always or almost always)

  EXAMPLE: HOW OFTEN have you been to the North Pole? . . . . . . . . ①  2  3  4  5

3. YES/NO TYPE

  EXAMPLE: Have you EVER filled out this questionnaire before? . . . . yes  (no)

4. BOX TYPE    ( )    CHECK ON THOSE BOXES THAT APPLY
                                - LEAVE ALL OTHER BOXES BLANK

  EXAMPLE: Have you EVER eaten any of the following foods:

|  | for breakfast | for lunch | for dinner |
|---|---|---|---|
| cereal | (✓) | ( ) | ( ) |
| pizza | ( ) | (✓) | (✓) |
| octopus | ( ) | ( ) | ( ) |
| fruit | (✓) | (✓) | (✓) |

5. X-RESPONSE

        Place an X beside any question that YOU DO NOT UNDERSTAND,
        or which does NOT APPLY TO YOU, or which CANNOT BE GIVEN A VALID ANSWER.

  EXAMPLE: Have you EVER had CAMPBELL'S DISEASE of the UTERUS? . . . . ✗  yes    no

        ( Patient responded with an X for two reasons:          )
        (    (a). He was a male.                             )
        (           and                             )
        (    (b). He did not know what CAMPBELL'S DISEASE is.    )

6. LITERAL RESPONSE

  EXAMPLE: What time do you usually go to work? . . . . . . . . . . . *8:30* (am) pm

*Appendix I*

INTRODUCTION

The questions enclosed in this booklet will help us to obtain a good understanding of your sleeping and waking behavior and problems. It is extremely important that you answer each question as completely and accurately as possible because, when you visit our clinic, a physician who is specially trained in the diagnosis and management of sleep disorders will discuss the answers with you in detail.

There are questions in this booklet that might be better answered by someone else (e.g. your spouse, bed-partner, or roommate). Certainly ask for help from such persons if they are available.

A FEW SIMPLE GUIDELINES

1. Do not spend too much time on any question. Your first impression is generally the best.

2. The time period of all the questions is THE PRESENT (which INCLUDES THE LAST SIX MONTHS), unless otherwise specified.

3. A "WEEKDAY" is any day on which you normally work. (For most people, it is 8 am to 5 pm, Monday through Friday.)

4. If you are engaged in shift work, or have any type of unusual sleep/wake schedule, then "DAYTIME" and "NIGHTTIME" refer to your own major waking and sleeping periods.

Now you're ready to answer the questions, so please turn to the next section.

REMEMBER:

1. Keep the RESPONSE SHEET examples along side you to remind you how to answer the questions.

2. The questions are on BOTH SIDES of the paper.

*Appendix I*

GENERAL

Do you feel that you:

1. - get too little sleep at night? . . . . . . . . . . . . . . . . .  yes   no
2. - get too much sleep at night? . . . . . . . . . . . . . . . . . .  yes   no
3. Have you EVER had a poor night's sleep? . . . . . . . . . . . .  yes   no

HOW GREAT a problem do you have:

4. - with getting to sleep at night? . . . . . . . . . . . . . . .  1 2 3 4 5
5. - because of waking up during the night? . . . . . . . . . . . .  1 2 3 4 5
6. - with waking up and getting up in the morning? . . . . . . . .  1 2 3 4 5
7. - with non-restorative sleep (that is, no matter how much sleep you get, you don't wake up feeling rested)? . . . . . . . . . . . . . . . . . . . .  1 2 3 4 5
8. HOW GREAT a problem do you have with SLEEPINESS (feeling sleepy, or struggling to stay awake) in the daytime? . . . . . . . . . . . . . . . . .  1 2 3 4 5
9. HOW GREAT a problem do you have with FATIGUE (tiredness, exhaustion, lethargy) even when you are NOT sleepy? . . . . . . . . . . . . . . . . .  1 2 3 4 5

SLEEP ONSET

10. HOW MUCH does your bedtime vary? . . . . . . . . . . . . . . . .  1 2 3 4 5
11. What time do you usually go to bed on WEEKDAYS? . . . . . . . .  ____ am / pm
12. How long after going to bed do you usually decide to go to sleep? . . . . . . . . . . . . . . . . . . . .  __ __ hr __ __ min
13. How long does it usually take you to fall asleep after deciding to go to sleep? . . . . . . . . . . . . . . . . . . . . . . . . . . . . . .  __ __ hr __ __ min
14. Have you EVER had difficulty falling asleep? . . . . . . . . . .  yes   no

When falling asleep at the beginning of the night, HOW OFTEN do you:

15. - have thoughts racing through your mind? . . . . . . . . . . .  1 2 3 4 5
16. - feel sad and depressed? . . . . . . . . . . . . . . . . . . .  1 2 3 4 5
17. - have anxiety (worry about things)? . . . . . . . . . . . . . .  1 2 3 4 5
18. - feel muscular tension? . . . . . . . . . . . . . . . . . . . .  1 2 3 4 5
19. - feel afraid of not being able to get to sleep? . . . . . . . .  1 2 3 4 5
21. - feel unable to move (paralyzed)? . . . . . . . . . . . . . . .  1 2 3 4 5
22. - notice that parts of your body startle or jerk? . . . . . . . . . . . . . . . . . . . . . . . .  1 2 3 4 5
23. - experience restless legs (crawling or aching feelings, and inability to keep legs still)? . . . . . . . . . .  1 2 3 4 5
24. - experience vivid, dream-like scenes (hallucinations) even though you know that you are awake? . . . . . . . . . . . . . . . . . . . . . . .  1 2 3 4 5
25. - experience any kind of pain or physical discomfort? . . . . . . . . . . . . . . . . . . . . .  1 2 3 4 5

*Appendix I*

|     | HOW MUCH are you afraid: | | | | | |
|---|---|---|---|---|---|---|
| 26. | - of the dark? | 1 | 2 | 3 | 4 | 5 |
| 27. | - to go to sleep? | 1 | 2 | 3 | 4 | 5 |

When you go to bed, HOW OFTEN do you:

| | | | | | | |
|---|---|---|---|---|---|---|
| 28. | - wear ear plugs? | 1 | 2 | 3 | 4 | 5 |
| 29. | - wear eye shades? | 1 | 2 | 3 | 4 | 5 |
| 30. | - go to sleep with music or some other sound? | 1 | 2 | 3 | 4 | 5 |
| 31. | - go to sleep with the light on? | 1 | 2 | 3 | 4 | 5 |
| 32. | - use some special routine (ritual)? | 1 | 2 | 3 | 4 | 5 |

DURING THE NIGHT
(that period of an average day during which you normally sleep)

33. What is the total number of hours of sleep that you usually get at night (DO NOT INCLUDE time that you spend awake in bed during the night)? ...... __ __ hr __ __ min

34. Have you EVER awakened during the night? ...... yes   no

35. How many times do you wake up during a typical night's sleep? ...... ____ times

36. How long is the typical longest wake? ...... __ __ hr __ __ min

If you do awaken during a typical night (after you first fall asleep), which part(s) of your sleep period is it:

37. - first third? ...... yes   no
38. - middle third? ...... yes   no
39. - last third? ...... yes   no

40. How many times do you get out of bed during a typical night's sleep? ...... ____ times

41. How long is the typical longest out-of-bed? ...... __ __ hr __ __ min

42. HOW OFTEN do you have a fear of not being able to go to sleep once you have awakened during the night? ...... 1  2  3  4  5

HOW OFTEN do you:

| | | | | | | |
|---|---|---|---|---|---|---|
| 43. | - sleep with someone else in your room? | 1 | 2 | 3 | 4 | 5 |
| 44. | - sleep with someone else in your bed? | 1 | 2 | 3 | 4 | 5 |
| 45. | - sleep on a special surface (orthopedic mattress, bed-boards, floor, etc.)? | 1 | 2 | 3 | 4 | 5 |
| 46. | - have restless, disturbed sleep? | 1 | 2 | 3 | 4 | 5 |
| 47. | - disturb the sleep of your bed-partner? | 1 | 2 | 3 | 4 | 5 |
| 48. | - provide assistance or attention to someone (such as child, invalid, bed-partner) during the night? | 1 | 2 | 3 | 4 | 5 |
| 49. | - provide attention to something else (a pet, other animals, etc.) during the night? | 1 | 2 | 3 | 4 | 5 |

*Appendix I*

HOW OFTEN is your sleep disturbed during the night or at sleep onset because of:

50. – heat? . . . . . . . . . . . . . . . . . . . . . . . . . . . . 1 2 3 4 5
51. – cold? . . . . . . . . . . . . . . . . . . . . . . . . . . . . 1 2 3 4 5
52. – light? . . . . . . . . . . . . . . . . . . . . . . . . . . . 1 2 3 4 5
53. – any type of noise? . . . . . . . . . . . . . . . . . . . . . 1 2 3 4 5
54. – not being in your usual bed? . . . . . . . . . . . . . . . . 1 2 3 4 5
55. – noise or movement of your bed-partner? . . . . . . . . . . . 1 2 3 4 5
56. – some other environment factor? . . . . . . . . . . . . . . . 1 2 3 4 5

HOW OFTEN is your sleep disturbed because of:

57. – asthma? . . . . . . . . . . . . . . . . . . . . . . . . . . . 1 2 3 4 5
58. – a persistent cough? . . . . . . . . . . . . . . . . . . . . . 1 2 3 4 5
59. – being unable to breathe in a flat position because of shortness of breath? . . . . . . . . . . . . 1 2 3 4 5
60. – "gas" in your stomach, indigestion, dyspepsia, or heartburn? . . . . . . . . . . . . . . 1 2 3 4 5
61. – awakening from sleep because of regurgitation (or burning in the throat, choking, or gagging on stomach contents)? . . . . . . . . . . . . . . . . . . . . . . . 1 2 3 4 5
62. – awakening because you are hungry? . . . . . . . . . . . . . . 1 2 3 4 5
63. – awakening because you are thirsty? . . . . . . . . . . . . . 1 2 3 4 5
64. – awakening with an urgent desire to urinate? . . . . . . . . . . . . . . . . . . . . . . . . . . . . 1 2 3 4 5
65. HOW MANY TIMES do you usually get up during the night to urinate? . . . . . . . . . . . . . . . . . . 1 2 3 4 5

HOW OFTEN do you:

66. – have nasal congestion (stuffiness, nasal obstruction) during the night? . . . . . . . . . . . . . . 1 2 3 4 5
67. – use tablets, nasal spray, or other medication in order to deal with nighttime nasal congestion (or obstruction)? . . . . . . . . . . . . . . . 1 2 3 4 5
68. – snore in any way? . . . . . . . . . . . . . . . . . . . . . . 1 2 3 4 5
69. – snore loudly and disruptively? . . . . . . . . . . . . . . . 1 2 3 4 5
70. – hold your breath, or stop breathing during sleep? . . . . . . . . . . . . . . . . . . . . . . . . . 1 2 3 4 5
71. – suddenly wake up gasping for breath or unable to breathe? . . . . . . . . . . . . . . . . 1 2 3 4 5
72. – have some other breathing problem during sleep? . . . . . . . . . . . . . . . . . . . . . . 1 2 3 4 5
73. – notice that your heart pounds (beats strongly), beats rapidly, or beats irregularly (palpitations), during the night? . . . . . . . . . . . . . . . 1 2 3 4 5
74. – sweat excessively during the night? . . . . . . . . . . . . . 1 2 3 4 5

*Appendix I*

HOW OFTEN do you:

75. - walk in your sleep? . . . . . . . . . . . . . . . . . . . . . . . . . 1 2 3 4 5
76. - talk in your sleep? . . . . . . . . . . . . . . . . . . . . . . . . . 1 2 3 4 5
77. - grind your teeth during your sleep? . . . . . . . . . . . . . . . . 1 2 3 4 5
78. - bang your head (on the bed, pillow, or wall) during your sleep? . . . . . . . . . . . . . . . . . 1 2 3 4 5
79. - make rocking or rolling movements during sleep? . . . . . . . . . . . . . . . . . . . . . . . . . . . . 1 2 3 4 5
80. - fall out of bed while asleep? . . . . . . . . . . . . . . . . . . . 1 2 3 4 5
81. - awaken from sleep screaming, violent, and confused (night terrors)? . . . . . . . . . . . . . . . . . . . . . . 1 2 3 4 5
82. - wet your bed (as an adult)? . . . . . . . . . . . . . . . . . . . . 1 2 3 4 5
83. HOW OFTEN do your legs twitch or kick during the night, while you are asleep? . . . . . . . . . . . . . . 1 2 3 4 5
84. HOW OFTEN have you had a convulsion (fit, seizure, epilepsy) during sleep? . . . . . . . . . . . . . . . 1 2 3 4 5
85. HOW OFTEN do you have other unusual movements during the night? . . . . . . . . . . . . . . . . . . . . 1 2 3 4 5
86. HOW OFTEN is your sleep disturbed during the night by headaches? . . . . . . . . . . . . . . . . . . . 1 2 3 4 5
87. HOW OFTEN is your sleep disturbed because of pain in your neck, back, spine, muscles, joints, arms, or legs? . . . . . . . . . . . . . . . . . . . . . . . 1 2 3 4 5

HOW OFTEN is your sleep disturbed because of:

88. - intense heart pain (angina)? . . . . . . . . . . . . . . . . . . . 1 2 3 4 5
89. - any other chest pain? . . . . . . . . . . . . . . . . . . . . . . . 1 2 3 4 5
90. - stomach or abdominal pains? . . . . . . . . . . . . . . . . . . . . 1 2 3 4 5
91. - restless legs (crawling or aching feelings and inability to keep your legs still)? . . . . . . . . . . . . . . 1 2 3 4 5
92. - leg cramps (charley horses)? . . . . . . . . . . . . . . . . . . . 1 2 3 4 5
93. - paresthesia ("pins and needles") in your arms or legs? . . . . . . . . . . . . . . . . . . . . . . . . 1 2 3 4 5
94. - an itching sensation? . . . . . . . . . . . . . . . . . . . . . . . 1 2 3 4 5
95. - any other kinds of pain or intense discomfort? . . . . . . . . . . . . . . . . . . . . . . . . . 1 2 3 4 5

HOW OFTEN (AFTER you first fall asleep) is your sleep disturbed during the night because of:

96. - having thoughts racing through your mind? . . . . . . . . . . . 1 2 3 4 5
97. - feeling sad and depressed? . . . . . . . . . . . . . . . . . . . . 1 2 3 4 5
98. - anxiety (worry about things)? . . . . . . . . . . . . . . . . . . 1 2 3 4 5
99. - feeling muscular tension? . . . . . . . . . . . . . . . . . . . . . 1 2 3 4 5
100. - being afraid of not being able to get back to sleep after you wake up during the night? . . . . . . . . . . . . . . . . . . . . . . . . . . 1 2 3 4 5

*Appendix I*

DREAMING

HOW OFTEN do you:

102. - have a night full of intense, vivid dreams? . . . . . . . . . . . 1 2 3 4 5
103. - have nightmares (frightening dreams)? . . . . . . . . . . . . . . 1 2 3 4 5
104. - wake up from a dream? . . . . . . . . . . . . . . . . . . . . . . 1 2 3 4 5
105. - have racing thoughts during your sleep? . . . . . . . . . . . . . 1 2 3 4 5
107. - have a recurring dream that disturbs your sleep? . . . . . . . . . . . . . . . . . . . . . . . 1 2 3 4 5
109. - awaken from sleep at a predetermined time just by yourself (without alarm clocks)? . . . . . . . . . . . . . . . . . . . . . . . . . . . . . 1 2 3 4 5

AWAKENING AND GETTING UP IN THE MORNING

110. HOW MUCH does the time you get up in the morning vary? . . . . . . . . . . . . . . . . . . . . 1 2 3 4 5

At what time do you:

111. - have your USUAL final awakening on WEEKDAYS? . . . . . . . . . . ____ am / pm
112. - finally leave your bed after awakening on a typical WEEKDAY morning? . . . . . . . . . . . . . . . . . . . ____ am / pm

HOW OFTEN do you:

113. - depend on an alarm clock (or other artificial means) to wake up? . . . . . . . . . . . . . . . . . . 1 2 3 4 5
114. - "sleep-in" in the morning (longer than one hour past your usual getting-up time? . . . . . . . . . . . . 1 2 3 4 5
115. - notice that you are unusually difficult to wake up in the morning? . . . . . . . . . . . . . . . 1 2 3 4 5
116. - try to wake up and are extremely disoriented, confused, even violent? . . . . . . . . . . . . . . 1 2 3 4 5
117. - feel unable to move (paralyzed) when waking up? . . . . . . . . . . . . . . . . . . . . . . . . . . . 1 2 3 4 5
118. - have dream-like images (hallucinations) when awakening even though you know that you are not asleep? . . . . . . . . . . . . . . . . . . . 1 2 3 4 5
119. - cough up excessive amounts of material after waking up? . . . . . . . . . . . . . . . . . . . . . . . . 1 2 3 4 5
120. - wake up with pains (aching, "pins and needles," restlessness) in your arms or legs? . . . . . . . . . . . . . . . 1 2 3 4 5
121. - wake up with a morning headache? . . . . . . . . . . . . . . . . 1 2 3 4 5

SLEEP/WAKE BEHAVIOR DURING WEEKENDS AND HOLIDAYS

|  | weekends | holidays |
|---|---|---|
| 122. What time do you usually go to bed? . . . | ____ am / pm | ____ am / pm |
| 124. What time do you usually get up in the morning? . . . . . . . . . . . . . . . | ____ am / pm | ____ am / pm |

391

## Appendix I

FINAL COMMENTS ABOUT YOUR SLEEP

126. Do any of your SLEEP PROBLEMS seem to go in cycles or recur at regular intervals? . . . . . . . . . . . . yes  no

127. Does any problem with EXCESSIVE DAYTIME SLEEPINESS tend to go in cycles or recur at regular intervals? . . . . . . . . . . . . . . . . . . . yes  no

128. Have you EVER slept or been overwhelmingly sleepy for several days at a time? . . . . . . . . . . . . . . . yes  no

129. Have you EVER been unable to sleep at all for several days at a time? . . . . . . . . . . . . . . . . . . . yes  no

130. Do you feel that your sleep is abnormal? . . . . . . . . . . . . yes  no

131. Do you feel that you have insomnia? . . . . . . . . . . . . . . . yes  no

132. If you have (or have had) a sleep or sleepiness problem, was it worse at any time in the past? . . . . . . . . . yes  no

CHILDHOOD SLEEP

As a child, how much of a problem did you have with:

134. - getting to sleep at night? . . . . . . . . . . . . . . . . . . . . yes  no
135. - waking up during the night? . . . . . . . . . . . . . . . . . . . yes  no
136. - waking up and getting up in the morning? . . . . . . . . . . . yes  no
137. - non-restorative sleep (that is, no matter how much sleep you got, you didn't wake up feeling rested)? . . . . . . . . . . . . . . . . . . yes  no
138. - sleepiness during the day? . . . . . . . . . . . . . . . . . . . . yes  no
139. - fatigue during the day? . . . . . . . . . . . . . . . . . . . . . yes  no

HOW OFTEN did you have any of the following:

140. - thumb sucking? . . . . . . . . . . . . . . . . . . . . . . . . . . yes  no
141. - rocking yourself to go to sleep? . . . . . . . . . . . . . . . . yes  no
142. - head banging? . . . . . . . . . . . . . . . . . . . . . . . . . . . yes  no
143. - bed wetting? . . . . . . . . . . . . . . . . . . . . . . . . . . . yes  no
144. - sleep talking? . . . . . . . . . . . . . . . . . . . . . . . . . . yes  no
145. - sleep walking? . . . . . . . . . . . . . . . . . . . . . . . . . . yes  no
146. - nightmares? . . . . . . . . . . . . . . . . . . . . . . . . . . . . yes  no
147. - night terrors (awakening from sleep screaming and confused)? . . . . . . . . . . . . . . . . . . . . . . . . . . . yes  no
148. - convulsions during sleep? . . . . . . . . . . . . . . . . . . . . yes  no
149. - fear of the dark? . . . . . . . . . . . . . . . . . . . . . . . . yes  no
150. - fear of sleep? . . . . . . . . . . . . . . . . . . . . . . . . . . yes  no
151. - grinding your teeth while asleep? . . . . . . . . . . . . . . . yes  no
152. Were you hyperactive (hyperkinetic) as a child? . . . . . . . . . . . . . . . . . . . . . . . . . . . . . . . . . yes  no

*Appendix I*

DAYTIME FUNCTIONING

153. How long does it usually take you to "get going" after you get up out of bed? . . . . . . . . . . . . . __ __ hr __ __ min

154. HOW OFTEN do you feel extremely alert and energetic during the whole day? . . . . . . . . . . . . . . . . . 1  2  3  4  5

155. HOW GREAT a problem do you have with SLEEPINESS (feeling sleepy, or struggling to stay awake) in the daytime? . . . . . . . . . . . . . . . . 1  2  3  4  5

156. HOW GREAT a problem do you have with FATIGUE (tiredness, exhaustion, lethargy) even when you are NOT sleepy? . . . . . . . . . . . . . . . . . . 1  2  3  4  5

157. Have you EVER felt tired during the day? . . . . . . . . . . . . yes    no

During the past six months, have you had EITHER spontaneous episodes of falling asleep without intending to (SLEEP ATTACKS), OR severe sleepiness WITHOUT actually falling asleep (FIGHTING SLEEP, struggling to stay awake) in any of the following situations:

CHECK ONLY THOSE BOXES THAT APPLY

| | spontaneously falling asleep | fighting sleep |
|---|---|---|
| 158. - during intercourse? | ( ) | ( ) |
| 160. - eating food (meals)? | ( ) | ( ) |
| 162. - on the telephone? | ( ) | ( ) |
| 164. - in conversation with another person at WORK? | ( ) | ( ) |
| 166. - in conversation with another person at other times? | ( ) | ( ) |
| 168. - talking in a group (guests at home)? | ( ) | ( ) |
| 170. - traveling (car, bus, train . . . )? | ( ) | ( ) |
| 172. - attending a performance (lectures, films, operas, plays . . . )? | ( ) | ( ) |
| 174. - watching television? | ( ) | ( ) |
| 176. - listening to the radio or stereo? | ( ) | ( ) |
| 178. - reading a book (not in bed)? | ( ) | ( ) |
| 180. - reading a book in bed? | ( ) | ( ) |

182. HOW GREAT a problem do (did) you have with your education (e.g. bad grades) because of sleepiness or fatigue? . . . . . . . . . . . . . . . . . 1  2  3  4  5

183. HOW GREAT a problem do you have with your performance at WORK because of sleepiness or fatigue? . . . . . . . . . . . . . . . . . . . . . . . 1  2  3  4  5

184. HOW MANY TIMES have you EVER had accidents at WORK because of sleepiness or fatigue? . . . . . . . . . . . __ __ times

185. HOW MANY TIMES have you EVER been involved in automobile accidents? . . . . . . . . . . . . . . . . . . . . __ __ times

186. HOW MANY TIMES have your automobile accidents been caused by sleepiness? . . . . . . . . . . . . . . __ __ times

187. HOW MANY TIMES have you EVER had NEAR automobile accidents (driving off the shoulder of the road, etc.) because of sleepiness? . . . . . . . . . . . . . . __ __ times

188. HOW OFTEN do you have to make special provisions (or arrangements) in order to drive an automobile because of sleepiness? . . . . . . . . . . . . . . . . . . . . . . 1  2  3  4  5

*Appendix I*

HOW WELL do you function in the:

189. - morning? .................................... 1 2 3 4 5
190. - midday? ..................................... 1 2 3 4 5
191. - afternoon? .................................. 1 2 3 4 5
192. - later afternoon (early evening)? ............ 1 2 3 4 5
193. - evening? .................................... 1 2 3 4 5

194. HOW MANY naps (actually falling asleep for five minutes or more) do you take ON PURPOSE during a usual weekday? ............... __ __ times

195. HOW MANY rest periods (in which you lie down but DO NOT SLEEP) do you take in a usual weekday? ....... __ __ times

196. HOW MANY times (in a usual weekday) do you try to take a nap but can't fall asleep? ............ __ __ times

HOW LONG is your nap (daytime sleep) and rest period (without sleep) during the following parts of a usual day:

197. - morning? .................................... __ hr __ min  __ hr __ min
199. - midday? ..................................... __ hr __ min  __ hr __ min
201. - afternoon? .................................. __ hr __ min  __ hr __ min
203. - late afternoon (early evening)? ............. __ hr __ min  __ hr __ min
205. - evening? .................................... __ hr __ min  __ hr __ min

HOW MUCH do you usually feel restored (refreshed, alert) after:

207. - a nap? ...................................... 1 2 3 4 5
208. - a rest? ..................................... 1 2 3 4 5

HOW LONG do you usually remain restored (refreshed, alert) after:

209. - a nap? ...................................... __ __ hr __ __ min
210. - a rest? ..................................... __ __ hr __ __ min

211. HOW OFTEN do you experience vivid dream-like images (hallucinations) while falling asleep or awakening from a nap even though you know you are still awake? ........... 1 2 3 4 5

212. HOW OFTEN do you have vivid dreams during naps? ................................... 1 2 3 4 5

213. HOW OFTEN have you felt unable to move (paralyzed) while falling asleep or awakening from a nap? ........................ 1 2 3 4 5

*Appendix I*

OTHER DAYTIME BEHAVIOR

HOW OFTEN do you:

214. – discover that you have performed a complex act such as driving a car to the wrong destination, and not remember how you did it? . . . . . . . . . . . . . . . . . . . . . . 1 2 3 4 5

215. – find yourself doing things which make no sense (such as writing nonsense or mixing chocolate and gravy)? . . . . . . . . . . . . . . . . . . . 1 2 3 4 5

216. – get told that you were acting strangely without your being aware of it at the time? . . . . . . . . . . . . . . . . . . . . . 1 2 3 4 5

217. – have a feeling of "weak knees" when you laugh? . . . . . . . . . . . . . . . . . . . . . . . . . . 1 2 3 4 5

218. – have episodes of sudden muscular weakness (paralysis or inability to move) when laughing, angry, or in other emotional situations? . . . . . . . . . . . . . . . . . . . . . . . . . . . . . 1 2 3 4 5

219. Do you think you are excessively sleepy during the daytime? . . . . . . . . . . . . . . . . . . . . . . . . . 1 2 3 4 5

QUESTIONS ABOUT YOUR GENERAL HEALTH

What IS (or WAS) your body weight:

| | now | six months ago | two years ago | when aged 20 | when heaviest ever |
|---|---|---|---|---|---|
| 222. | ____lbs | ____lbs | ____lbs | ____lbs | ____lbs |

227. Have you had a substantial change in appetite during the past six months? . . . . . . . . . . . . . . . yes   no

Do you have any problems with:

228. – your eyes or vision? . . . . . . . . . . . . . . . . . . . . . . . yes   no

229. – your ears or hearing? . . . . . . . . . . . . . . . . . . . . . . yes   no

230. – nasal congestion, obstruction, or discharge? . . . . . . . . . . yes   no

231. – swallowing? . . . . . . . . . . . . . . . . . . . . . . . . . . . yes   no

232. – a lump or obstruction in your throat? . . . . . . . . . . . . . yes   no

248. Has your voice changed in the last year? . . . . . . . . . . . . . yes   no

249. Have you had any problems with your skin, hair, or nails? . . . . . . . . . . . . . . . . . . . . . . . . . . yes   no

Have you EVER had problems with your:

250. – stomach? . . . . . . . . . . . . . . . . . . . . . . . . . . . . . yes   no

251. – liver? . . . . . . . . . . . . . . . . . . . . . . . . . . . . . . yes   no

252. – kidneys? . . . . . . . . . . . . . . . . . . . . . . . . . . . . . yes   no

253. – bowels? . . . . . . . . . . . . . . . . . . . . . . . . . . . . . yes   no

254. – bladder? . . . . . . . . . . . . . . . . . . . . . . . . . . . . . yes   no

## Appendix I

Have you EVER had any problems with:

| | | | |
|---|---|---|---|
| 255. | - tumors (cancer)? | yes | no |
| 256. | - tonsils or adenoids? | yes | no |
| 257. | - sinusitis or nasal polyps? | yes | no |
| 258. | - thyroid gland (or goiter)? | yes | no |
| 259. | - low blood sugar (hypoglycemia)? | yes | no |
| 260. | - sugar in your urine (diabetes)? | yes | no |
| 261. | - high blood pressure? | yes | no |
| 262. | - heart disease? | yes | no |
| 263. | - chest (asthma, bronchitis, pneumonia, etc.)? | yes | no |
| 264. | Have you had your tonsils or adenoids removed? | yes | no |
| 265. | Have you EVER had an operation on your nose? | yes | no |
| 266. | Have you EVER had poliomyelitis or encephalitis? | yes | no |

HOW OFTEN do you get pains in your:

| | | |
|---|---|---|
| 267. | - neck, back, joints, or muscles? | 1 2 3 4 5 |
| 268. | - heart (angina)? | 1 2 3 4 5 |
| 269. | - chest? | 1 2 3 4 5 |
| 270. | - abdomen (stomach)? | 1 2 3 4 5 |
| 271. | - other? | 1 2 3 4 5 |
| 272. | Have you EVER had any head injuries? | 1 2 3 4 5 |
| 273. | Have you EVER been knocked unconscious? | 1 2 3 4 5 |

HOW OFTEN do you:

| | | |
|---|---|---|
| 274. | - have swelling in your ankles? | 1 2 3 4 5 |
| 275. | - suffer from uncomfortable feelings (numbness, "pins and needles") in your arms and legs (paresthesia)? | 1 2 3 4 5 |
| 276. | - have headaches during the day? | 1 2 3 4 5 |
| 277. | - suffer from dizzy spells? | 1 2 3 4 5 |
| 278. | - have episodes of loss of consciousness or fainting? | 1 2 3 4 5 |
| 279. | - have fits (convulsions, seizures, epilepsy)? | 1 2 3 4 5 |
| 280. | - have problems with relaxing your grip after you've grabbed something with your hand? | 1 2 3 4 5 |
| 281. | - have muscular weakness in any part of your body? | 1 2 3 4 5 |
| 282. | - have problems with clumsiness or incoordination? | 1 2 3 4 5 |
| 283. | - have shortness of breath? | 1 2 3 4 5 |
| 284. | - hold your breath or hyperventilate? | 1 2 3 4 5 |

*Appendix I*

HOW OFTEN do you:

285. - have heart flutters (irregular heart rhythm, palpitations) or rapid heart rate? ............ 1 2 3 4 5
286. - have an unusual sensitivity to heat? ............... 1 2 3 4 5
287. - have an unusual sensitivity to cold? ............... 1 2 3 4 5
288. - have allergies to food? ...................... 1 2 3 4 5
289. - have allergies to medication? .................. 1 2 3 4 5
290. - have any other allergies (skin rashes, hay fever, asthma, etc.)? .................... 1 2 3 4 5

FOR WOMEN

291. Are your menstrual periods in any way abnormal or irregular? ...................... yes no
292. Are you pregnant? ........................... yes no
293. Have you EVER taken birth control pills (oral contraceptives)? ..................... yes no
294. Are you past menopause (change of life)? ............ yes no
295. Are you having menopausal symptoms at present? ......... yes no

SEX

296. Do you feel that you have a sexual problem (concern)? ........................ yes no
297. Do you feel that your desire for sex, or interest in sex, is less than it used to be? .......... yes no

HOW OFTEN do you:

298. - have problems reaching an orgasm (climax)? ............ 1 2 3 4 5
299. - have pain or discomfort during intercourse? .......... 1 2 3 1 5

Do you find that you sleep better after:

300. - having sex? ............................. yes no
301. - masturbating? ........................... yes no
302. Does some sleep problem or sleep schedule interfere with your sex life? .................. yes no

FOR MEN

HOW OFTEN do you have problems with:

303. - obtaining an erection? ...................... 1 2 3 4 5
304. - maintaining an erection? ..................... 1 2 3 4 5
305. - ejaculating (e.g. premature ejaculation or inability to ejaculate)? .................. 1 2 3 4 5
306. - physically distorted erections? ................. 1 2 3 4 5
307. - painful erections during the night? ............... 1 2 3 4 5
309. - HOW OFTEN do you awaken with an erection during the night or in the morning? ............... 1 2 3 4 5

*Appendix I*

EMOTIONAL AND SOCIAL ASSESSMENT

310. Place a mark on the line somewhere between 0 (low) and 100 (high) that indicates your general level of well-being at the present moment:
0 _____ 100

311. HOW MUCH stress do you have at the present time? . . . . . . . . . . . . . . . . . . . . . . . 1 2 3 4 5

312. HOW OFTEN do you feel that your personality has changed (e.g., that you just weren't yourself), or that you have become noticeably more irritable? . . . . . . . 1 2 3 4 5

LIFE DISSATISFACTIONS

To what degree are you dissatisfied (unhappy or have a problem) with the following:

313. - your leisure time and social life? . . . . . . . . . . . . . . . 1 2 3 4 5
314. - your lifestyle? . . . . . . . . . . . . . . . . . . . . . . . . 1 2 3 4 5
315. - your living arrangements? . . . . . . . . . . . . . . . . . . . 1 2 3 4 5
316. - your relationship with your parents? . . . . . . . . . . . . . 1 2 3 4 5
317. - your family situation and relationships? . . . . . . . . . . . 1 2 3 4 5
318. - your love relationship(s)? . . . . . . . . . . . . . . . . . . 1 2 3 4 5
319. - your sex life? . . . . . . . . . . . . . . . . . . . . . . . . 1 2 3 4 5
320. - your finances? . . . . . . . . . . . . . . . . . . . . . . . . 1 2 3 4 5
321. - your job? . . . . . . . . . . . . . . . . . . . . . . . . . . . 1 2 3 4 5
322. - your education? . . . . . . . . . . . . . . . . . . . . . . . . 1 2 3 4 5
323. - your physical health? . . . . . . . . . . . . . . . . . . . . . 1 2 3 4 5
324. - your sleep? . . . . . . . . . . . . . . . . . . . . . . . . . . 1 2 3 4 5
325. - your religious activities? . . . . . . . . . . . . . . . . . . 1 2 3 4 5
326. - your political, civic, or volunteer work? . . . . . . . . . . . 1 2 3 4 5
327. - your behavior? . . . . . . . . . . . . . . . . . . . . . . . . 1 2 3 4 5
328. - your emotional or mental state? . . . . . . . . . . . . . . . . 1 2 3 4 5
329. - yourself? . . . . . . . . . . . . . . . . . . . . . . . . . . . 1 2 3 4 5

330. Are you dissatisfied or do you have a problem with any other areas not mentioned? . . . . . . . . . . . . . . . . yes    no

331. HOW OFTEN have you considered or attempted suicide? . . . . . . . . . . . . . . . . . . . . . . . 1 2 3 4 5

332. Have you EVER seen a clinical psychologist or a psychiatrist? . . . . . . . . . . . . . . . . . . . . . . . . . yes    no

333. Have you EVER been admitted to a psychiatric ward or hospital? . . . . . . . . . . . . . . . . . . . yes    no

KDS SCALE

| | | | |
|---|---|---|---|
| 334. | I feel downhearted and blue | yes | no |
| 335. | My mornings used to be my best hours | yes | no |
| 336. | When I meet people I feel I have nothing to say | yes | no |
| 337. | I am going to enjoy my food today | yes | no |
| 338. | I feel that things are looking up and that I can accomplish great things I never could do before | yes | no |
| 339. | I am scared of going to new places or meeting new people | yes | no |
| 340. | I simply don't have the energy to do things the way I used to | yes | no |
| 341. | I find that my thinking has slowed down recently | yes | no |
| 342. | I feel restless and I cannot keep still | yes | no |
| 343. | Often the silliest thoughts come to my mind and I can't keep them out | yes | no |
| 344. | I find it increasingly difficult to make decisions | yes | no |
| 345. | I feel I am useful and needed | yes | no |
| 346. | I am dreaming now more than I usually do | yes | no |
| 347. | If I watch very carefully, I can hear or see things other people don't | yes | no |
| 348. | I feel that others would be better off if I were dead | yes | no |
| 349. | I somehow have a feeling that people are against me | yes | no |
| 350. | I feel my thoughts are racing | yes | no |
| 351. | I am having very strange and peculiar experiences | yes | no |
| 352. | I now have more sexual desires than I have had in some time | yes | no |
| 353. | When I am talking to somebody, the slightest thing distracts me, even if a person only crosses his legs | yes | no |
| 354. | I recently have had more trouble expressing my thoughts or saying what I want to say | yes | no |
| 355. | I have been waking up earlier than I used to | yes | no |
| 356. | I am troubled because I have to repeat things over and over again | yes | no |
| 357. | I started to avoid riding trains, elevators, bridges, or being in enclosed areas or high places | yes | no |
| 358. | I am sleeping more than I used to | yes | no |
| 359. | Nowadays I feel worse in the morning | yes | no |
| 360. | My memory is not as sharp as it used to be | yes | no |
| 361. | Lately I find myself losing my temper | yes | no |
| 362. | Nowadays when I get anxious, my heart starts to beat fast | yes | no |
| 363. | I had trouble getting to sleep | yes | no |
| 364. | I woke up during the night more than once | yes | no |

*Appendix I*

PAST MEDICAL HISTORY

373. Previous illness:

| year of onset | name of illness |
|---|---|
| _____ | _____ |
| _____ | _____ |
| _____ | _____ |
| _____ | _____ |
| _____ | _____ |

374. Previous injuries:

| year of injury | type of injury |
|---|---|
| _____ | _____ |
| _____ | _____ |
| _____ | _____ |

375. Previous hospital admission (include surgical operations and psychiatric admissions):

| month | year | location | reason for admission |
|---|---|---|---|
| ____ | ____ | _____ | _____ |
| ____ | ____ | _____ | _____ |
| ____ | ____ | _____ | _____ |
| ____ | ____ | _____ | _____ |

376. Previous sleep recordings or EEGs:

| month | year | location | reason for recording |
|---|---|---|---|
| ____ | ____ | _____ | _____ |
| ____ | ____ | _____ | _____ |
| ____ | ____ | _____ | _____ |

*Appendix I*

FAMILY TREE

|      |          |          |       | mother |     |       | father |       |       |
|------|----------|----------|-------|--------|-----|-------|--------|-------|-------|
| 377. |          |          |       | ( )    |     |       | ( )    |       |       |

|      | sisters |     |     |     | (   )    |     | brothers |     |     |
|------|---------|-----|-----|-----|----------|-----|----------|-----|-----|
| 378. | ( )     | ( ) | ( ) | ( ) | yourself | ( ) | ( )      | ( ) | ( ) |

|      | daughters |     |     |     |  |     | sons |     |     |
|------|-----------|-----|-----|-----|--|-----|------|-----|-----|
| 379. | ( )       | ( ) | ( ) | ( ) |  | ( ) | ( )  | ( ) | ( ) |

Identify each living family member by placing their PRESENT AGE (in years) in an appropriate block. INCLUDE ONLY BLOOD RELATIVES.

If a family member is deceased, then write:

    (a). The DATE (year only) of their death.    *1964* EXAMPLE

    (b). their AGE (in years) at the time of their death.    (*17*)

FAMILY HISTORY

Does anyone in your family (NOT including yourself) have:

| | CHECK ONLY THOSE BOXES THAT APPLY | insomnia or sleep problems | sleepiness during the daytime | emotional or psychiatric problems |
|---|---|---|---|---|
| 380. | son | ( ) | ( ) | ( ) |
| 383. | daughter | ( ) | ( ) | ( ) |
| 386. | grandchildren | ( ) | ( ) | ( ) |
| 389. | brother | ( ) | ( ) | ( ) |
| 392. | sister | ( ) | ( ) | ( ) |
| 395. | father | ( ) | ( ) | ( ) |
| 398. | mother | ( ) | ( ) | ( ) |
| 401. | uncles | ( ) | ( ) | ( ) |
| 404. | aunts | ( ) | ( ) | ( ) |
| 407. | paternal grandfather | ( ) | ( ) | ( ) |
| 410. | paternal grandmother | ( ) | ( ) | ( ) |
| 413. | maternal grandfather | ( ) | ( ) | ( ) |
| 416. | maternal grandmother | ( ) | ( ) | ( ) |
| 419. | cousins | ( ) | ( ) | ( ) |

## Appendix I

Has anyone in your family (NOT including yourself):

| | | |
|---|---|---|
| 422. | – died suddenly in their sleep? | yes  no |
| 423. | – had trouble with restless (twitchy) legs while sleeping (or trying to sleep)? | yes  no |
| 424. | – had breathing problems at night? | yes  no |
| 425. | – had loud snoring at night? | yes  no |
| 426. | – been troubled by sudden attacks of weakness (inability to move) when overexcited (angry, laughing, etc.)? | yes  no |
| 427. | – died from "cot-death" (crib death, sudden infant death syndrome)? | yes  no |
| 428. | – been hyperactive (or hyperkinetic) as children or teenagers? | yes  no |
| 429. | – had electroconvulsive shock therapy? | yes  no |
| 430. | – had a nervous breakdown and/or hospitalization for emotional illness? | yes  no |
| 431. | Does a tendency to worry run in your family? | yes  no |
| 432. | Does nervousness seem to run in your family? | yes  no |

Has anyone in your family (NOT including yourself) had:

| | | |
|---|---|---|
| 433. | – diabetes? | yes  no |
| 434. | – low blood sugar (hypoglycemia)? | yes  no |
| 435. | – unusual obesity (overweight)? | yes  no |
| 436. | – allergies or asthma? | yes  no |
| 437. | – high blood pressure? | yes  no |
| 438. | – heart disease? | yes  no |
| 439. | – stroke? | yes  no |
| 440. | – arthritis? | yes  no |
| 441. | – stomach ulcers or bowel problems? | yes  no |
| 442. | – thyroid problems? | yes  no |
| 443. | – cancer? | yes  no |

LIST any other disease or disorder which is common among your family and relatives

_____

_____

*Appendix I*

MEALS

444. How many times do you eat (including snacks) during a usual 24-hour period? . . . . . . . . . . . . . __ __ times

445. At what time do you usually have the main meal of the weekday? . . . . . . . . . . . . . . . . . . . ___ am / pm

HOW OFTEN do you have something to eat (including snacks):

446. - within two hours of trying to go to sleep? . . . . . . . . . 1 2 3 4 5
447. - during the night? . . . . . . . . . . . . . . . . . . . . . 1 2 3 4 5
448. Is there anything unusual about your diet? . . . . . . . . . . yes   no

FLUIDS

HOW MUCH of these fluids do you drink?

|  | during a usual 24-hour period | within two hours of going to sleep | during the night |
|---|---|---|---|
| 449. - coffee? | __ __ cups | __ __ cups | __ __ cups |
| 452. - tea? | __ __ cups | __ __ cups | __ __ cups |
| 455. - cola drinks? | __ __ bottles | __ __ bottles | __ __ bottles |
| 458. - some other fluid? |  |  | __ __ cups |

HOW MANY alcoholic drinks do you have during a usual 24-hour period?

|  | weekday | weekend day |
|---|---|---|
| 459. - bottles (cans) of beer? | __ __ drinks | __ __ drinks |
| 461. - glasses of wine? | __ __ drinks | __ __ drinks |
| 463. - shots of liquor? | __ __ drinks | __ __ drinks |

HOW OFTEN do you drink alcoholic beverages:

465. - within two hours of trying to go to sleep? . . . . . . . . . 1 2 3 4 5
466. - during the night? . . . . . . . . . . . . . . . . . . . . . 1 2 3 4 5
467. Do you consume significantly LESS alcohol NOW than you did in the PAST? . . . . . . . . . . . . . . . . . yes   no

HOW OFTEN have you:

468. - used alcohol in order to get to sleep? . . . . . . . . . . . 1 2 3 4 5
469. - used alcoholic beverages within a few hours of awakening (e.g. a morning drink)? . . . . . . . . . . . 1 2 3 4 5
470. - used alcoholic beverages to steady your nerves? . . . . . . 1 2 3 4 5
471. - "gone on the wagon"? . . . . . . . . . . . . . . . . . . . . 1 2 3 4 5
472. - gotten sick from drinking alcoholic beverages? . . . . . . . 1 2 3 4 5
473. - had blackouts associated with alcoholic beverages? . . . . . . . . . . . . . . . . . . . . . . . . . . . 1 2 3 4 5
474. - had violent or overexcited behavior associated with drinking alcoholic beverages? . . . . . . . . . 1 2 3 4 5
475. - been under the influence of alcohol and carried out actions without being aware of what you were doing? . . . . . . . . . . . . . . . . . . . . 1 2 3 4 5

## Appendix I

HOW OFTEN have you:

476. – had DT's, rumfits, shakes, or hallucinations associated with drinking alcoholic beverages? . . . . . . . . . . . . . . . . . . . . . . 1  2  3  4  5

477. – received complaints from your family about your drinking? . . . . . . . . . . . . . . . . . . . . . . . . 1  2  3  4  5

478. – had a personal concern about your drinking? . . . . . . . . . 1  2  3  4  5

479. – missed or been late for work or appointments because of drinking alcoholic beverages? . . . . . . . . . . . . . . . . . . . . . . . . 1  2  3  4  5

480. – had problems with driving a vehicle because of drinking alcoholic beverages? . . . . . . . . . . . . 1  2  3  4  5

481. – had detoxification or other treatment for excessive drinking? . . . . . . . . . . . . . . . . . . . . . 1  2  3  4  5

TOBACCO AND STREET DRUGS

482. How many years were you a smoker? . . . . . . . . . . . . . . .  __ __ years

HOW MUCH tobacco do you smoke during a usual 24-hour period?:

                                                                       the past   now

483. packs of cigarettes? . . . . . . . . . . . . . . . . . . . . . .  __ __   __ __

485. cigars? . . . . . . . . . . . . . . . . . . . . . . . . . . . .  __ __   __ __

487. (pipe) bowls? . . . . . . . . . . . . . . . . . . . . . . . . . __ __   __ __

HOW OFTEN do you smoke tobacco:

489. – within two hours of sleep? . . . . . . . . . . . . . . . . . . 1  2  3  4  5

490. – during the night? . . . . . . . . . . . . . . . . . . . . . . 1  2  3  4  5

HOW OFTEN have you used:

491. – marijuana (or THC)? . . . . . . . . . . . . . . . . . . . . . 1  2  3  4  5

492. – cocaine? . . . . . . . . . . . . . . . . . . . . . . . . . . . 1  2  3  4  5

493. – hallucinogenic drugs (LSD, mescaline, angel dust (PCP), peyote)? . . . . . . . . . . . . . . . . . . . 1  2  3  4  5

494. – stimulants (uppers)? . . . . . . . . . . . . . . . . . . . . . 1  2  3  4  5

495. – depressants (downers)? . . . . . . . . . . . . . . . . . . . . 1  2  3  4  5

496. – narcotics (heroin, morphine, opium)? . . . . . . . . . . . . . 1  2  3  4  5

497. – other (e.g. glue sniffing, etc.)? . . . . . . . . . . . . . . 1  2  3  4  5

HOW OFTEN have you used any of the following to HELP YOU GO TO SLEEP:

498. – tobacco? . . . . . . . . . . . . . . . . . . . . . . . . . . . 1  2  3  4  5

499. – marijuana? . . . . . . . . . . . . . . . . . . . . . . . . . . 1  2  3  4  5

500. – narcotics? . . . . . . . . . . . . . . . . . . . . . . . . . . 1  2  3  4  5

501. HOW OFTEN have you been exposed to toxic (radioactive, or cancer-producing) chemicals or agents? . . . . . . . . . . . . . . . . . . . . . . . . . . . . 1  2  3  4  5

*Appendix I*

MEDICINES

Do you take any type of medication at the PRESENT TIME to help you with:

502. - a problem with your sleep? . . . . . . . . . . . . . . . . . . . . . . . yes  no

503. - a problem with daytime sleepiness (staying awake and alert) or fatigue? . . . . . . . . . . . . . . . . . . . . . yes  no

Have you EVER obtained a prescription for medication from a physician to help you with:

504. - a problem with your sleep? . . . . . . . . . . . . . . . . . . . . . . . yes  no

505. - a problem with daytime sleepiness (staying awake and alert) or fatigue? . . . . . . . . . . . . . . . . . . . . . yes  no

CHECK ONLY THOSE BOXES THAT APPLY

Have you EVER taken any of the following medications:

| | to aid sleep | to combat sleepiness | any other reason |
|---|---|---|---|
| 506. - aspirin? | ( ) | ( ) | ( ) |
| 509. - other analgesics (for example: Darvon, Tylenol, codeine)? | ( ) | ( ) | ( ) |
| 512. - dyspepsia medication (for example: Maalox, Riopan, Rolaids, Tums)? | ( ) | ( ) | ( ) |
| 515. - nasal decongestants (pills, sprays)? | ( ) | ( ) | ( ) |
| 518. - tranquillizers and muscle relaxants (for example: Valium, Librium, Meprobamate (Miltown, Equanil), Mellaril, Thorazine, Stelazine, Haldol, Navane, Prolixin)? | ( ) | ( ) | ( ) |
| 521. - antidepressant medication (for example: Elavil, Tofranil, Sinequan)? | ( ) | ( ) | ( ) |
| 524. - barbiturate sedatives (sleeping pills, for example: Seconal, Tuinal, Nembutal, Phenobarbital)? | ( ) | ( ) | ( ) |
| 527. - nonbarbiturate sedatives (sleeping pills, for example: Placidyl, Quaalude, Noludar, Dalmane, chloral hydrate, Benadryl)? | ( ) | ( ) | ( ) |
| 530. - pharmacy NONprescription sleeping pills (for example: Nytol, Compoz, Dormin, Sominex)? | ( ) | ( ) | ( ) |
| 533. - antiallergy medications (for example: Tedral, Aminophyllin, antihistamines, cortisone)? | ( ) | ( ) | ( ) |
| 536. - stimulants (for example: Ritalin, amphetamines, diet pills)? | ( ) | ( ) | ( ) |
| 539. - MILD stimulants (coffee, tea)? | ( ) | ( ) | ( ) |
| 542. pharmacy NONprescription stimulants (for example: No-Doz, Vivarin, caffeine tablets, eye-openers, Tirend, Ban-Drowz)? | ( ) | ( ) | ( ) |
| 545. - anticonvulsants (for example: Dilantin)? | ( ) | ( ) | ( ) |
| 548. - any other medications? | ( ) | ( ) | ( ) |

## Appendix I

Have you EVER taken:

| | | | |
|---|---|---|---|
| 550. | - insulin? | yes | no |
| 551. | - cardiac drugs? | yes | no |
| 552. | - cancer chemotherapy? | yes | no |
| 553. | - thyroid medications? | yes | no |
| 554. | - steroids (Cortisone, Prednisone)? | yes | no |
| 555. | - sex hormones (testosterone, estrogen)? | yes | no |
| 556. | - drugs to treat Parkinson's disease (L-Dopa)? | yes | no |

Please list all current medications (including oral contraceptives and aspirin, etc.).

557.   name                dosage per day
       _____  _____
       _____  _____
       _____  _____
       _____  _____
       _____  _____

OTHER SLEEP AIDS

HOW OFTEN do you use the following nondrug techniques to help you sleep?:

| | | |
|---|---|---|
| 558. | - medication? | 1 2 3 4 5 |
| 559. | - biofeedback? | 1 2 3 4 5 |
| 560. | - hypnosis (tapes, etc.)? | 1 2 3 4 5 |
| 561. | - mental imagery (counting sheep, etc.)? | 1 2 3 4 5 |
| 562. | - relaxation techniques? | 1 2 3 4 5 |
| 563. | - baths (hot tubs, steam baths, Jacuzzi, saunas)? | 1 2 3 4 5 |
| 564. | - massage? | 1 2 3 4 5 |
| 565. | - exercise? | 1 2 3 4 5 |
| 566. | - acupuncture? | 1 2 3 4 5 |
| 567. | - electro sleep? | 1 2 3 4 5 |
| 568. | - special diets, foods, drinks, or vitamins? | 1 2 3 4 5 |
| 569. | Have you used any other nondrug techniques? | 1 2 3 4 5 |

*Appendix I*

|  | Have you EVER consulted with any of the following to help you with a sleep problem or daytime sleepiness: | | CHECK ONLY THOSE BOXES THAT APPLY | |
|---|---|---|---|---|
| 570. | - general practitioner? | ( ) | - chiropractor? | ( ) |
| 572. | - obstetrics/gynecology? | ( ) | - osteopath? | ( ) |
| 574. | - cardiologist? | ( ) | - homeopaths? | ( ) |
| 576. | - other internists? | ( ) | - counselor? | ( ) |
| 578. | - psychiatrist? | ( ) | - social worker? | ( ) |
| 580. | - other physician? | ( ) | - nurse? | ( ) |
| 582. | - clinical psychologist? | ( ) | - clergyman? | ( ) |

EXERCISE

584. How many times in a usual week do you participate in a sport or partake in some other form of physical exercise? . . . . . . . . . . . . . . . . . . . . . . ___ ___ times

WHAT TIME of the day do you exercise or take part in a regular social or recreational activity (e.g. music, theater):

CHECK ONLY THOSE BOXES THAT APPLY

|  |  | exercise | social or recreational activity |
|---|---|---|---|
| 585. | - in the morning? | ( ) | ( ) |
| 587. | - midday? | ( ) | ( ) |
| 589. | - afternoon? | ( ) | ( ) |
| 591. | - late afternoon (early evening)? | ( ) | ( ) |
| 593. | - late evening? | ( ) | ( ) |

595. Briefly describe the type of physical exercise:

_____

_____

CHILDHOOD FAMILY

596. Were you born as a part of a multiple birth (twins, triplets, etc.)? . . . . . . . . . . . . . . . yes  no

597. What was your birth weight? . . . . . . . . . . . . . . . . . . . . . ___ ___ lbs

598. Were there any unusual conditions of pregnancy or delivery (complications, premature birth, birth trauma, blue baby, etc.)? . . . . . . . . . . . . . . yes  no

*Appendix I*

With whom did you live for most of the time until you were 18 years of age?:

| | | | |
|---|---|---|---|
| 599. | - natural mother? | yes | no |
| 600. | - stepmother? | yes | no |
| 601. | - adoptive mother? | yes | no |
| 602. | - foster mother? | yes | no |
| 603. | - natural father? | yes | no |
| 604. | - stepfather? | yes | no |
| 605. | - adoptive father? | yes | no |
| 606. | - foster father? | yes | no |
| 607. | - siblings (brothers and/or sisters)? | yes | no |
| 608. | - other relative(s)? | yes | no |
| 609. | - an institution? | yes | no |
| 610. | - other? | yes | no |
| 611. | How close was your family during your childhood? | | 1 2 3 4 5 |
| 612. | How well did your parents get along with each other while you were growing up? | | 1 2 3 4 5 |

What were your parents' occupations while you were growing up:

614. - mother? _____

615. - father? _____

616. Have you had any serious disciplinary action taken against you while you were in school? .................................... yes no

617. Have you had any legal action taken against you other than minor traffic violations? ........................................ yes no

EDUCATION

HOW MUCH formal education have you and your parents had:     CHECK ONLY THOSE BOXES THAT APPLY

| | | yourself | mother | father |
|---|---|---|---|---|
| 618. | - less than an 8th-grade education? | ( ) | ( ) | ( ) |
| 621. | - completed 8th grade but did not graduate from high school? | ( ) | ( ) | ( ) |
| 624. | - high-school graduate or equivalent? | ( ) | ( ) | ( ) |
| 627. | - one to three years of college, business, or trade school (AA degree)? | ( ) | ( ) | ( ) |
| 630. | - four-year college graduate (BA, BS, etc.)? | ( ) | ( ) | ( ) |
| 633. | - completed graduate school (MA, MS, MD, PhD, etc.)? | ( ) | ( ) | ( ) |

*Appendix I*

OCCUPATION

636. What is your present occupation? .......... _____

Your present work situation is best described as:

637. - employed? ................................. yes no
638. - self-employed? ............................ yes no
639. - laid off? ................................. yes no
640. - suspended or dismissed from job? .......... yes no
641. - retired? .................................. yes no
642. - unemployed? ............................... yes no
643. - part-time work? ........................... yes no
644. - temporary job? ............................ yes no
645. - homemaker, no outside employment? ......... yes no
646. Do you work variable (rotating) shifts? ..... yes no
647. Do you work split shifts (working day broken up into two or more separate work periods)? ... yes no
648. Does your job involve working on weekends? .. yes no
649. At the present time, do you work at more than one job? ............................... yes no
650. How many hours per week do you work? ........ __ __ hrs

What are the hours:

651. - from? .................................... ____ am / pm
652. - to? ...................................... ____ am / pm
653. HOW OFTEN do you travel across time zones? ..................................... 1  2  3  4  5
654. How long does it take you to adjust after traveling across time zones? ......... __ __ days
655. Have you been in the military? .............. yes no
656. - What was your rank? ...................... _____
657. - How long were you in? .................... __ __ years __ __ months
658. - What was your job? ....................... _____
659. - Were you EVER in active combat? .......... yes no
660. What is the best job you EVER had? .......... _____
661. Have you EVER had a job which involved working at unusual times (e.g. not a "9 am to 5 pm" job)? ......... yes no
662. What is (or was) your spouse's occupation? ................................. _____

*Appendix I*

PRESENT LIVING SITUATION

What is your present living situation:

| | | |
|---|---|---|
| 663. | - a house?............................................. | yes  no |
| 664. | - an apartment?....................................... | yes  no |
| 665. | - a dormitory?........................................ | yes  no |
| 666. | - an institution?..................................... | yes  no |

HOW MANY people live in your present household:

| | | |
|---|---|---|
| 667. | - spouse or living companion?......................... | __ __ people |
| 668. | - your children?...................................... | __ __ people |
| 669. | - brothers or sisters?................................ | __ __ people |
| 670. | - own parent(s)?...................................... | __ __ people |
| 671. | - other relative(s)?.................................. | __ __ people |
| 672. | - roommate(s)?........................................ | __ __ people |
| 673. | - companion(s)?....................................... | __ __ people |
| 674. | - fellow inmates or patients?......................... | __ __ people |
| 675. | - other people?....................................... | __ __ people |
| 676. | How many times have you been married?................. | __ __ times |
| 677. | What was your age at the time of your first marriage?........................................ | __ __ years |
| 678. | What is the longest period of time that you have lived with your present spouse or living companion without any major separations?.......................................... | __ __ years __ __ months |
| 679. | How well do you and your spouse or living companion get along?............................. | 1  2  3  4  5 |
| 680. | How many adopted or step children have you had?....... | _____ children |

RELIGION

What is your religious affiliation?

| | | |
|---|---|---|
| 681. | - Catholic?........................................... | yes  no |
| 682. | - Protestant?......................................... | yes  no |
| 683. | - Jewish?............................................. | yes  no |
| 684. | - no religious affiliation at present?................ | yes  no |
| 685. | - other?........................................yes  no ... if yes, please specify _____ | |
| 686. | HOW MUCH importance does religion have in your daily life?..................................... | 1  2  3  4  5 |

*Appendix I*

MAKES BETTER-WORSE LIST      (1)

How do the following factors affect your sleep?
(CHECK ONLY THOSE BOXES THAT APPLY)

|      |                              | makes better | no change | makes worse |
|------|------------------------------|:---:|:---:|:---:|
| 687. | some specific food?          | ( ) | ( ) | ( ) |
| 690. | any type of food?            | ( ) | ( ) | ( ) |
| 693. | coffee?                      | ( ) | ( ) | ( ) |
| 696. | tea?                         | ( ) | ( ) | ( ) |
| 699. | cola drink?                  | ( ) | ( ) | ( ) |
| 702. | alcoholic beverage?          | ( ) | ( ) | ( ) |
| 705. | physical exercise?           | ( ) | ( ) | ( ) |
| 708. | mental stress?               | ( ) | ( ) | ( ) |
| 711. | anxiety or worry?            | ( ) | ( ) | ( ) |
| 714. | fatigue?                     | ( ) | ( ) | ( ) |
| 717. | daytime nap?                 | ( ) | ( ) | ( ) |
| 720. | daytime rest?                | ( ) | ( ) | ( ) |
| 723. | certain kinds of weather?    | ( ) | ( ) | ( ) |
| 726. | heat?                        | ( ) | ( ) | ( ) |
| 729. | cold?                        | ( ) | ( ) | ( ) |
| 732. | noise?                       | ( ) | ( ) | ( ) |
| 735. | shift work?                  | ( ) | ( ) | ( ) |
| 738. | seasons?                     | ( ) | ( ) | ( ) |
| 741. | air travel?                  | ( ) | ( ) | ( ) |
| 744. | not being in your usual bed? | ( ) | ( ) | ( ) |
| 747. | adolescence?                 | ( ) | ( ) | ( ) |
| 750. | menstrual cycle?             | ( ) | ( ) | ( ) |
| 753. | during pregnancy?            | ( ) | ( ) | ( ) |
| 756. | following pregnancy?         | ( ) | ( ) | ( ) |
| 759. | during menopause?            | ( ) | ( ) | ( ) |
| 762. | following menopause?         | ( ) | ( ) | ( ) |
| 765. | weekends?                    | ( ) | ( ) | ( ) |
| 768. | holidays?                    | ( ) | ( ) | ( ) |
| 771. | some type of illness?        | ( ) | ( ) | ( ) |

*Appendix I*

MAKES BETTER-WORSE LIST     (2)

How do the following factors affect your sleepiness in the daytime?
(CHECK ONLY THOSE BOXES THAT APPLY)

|  |  | makes better | no change | makes worse |
|---|---|---|---|---|
| 774. | some specific food? | ( ) | ( ) | ( ) |
| 777. | any type of food? | ( ) | ( ) | ( ) |
| 780. | coffee? | ( ) | ( ) | ( ) |
| 783. | tea? | ( ) | ( ) | ( ) |
| 786. | cola drink? | ( ) | ( ) | ( ) |
| 789. | alcoholic beverage? | ( ) | ( ) | ( ) |
| 792. | physical exercise? | ( ) | ( ) | ( ) |
| 795. | mental stress? | ( ) | ( ) | ( ) |
| 798. | anxiety or worry? | ( ) | ( ) | ( ) |
| 801. | fatigue? | ( ) | ( ) | ( ) |
| 804. | daytime nap? | ( ) | ( ) | ( ) |
| 807. | daytime rest? | ( ) | ( ) | ( ) |
| 810. | certain kinds of weather? | ( ) | ( ) | ( ) |
| 813. | heat? | ( ) | ( ) | ( ) |
| 816. | cold? | ( ) | ( ) | ( ) |
| 819. | noise? | ( ) | ( ) | ( ) |
| 822. | shift work? | ( ) | ( ) | ( ) |
| 825. | seasons? | ( ) | ( ) | ( ) |
| 828. | air travel? | ( ) | ( ) | ( ) |
| 831. | not being in your usual bed? | ( ) | ( ) | ( ) |
| 834. | adolescence? | ( ) | ( ) | ( ) |
| 837. | menstrual cycle? | ( ) | ( ) | ( ) |
| 840. | during pregnancy? | ( ) | ( ) | ( ) |
| 843. | following pregnancy? | ( ) | ( ) | ( ) |
| 846. | during menopause? | ( ) | ( ) | ( ) |
| 849. | following menopause? | ( ) | ( ) | ( ) |
| 852. | weekends? | ( ) | ( ) | ( ) |
| 855. | holidays? | ( ) | ( ) | ( ) |
| 858. | some type of illness? | ( ) | ( ) | ( ) |

*Appendix I*

CONCLUSION

861. Now that you completed this questionnaire,
do you feel that your sleep OR daytime
alertness is abnormal in any way? . . . . . . . . . . . . . . . . . . . . . yes  no

862. What is your personal interpretation as to why you have
your particular sleep/wake problem?

_____

_____

_____

_____

IS THERE ANYTHING ELSE?

863. If your sleep/wake behavior is not adequately covered by the above
questions, briefly describe the nature of your sleep/wake behavior
and list anything else (not yet covered) which especially interferes
with your sleep or wakefulness:

_____

_____

_____

_____

PLEASE CHECK THROUGH THE QUESTIONNAIRE TO SEE
IF YOU HAVE ANSWERED ALL THE QUESTIONS ON BOTH
SIDES OF THE PAPER.

# APPENDIX II

CHRISTIAN GUILLEMINAULT
MARIANNE SOUQUET

During the first years of life, infants develop clearly identifiable sleep stages. Researchers and clinicians often use the criteria outlined in the *Manual of Standardized Terminology, Techniques, and Criteria for the Scoring of States of Sleep and Wakefulness in Newborn Infants* (Anders et al., 1971) *(1)*; however, since this manual was originally developed to score sleep in newborns, it does not take into consideration the obvious maturational progression that occurs in infants during the first six months of life. In 1979, we published a scoring system that has been used at Stanford for the past five years and has been validated by over 400 infant recordings (nocturnal or 24-hour) *(2)*. This scoring system uses an epoch-by-epoch approach based on the Rechtschaffen and Kales (1968) *(3)* scoring system. An "epoch" is defined as "30 seconds of continuous polygraphic activity." The most notable change is the criterion for delta waves—a delta wave being a wave of 2 Hz or slower with an amplitude of at least 150 μV. For full-term infants up to approximately six weeks of age, we found Anders's manual *(1)* entirely satisfactory; for older infants, however, the manual overlooks much information contained in the EEG. Our proposed classification allows better definition of sleep stages; like all attempts at classification, it has its own merits and faults. It is reproduced with permission from a previous publication. *(2)*.

*Appendix II*

# Scoring Criteria

## A. Three-month-old infant:

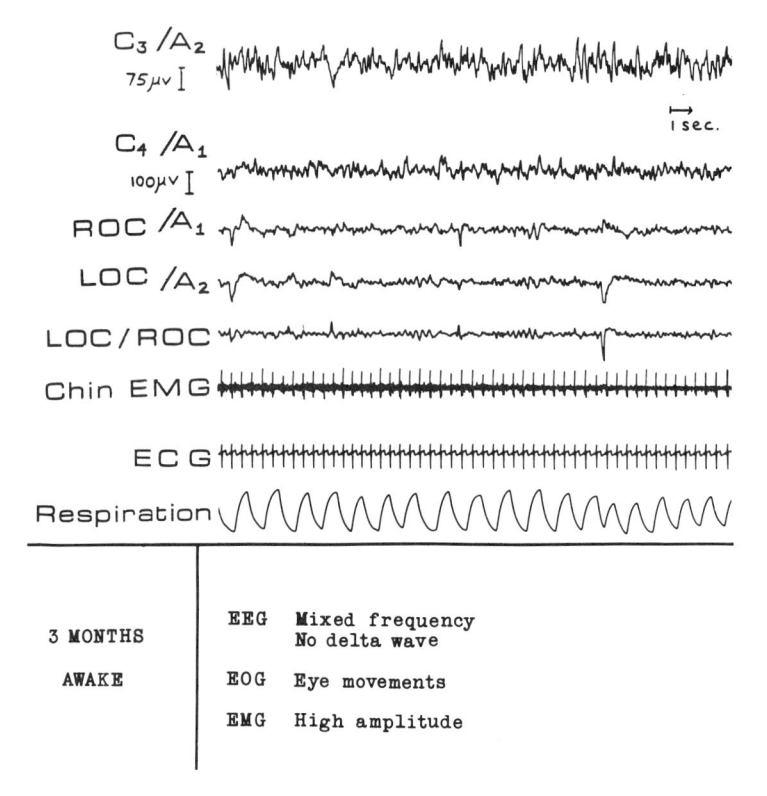

```
C₃/A₂   [EEG trace]
75μV

C₄/A₁   [EEG trace]
100μV

ROC/A₁  [EOG trace]
LOC/A₂  [EOG trace]
LOC/ROC [EOG trace]
Chin EMG [EMG trace]
ECG     [ECG trace]
Respiration [respiration trace]
```

| 3 MONTHS<br>AWAKE | EEG | Mixed frequency<br>No delta wave |
|---|---|---|
| | EOG | Eye movements |
| | EMG | High amplitude |

**Figure AII–1—stage wakefulness:** Stage wakefulness is characterized by mixed-frequency EEG with no delta waves; the voltage is relatively low (less than 75 μV). It is usually accompanied by a relatively high tonic EMG and often by rapid eye movements. The eyes are usually open, but may be closed.

**Movement Time (MT):** An epoch is scored "MT" if movement artifact obscures the EEG and EOG tracings in one-half or more of the epoch.

*Appendix II*

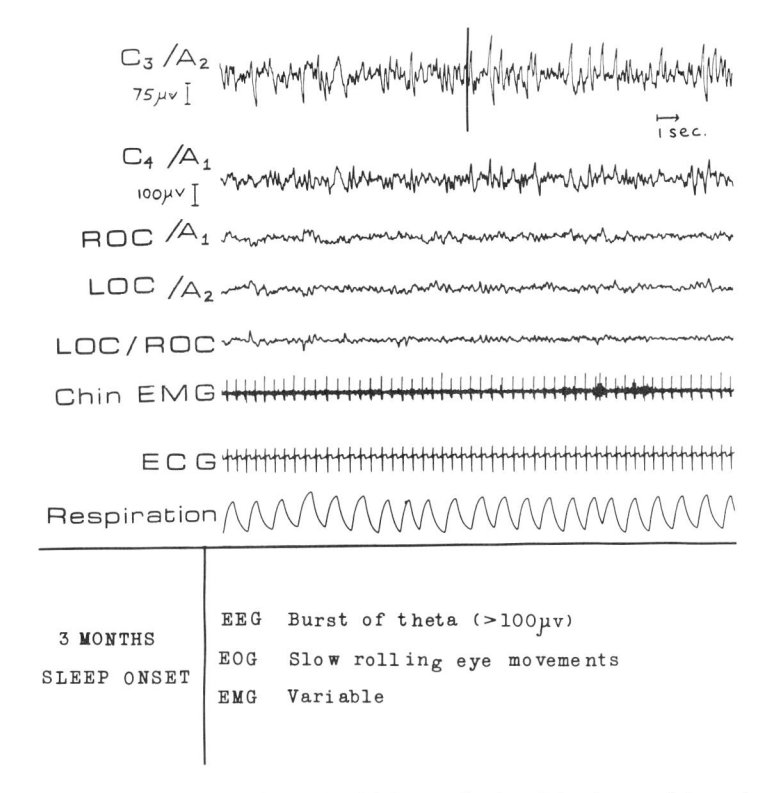

```
C₃/A₂
75μV

C₄/A₁
100μV

ROC/A₁

LOC/A₂

LOC/ROC

Chin EMG

ECG

Respiration
```

|  |  |  |
|---|---|---|
| 3 MONTHS SLEEP ONSET | EEG | Burst of theta (>100μv) |
| | EOG | Slow rolling eye movements |
| | EMG | Variable |

**Figure AII-2—sleep onset.** Note the high amplitude of the burst of theta (over 100 μV).

*Appendix II*

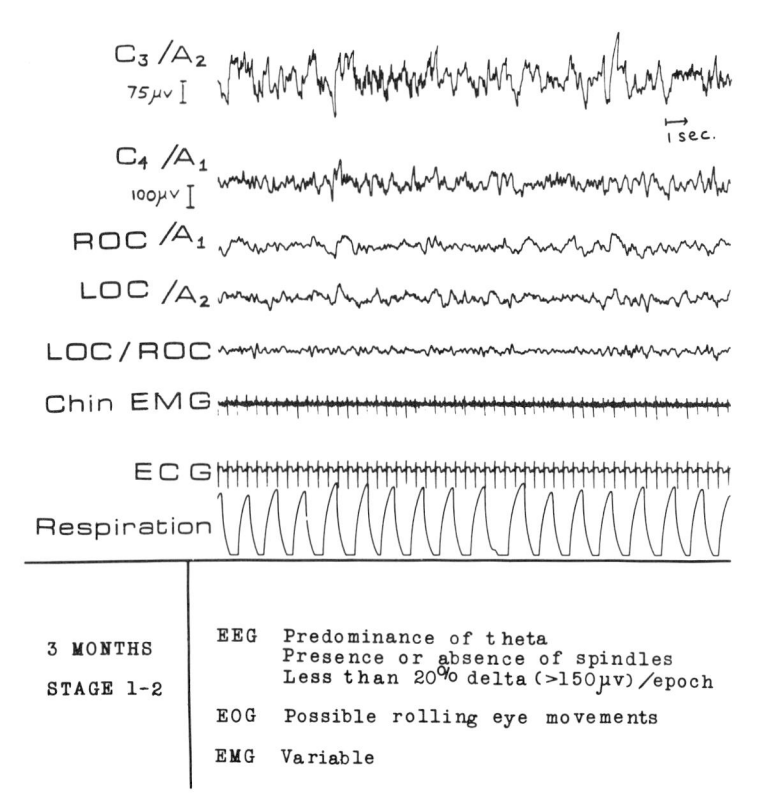

```
C₃/A₂   75μV
C₄/A₁   100μV
ROC/A₁
LOC/A₂
LOC/ROC
Chin EMG
ECG
Respiration
                                                         1 sec.
```

| 3 MONTHS<br>STAGE 1-2 | EEG | Predominance of theta<br>Presence or absence of spindles<br>Less than 20% delta (>150μv)/epoch |
|---|---|---|
| | EOG | Possible rolling eye movements |
| | EMG | Variable |

**Figure AII–3—stage 1–2:** Stage 1–2 is defined by mixed-frequency EEG (1 to 15 Hz) with less than 20% delta waves (greater than 150 μV). Sleep spindles often are not present; if they are present, stage 2 is defined as a separate entity. Background theta activity disappears as delta activity becomes prominent. There may be some slow rolling eye movements; rapid eye movements are absent. The EMG usually is of lower amplitude than during quiet wakefulness. The behavior generally is quiet but may show sucking, body movements, startles, jerks, and/or sighs.

*Appendix II*

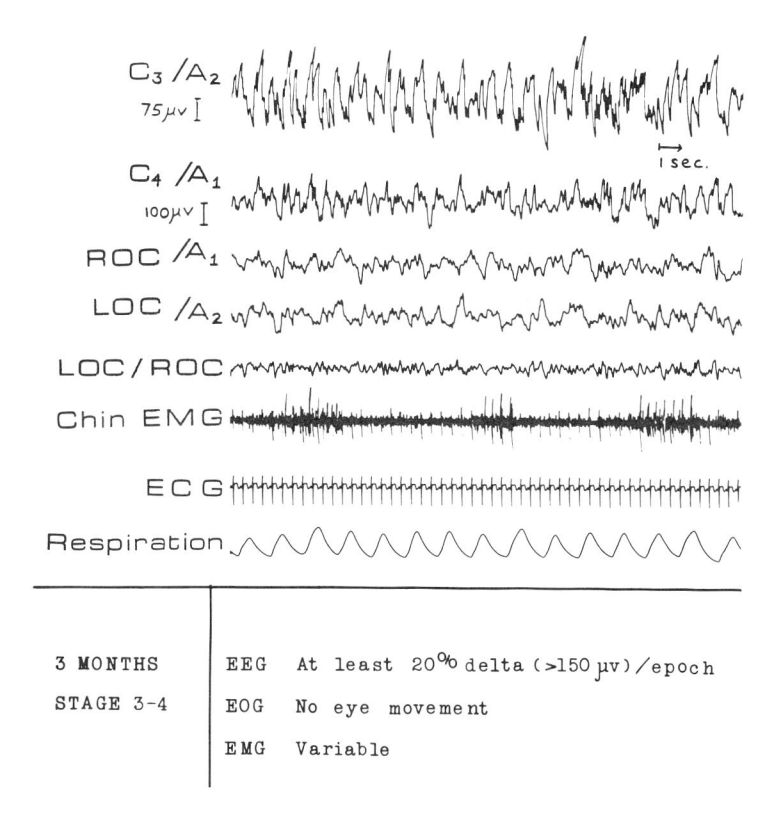

```
C₃/A₂
 75μV
C₄/A₁
100μV
ROC/A₁
LOC/A₂
LOC/ROC
Chin EMG
ECG
Respiration
```

|  |  |  |
|---|---|---|
| 3 MONTHS | EEG | At least 20% delta (>150 μV)/epoch |
| STAGE 3-4 | EOG | No eye movement |
|  | EMG | Variable |

**Figure AII–4—stage 3–4:** Stage 3–4 is defined by an EEG containing at least 20% delta waves (greater than 150 μV). Sleep spindles usually are not present. It is interesting to note that background theta activity appears to decrease as delta activity becomes prominent, and may be virtually absent just prior to REM. Behavior is predominantly quiet, but may show occasional sighs. Active sucking disappears. Usually, no distinction is made between stage 3 and stage 4.

Appendix II

```
C₃/A₂
75μV
                                                    ⟶
                                                  1 sec.
C₄/A₁
100μV

ROC/A₁

LOC/A₂

LOC/ROC

Chin EMG

ECG

Respiration
```

| 3 MONTHS<br>REM SLEEP | EEG | Predominance of theta |
|---|---|---|
| | EOG | Rapid eye movements |
| | EMG | Low amplitude |

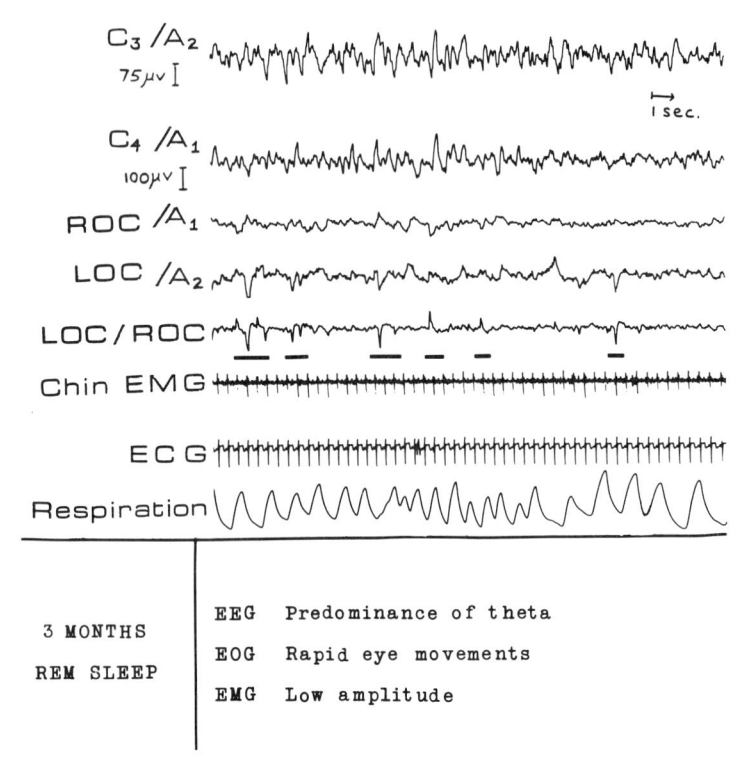

**Figure AII–5—stage REM:** Stage REM is defined by episodic rapid eye movements, a tonically suppressed EMG, and mixed-frequency EEG (1 to 12 Hz) with a predominance of theta activity (3 to 7 Hz). Behavior is characterized by twitches, jerks, sucking, smiles, vocalization, sighs, irregular respiration, and eyes open for short periods. Note: The rules for starting and ending stage REM are the same as those recommended in the international manual for scoring sleep in adults (Rechtschaffen and Kales, 1968).

*Appendix II*

## B. Six-month-old infant:

(These criteria can be used for infants from four and one-half weeks to one year of age.)

**Stage Wakefulness (W):**  Same as criteria for three-month-old infant.

**Movement Time (MT):**  Same as criteria for three-month-old infant.

| 6 MONTHS STAGE 1 | EEG | Predominance of theta<br>Absence of spindles<br>Absence of delta (>150 μv) |
|---|---|---|
| | EOG | Possible rolling eye movements |
| | EMG | Variable |

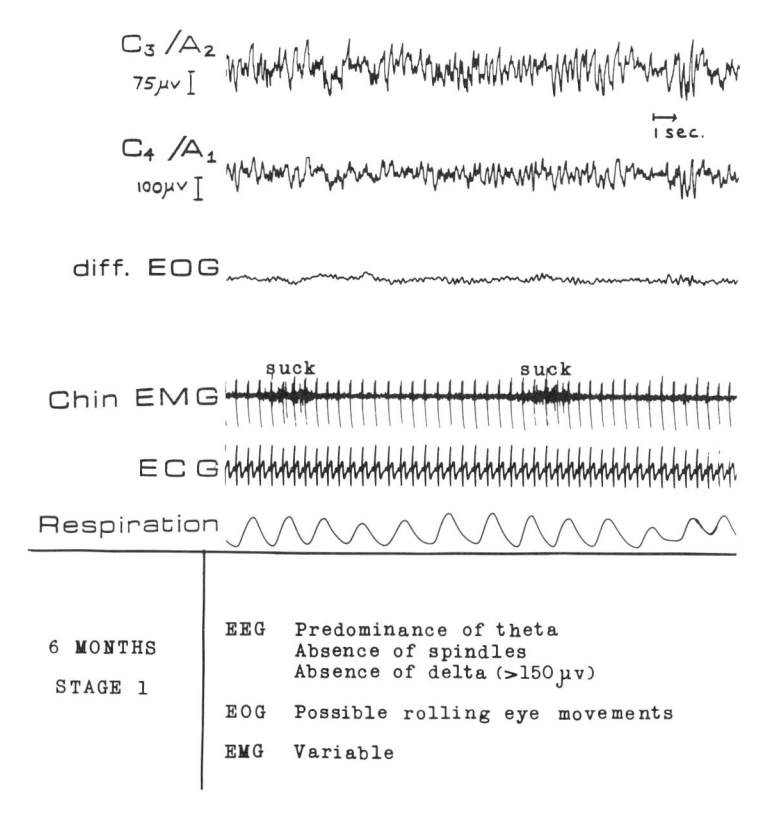

**Figure AII–6—stage 1:**  Stage 1 is defined by mixed-frequency EEG (1 to 12 Hz) with a predominance of theta activity (3 to 7 Hz), absence of sleep spindles, and less than 20% delta waves (greater than 150 μV). At sleep onset, stage 1 is frequently characterized by a burst of regular high-amplitude theta waves and slow rolling eye movements. Rapid eye movements are absent. The EMG usually is of lower amplitude than during quiet wakefulness. Behavior generally is quiet, but there may be sucking, body movements, startles, jerks, and/or sighs.

*Appendix II*

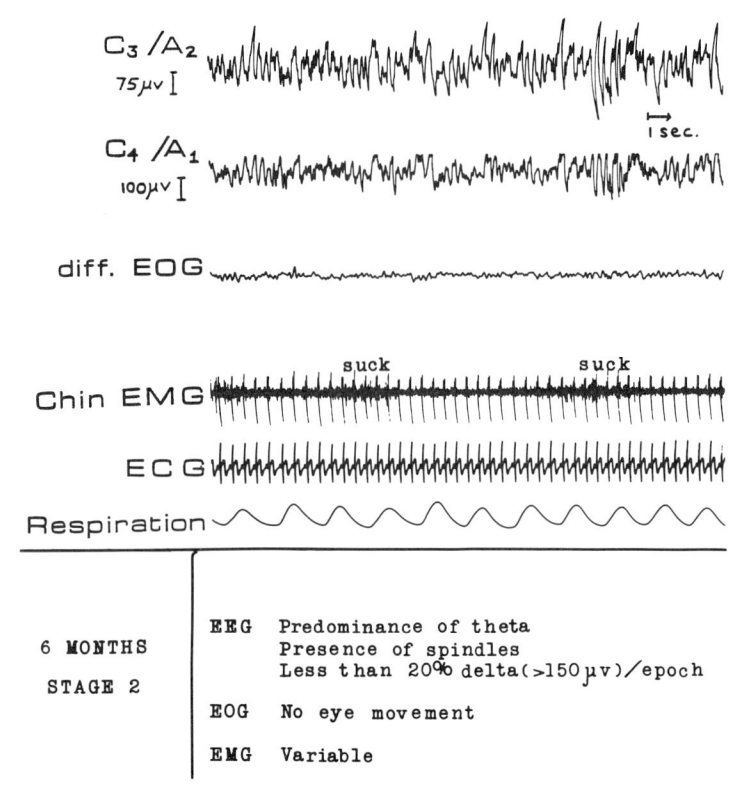

|  |  |  |
|---|---|---|
| 6 MONTHS<br>STAGE 2 | EEG | Predominance of theta<br>Presence of spindles<br>Less than 20% delta(>150 μv)/epoch |
|  | EOG | No eye movement |
|  | EMG | Variable |

**Figure AII–7—stage 2:** Stage 2 is defined by the presence of sleep spindles (12 to 14 Hz), and less than 20% delta waves (greater than 150 μV). (Stage 2 is scored unless the spindle-to-spindle interval is greater than five minutes.) Behavior generally is quiet, but there may be sucking, startles, jerks, and/or sighs.

*Appendix II*

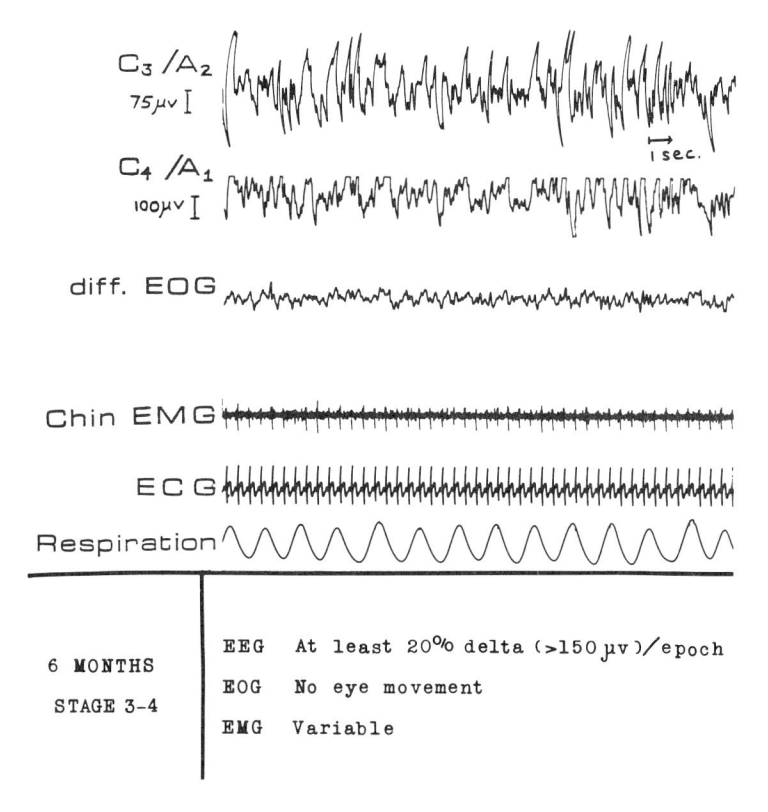

|  |  |  |
|---|---|---|
| 6 MONTHS<br>STAGE 3-4 | EEG | At least 20% delta (>150 μv)/epoch |
|  | EOG | No eye movement |
|  | EMG | Variable |

**Figure AII-8—stage 3-4:** Same criteria as for three-month-old infant.

C₃/A₂ 75μV

C₄/A₁ 100μV

1 sec.

diff. EOG

Chin EMG

ECG

Respiration

| 6 MONTHS | EEG | Predominance of theta |
| REM SLEEP | EOG | Rapid eye movements |
|  | EMG | Low amplitude |

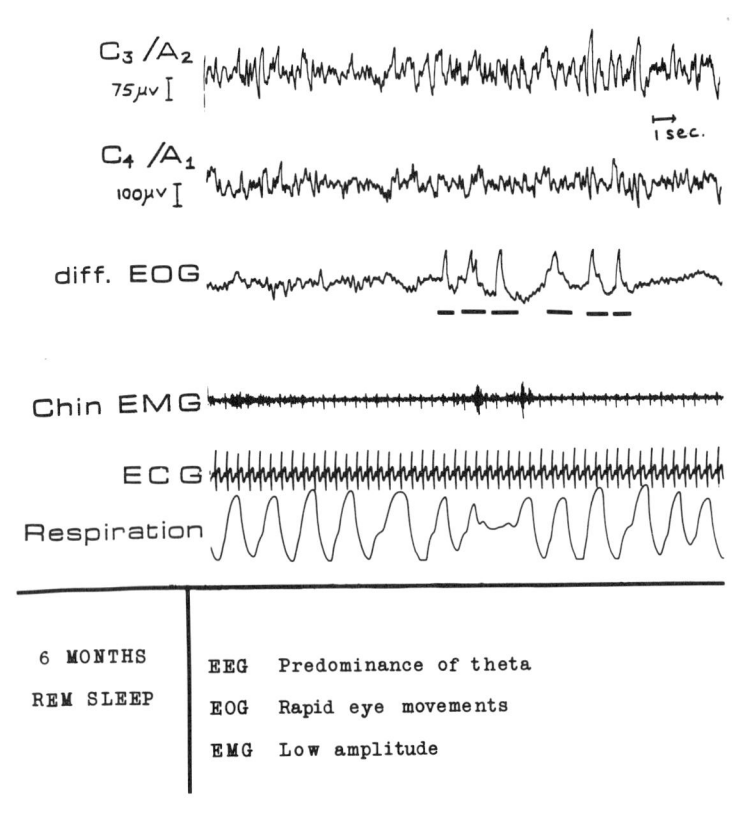

**Figure AII–9—stage REM:** Same criteria as for three-month-old infant. Behavior is characterized by twitches, sighs, and irregular respiration, but the infant is quieter than at a younger age. REM onset is frequently announced by a burst of very regular high-amplitude (over 200 μV) delta discharge.

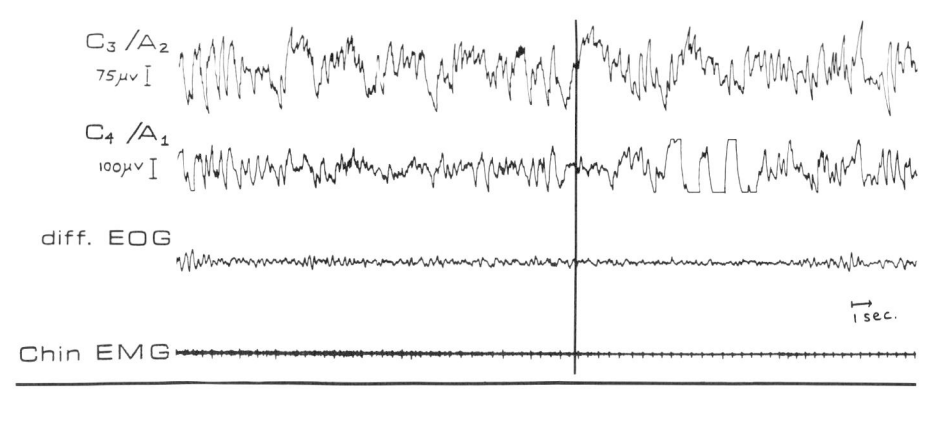

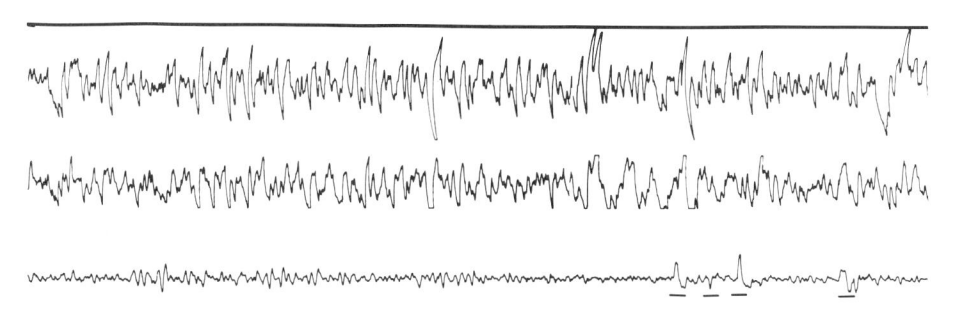

**Figure AII–10—transition to stage REM:** For infants over one year of age, the Rechtschaffen and Kales international adult scoring system is applicable and gives valid results. The lower section is a continuation of the upper. REM sleep should be scored from the vertical line where both the EEG and the EMG change. Note the long heartbeat at the entry into REM sleep.

# TECHNIQUES OF RECORDING

### A. EEG Recording:

The paper speed is 10 mm/sec. The derivations used are $C_4/A_1$ and $C_3/A_2$. The low-frequency filter is set at 0.3 Hz, the high-frequency filter at 30 Hz. The gains are 75 µV/cm.

### B. Eye Movement Recording:

The derivation used is left eye to right eye, using the differential eye technique. This derivation is recorded on one channel using two double electrodes placed on the outer canthus of each eye and above the opposite eye. The low-frequency filter is set at 0.3 Hz and the high-frequency filter at 30 Hz. The gains are 73 µV/cm.

*Appendix II*

## C. EMG Recording:

Electrodes are placed submentally for the EMG recording; three electrodes are used, one as a spare. The gain is at least 20 μV/cm. The low-frequency filter is set at 10 Hz, the high-frequency filter at 60 Hz.

## D. Behavioral Observations:

Coded behavioral observations are noted continuously on the recording chart. These include: eyes open, eyes closed, eye movements, body movements, jerks and twitches (including the part of the body involved), startles, vocalizations, respiratory irregularities (sighs, pauses, etc.), and infant quiet.

# REFERENCES

1. Anders T, Emde R, Parmalee A, eds. A manual of standardized terminology, techniques, and criteria for scoring of states of sleep and wakefulness in newborn infants. Los Angeles: UCLA Brain Information Service/Brain Research Institute, 1971.
2. Guilleminault C, Souquet M. Sleep states and related pathology. In: Korobkin R, Guilleminault C, eds. Advances in perinatal neurology, vol. 1. New York: Spectrum, 1979.
3. Rechtschaffen, A, Kales A, eds. A manual of standardized terminology, techniques and scoring system for sleep stages of human subjects. Los Angeles: UCLA Brain Information Service/Brain Research Institute, 1978.

---

Figures AII–1 through AII–10 are reproduced from Guilleminault C, Souquet M, "Sleep states and related pathology," in: Korobkin R, Guilleminault C, eds., *Advances in Perinatal Neurology, Volume 1,* New York: Spectrum, 1979.

# INDEX

Abdominal respiratory effort, 188–189, 196–200, 213–222. *See also* Diaphragm
Acid clearance test, and gastroesophageal reflux, 334
Acromegaly, and sleep apnea, 171
Active sleep (REM sleep), in infants, 80, 83, 84, 86, 88, 91. *See also* Rapid eye movement sleep
Adenoids in children, 171, 177–179
Adolescence
 bedtimes in, 100–101, 105–106, 107
 changes in sleep patterns during, 103–104, 107, 109, 117
 and drug ingestion, 113
 hormonal changes during, 99, 104, 114–115
 and narcolepsy, 99, 109, 116–117
 and sleep, 99–122 *passim*
 sleep disorders in, 99, 102–103, 109, 111, 113, 116–117
 sleep habits during, 100–103
 and sleep latency, 103, 106, 109–111, 112, 113, 146
Advanced sleep phase syndrome, 301. *See also* Chronobiology; Chronotherapy
Affective disorders and sleep, 245–261 *passim*. *See also* Depression
Age
 and circadian rhythms, 301

 and depression, 255–256, 257, 260–261
 and insomnia, 225, 233
 and nocturnal penile tumescence, 345, 346
 and periodic movements in sleep, 270
 sleep changes related to, 157, 158, 159
 *See also* Elderly patients
Airflow
 cessation, 159
 dynamics of, 168–169
 in evaluation of insomnia, 239
 monitoring of, 160, 161–162, 165
 at nose and mouth, 188, 189, 196, 198, 199, 200
 reduction of, 160
 and sleep apnea, 166, 213–215
Airway, upper
 compromised, 170
 obstruction of, 158, 159, 160, 164, 166, 175, 176, 195, 215, 218, 222
 patency of, 168, 171
Alcohol ingestion
 in adolescents, 113
 effect on sleep, 157, 246
 and hypnotic medication, 228
 and insomnia, 236
 and nocturnal penile tumescence, 346, 362
 and sleep hygiene, 229
Allergies, and sleep disorders, 156, 228, 230
Alpha-delta sleep, 238
Alpha motoneuron, 172
Alpha rhythm (in EEG), 2, 3, 8, 12, 158, 197, 199
Alzheimer disease, 260–261

Ambulatory monitoring
 of activity, 241–242, 304, 316
 of body temperature, 310–311, 315–316
 of electrocardiogram, 163, 164, 165, 178, 184, 192–195, 211
 with Medilog recorder, 287–291
 with Solicorder, 304, 315–316
Aminophylline, for preventing apnea, 17
Amyloidosis, and restless legs syndrome, 269
Anticonvulsant drugs, 374, 375
Antidepressant drugs, 231, 249, 259, 260, 261, 276
Antihistamines, effect on sleep, 156
Antihypertensive drugs, effects on sleep, 231
Anxiety, effect on sleep, 158, 230, 235–236, 237, 259, 260
Anxiety disorders, 259, 260
Apnea
 caused by head or neck trauma, 176–177
 central, 159, 160, 165–171 *passim*, 188, 195–197, 200, 213–215, 259
 characteristics of, 37
 in congenital central hypoventilation syndrome, 175
 and depression, 170, 247, 258–259, 261
 and gastroesophageal reflux, 20, 195
 identification of, 20–21, 37, 50, 239

427

*Index*

Apnea *(cont.)*
  in infants, 17, 18, 20–31 *passim*, 36–39, 40, 45, 50, 87, 89–93, 159, 162
  in insomnia, 227, 232, 237, 239
  mixed, 159, 171, 199
  and nocturnal myoclonus (periodic movements in sleep), 270, 271, 275, 286
  normative data (in infants), 24, 29–31
  obstructive, 159–171 *passim*, 188, 195–199, 213, 215, 222, 258, 259
  polygraphic tracings, 22–23, 87, 89–91
  and respiratory rate, 45, 50
  and snoring, 161, 168, 170
  *See also* Hypopnea; Respiration; Sleep apnea syndromes
Apnea Index (AI), 159, 162
Apnea monitors
  failure of, 20–21
  at home, 39
  and hypoxemia, 20
  in neonatal intensive care units, 18
Apnea plus Hypopnea Index [(A+H)I], 162, 166, 196
Arousal from sleep
  definition of, 157–159
  EEG changes during, 158
  with hypoxemia, 173
  and periodic movements in sleep (nocturnal myoclonus), 269, 271, 272, 273, 282, 290
  and sleep apnea, 170, 196, 200, 201
Arousal index, 273
Arousal response, 175
Artifact
  blink, 11
  cable-movement, 280
  definition, 12
  ECG, 6, 280
  faulty electrodes, 280
  movement, 81, 84, 89, 92, 197, 198, 199, 200, 201, 281, 282, 287, 335, 348
  in MSLT, 150
  muscle, 11, 199
  in NPT monitoring, 356–357, 358, 361, 362
  in pupillography, 138, 139, 140, 141, 142

  respiratory, 280
  sweat, 9, 115
Association of Sleep Disorders Centers (ASDC)
  nosology, 233–239, 245, 258, 261, 270–274 *passim*
  survey of patient population, 160
Asthma, and sleep, 172
Atropine sulfate, and sleep apnea, 163
Auditory evoked potentials, in infants, 18, 21, 24, 32–34, 38, 62, 73–74, 84, 89, 92
Automatic behavior, and sleep apnea, 161
Autonomic nervous system
  and arousal from sleep, 157–158
  and congenital central hypoventilation syndrome, 176
  and rapid eye movement sleep, 162, 183
  and respiration, 164
  and sleep-wakefulness cycle, 127, 128
Avitaminosis, and restless legs syndrome, 269

Baclofen, and periodic movements in sleep, 276
BAEP. *See* Auditory evoked potentials
Bed partner, 227, 269
Bedtimes, in adolescence, 100–101, 105–106, 107
Bed-wetting. *See* Enuresis
Berger, Hans, 1–2
Bernoulli effect, 168
Beta rhythm (in EEG)
  definition, 12
  and mu rhythm, 14
Bird-like face syndrome (micrognathia), and sleep apnea, 171
Blindness, and circadian rhythms, 301
Blistering of skin, with tcPO$_2$ electrodes, 62, 70, 71
Blood pressure, 184, 196
  and excessive daytime sleepiness, 258
  and obstructive sleep apnea syndrome, 161, 163, 166, 167
Blood sampling technique (in

Human Chronophysiology Lab), 311–313
Body temperature
  ambulatory monitoring of, 310–311, 315–316
  and circadian rhythm, 298, 304–305, 310, 314, 318, 319, 322–323
  periodicity, 148
Bradycardia
  in chronic obstructive lung disease, 173
  in infants, 18, 20, 37, 38, 40
  and obstructive sleep apnea syndrome, 163, 164
  *See also* Cardiac arrhythmia
Breast-feeding, during infant monitoring, 63–64, 71
Breathing. *See* Respiration
Breathing pauses, in infants, 20–36 *passim*
  normative data for, 29–31
  polygraphic tracings of, 22–23
  *See also* apnea
Bronchiectasis, and gastroesophageal reflux, 332

Caffeine
  and apnea, 17
  effect on sleep, 246
  and insomnia, 229
  and nocturnal penile tumescence, 362
  withdrawal from, and restless legs syndrome, 269
Calibration
  of polygraph, 10–12
  of Respitrace, 218–222
Canthus, 5, 12, 185
Carbamazepine, and restless legs syndrome, 269
Carbon dioxide
  end-tidal, 20, 21, 35, 175
  excessive (hypercapnia), 157, 161, 170, 171, 175, 176, 195
  expired, 77, 79, 89–91, 92, 184, 195
  transcutaneous monitoring of, 17, 18, 20, 21, 35, 36, 39, 40, 50, 62–92 *passim*
Carcinoma, and restless legs syndrome, 269
Cardiac arrhythmia
  bradycardia, 18, 20, 37, 38, 40, 163, 164, 173

428

*Index*

in central alveolar hypoventilation, 176
in chronic obstructive lung disease, 173
in infants and children, 18–20, 37–40, 176, 178
in rapid eye movement sleep, 173, 174
in sleep apnea, 163–165, 170, 171, 172, 192–195, 198
tachycardia, 18, 50, 158, 163
*See also* Electrocardiogram; Heart rate
Cardiac disorders, and sleep complaints, 172
Cardiac evaluation, and insomnia, 230
Cardiac output, 184, 196
Cataplexy, in narcolepsy, 117, 134
Catheter tip pressure transducer, 195. *See also* Transducers
Caton, Richard, 1
Cavernography, 364–367
CCHS (Congenital central hypoventilation syndrome), 175–176
Central nervous system, 17, 18, 24, 127, 168, 170, 175, 176
Central (Primary) Alveolar Hypoventilation Syndrome (Ondine's Curse), 172, 175–177
Central sleep apnea, 159, 160, 165–171 *passim*, 188, 195–197, 200, 213–215, 259. *See also* Apnea; Sleep apnea syndromes
Chemoreceptors, 170, 175, 176
Children
assessment of sleep disorders in, 111–112, 115–117
and circadian rhythm, 184
EEG during arousal, 158
and epilepsy, 373
and insomnia, 237
narcolepsy in, 116–117
respiratory problems during sleep, 172
and sleep apnea, 159, 170
sleep patterns of, 103–104, 109, 146
and sleep recording, 233
and snoring, 164, 170, 177–179
*See also* Adolescents; Infants
Chlorimipramine hydrochloride,

and periodic movements in sleep, 271
Chronic obstructive lung disease, 160, 171, 172, 173
Chronobiology, 297–325 *passim*. *See also* Circadian rhythms
Chronotherapy, 299, 300, 304, 307, 308
Circadian rhythms, 41–43, 162, 184, 297–325 *passim*
Clonazepam, and periodic movements in sleep, 276
Collodian-sealed electrodes, 4, 8, 377
Congenital central hypoventilation syndrome (CCHS), 175–176
Congestive heart failure, 176
Cortisol level, and circadian rhythm, 318–319, 324
Crib death. *See* Sudden infant death syndrome
Cyanosis, in CCHS, 175. *See also* Hypoxemia
Cystic fibrosis, and sleep, 172

Delayed sleep phase syndrome, 271, 298–307 *passim*. *See also* Chronobiology; Chronotherapy
Delta rhythm (in EEG), 13, 233, 247, 248, 249, 250
Delta sleep (slow-wave sleep; stages 3 + 4), 13, 250, 251, 252, 253, 254, 257. *See also* Slow-wave sleep
De Mairan, 297
Dementia, in old age, 206–261
Depression
and age, 255–256, 257, 260–261
and ASDC nosology, 245, 258, 261
and chronotherapy, 299
and DIMS, 230, 237, 242, 245, 258, 261
and DOES, 245, 253, 258, 261
and EEG sleep variables, 255–257
and nocturnal myoclonus, 247, 258, 261
and periodic movements in sleep, 276
primary vs. secondary, 251–255
and restless legs syndrome, 268

and sleep apnea, 170, 247, 258–259, 261
and sleep latency, 245, 249–256 *passim*
treatment of, 259–261
Desynchronized sleep. *See* Rapid eye movement sleep
Diabetes, 269, 346, 364
Diaphragm
activity during sleep apnea, 159, 160, 165, 167, 168–169, 171
fatigue of, 195
pacing of, 195
*See also* Abdominal respiratory effort
Digital recording, 242
Disorders of excessive sleepiness (DOES). *See* Excessive daytime sleepiness
Disorders of initiating and maintaining sleep (DIMS), 225–242 *passim*
classification according to ASDC nosology, 233–239
and depression, 230, 237, 242, 245, 258, 261
prevalence of, 160
and sleeping pill ingestion, 225–226, 228–229, 231–232. *See also* Hypnotic medication
without objective findings, 238–239
*See also* Insomnia
Dreaming, and eye movement, 2, 5 127. *See also* Eye movements during sleep; Rapid eye movement sleep
Drug ingestion
in adolescents, 113
effect on sleep of, 156, 157, 246, 258
and insomnia, 225–229, 231–232, 236, 238
and nocturnal penile tumescence, 362, 365, 368
and periodic movements in sleep, 276
*See also* Hypnotic medication; Stimulant medication

Edinger-Westphal nucleus, 128, 133
Edrophonium hydrochloride, in obstructive sleep apnea syndrome, 163

429

*Index*

Elderly patients
 and depression, 255–256, 257, 260–261
 and excessive daytime sleepiness, 233
 and periodic movements in sleep (nocturnal myoclonus), 233, 270
 and sleep apnea, 233
Electrocardiogram (ECG)
 artifacts in, 6, 280
 Holter (ambulatory) monitoring of, 163, 164, 165, 178, 184, 192–195, 211
 in infants, 17, 18, 19–20, 62, 63, 65–66, 81, 84, 92
 R-R interval in, 164, 165, 178, 192–195
 in sleep apnea, 183, 184–185, 192–195, 198, 199, 201, 214
 *See also* Cardiac arrhythmia; Heart rate
Electrocorticogram (ECoG), 13
Electrodes
 ground, 65, 67, 185, 186, 187, 288, 333
 impedance, 6–8, 67–68, 69, 84, 89, 185
 for infant monitoring, 62–81 *passim*
 International 10-20 placement system, 158, 185, 377
 nasopharyngeal leads, 376, 377, 378
 placement of, for sleep monitoring, 3–8
 sphenoidal, 376, 377, 378
Electroencephalogram (EEG)
 changes in, during arousal, 158
 and epilepsy, 3, 373–376
 high-amplitude waves, 2, 3
 in infants, 18, 32–34, 37–38, 62, 63, 71–73, 80, 81, 83–84, 92, 378
 and insomnia, 230, 232, 237, 239, 240
 and low-frequency filter, 115
 and rapid eye movement sleep, 148
 sharp waves in, 373
 and sleep apnea, 183, 184–185, 186, 187, 188, 197, 200, 201
 in sleep recording, 1–4, 6–9
 terminology for, 12–15

 *See also* Alpha rhythm; Beta rhythm; Delta rhythm
Electromyogram (EMG)
 in adolescents, 105
 anterior tibialis, 5, 11, 266, 271, 272, 273, 276–291
 chin, 5, 6, 8, 9, 18
 in DIMS, 236, 237, 239, 240–241
 in infants, 62, 63, 74–76, 83–84, 86, 87, 92
 intercostal, 5–7, 157, 160, 168, 172, 173, 174
 in sleep apnea, 168–169, 183, 184–185, 186, 187, 188, 199, 201
 in sleep research, 3, 5–7, 8, 11, 13
Electronic pupillography (EPG). *See* Pupillography
Electro-oculogram (EOG)
 in adolescents, 105
 definition, 13
 electrode placement, 4–5, 6–7
 first used in sleep research, 2–3
 in infants, 80–81
 in multiple sleep latency test, 150
 in sleep apnea, 183, 184–185, 186, 187, 188
 *See also* Eye movements during sleep; Rapid eye movement sleep
Encephalitis, 176
Endocrine conditions
 and depression, 246
 and DIMS, 228, 230
 and sleep apnea, 159, 171
Entrainment, 297, 298, 301, 304, 317, 324, 325. *See also* Chronobiology; Chronotherapy
Enuresis
 in adolescents, 100
 in children, 177
 and epilepsy, 375
 in sleep apnea syndrome, 161
Environmental factors, and sleep, 157
Epilepsy
 diagnostic error, 116
 EEG evaluation of, 3, 373–376
 myoclonic, 267, 276
 nocturnal, 176, 232, 373, 375–376

 and periodic movements in sleep, 265, 266, 267, 271
 polygraphic monitoring of, 3, 376–380
 and sleep, 373–380
 *See also* Seizures
Esophageal monitoring
 in children, 178
 of pH, 184, 195, 333–335
 with pressure balloons, 160, 195
 and sleep apnea, 168–169, 184, 185, 195, 199
Esophagitis
 and GER, 331, 332, 334
 and sleep apnea, 195
Excessive daytime sleepiness, 155–161 *passim*, 171, 172, 176, 177, 261
 in adolescence, 99, 102–103, 109, 116
 and allergies, 156
 and depression, 245, 253, 258, 261
 in elderly patients, 233
 and epilepsy, 375
 and multiple sleep latency tests, 145, 146, 147, 148, 150
 and periodic movements in sleep, 270, 271, 272, 274
 prevalence of, 160
 and sleep apnea, 160, 161
 without objective findings, 148–149
Eye movements during sleep, monitoring of
 electrode placement, 4–5, 6–7
 historical work, 2–3
 in infants, 18, 50, 62, 63, 79–84, 88
 *See also* Electro-oculogram; Rapid eye movement sleep

Fast sleep. *See* Rapid eye movement sleep
Fibrositis, 238
Finger pulse, as index of arousal, 158
First-night effects, 104, 107, 231, 232, 250, 347
Focal activity, 3, 373. *See also* Electroencephalogram; Epilepsy; Seizures
Folic acid deficiency, and restless legs syndrome, 269

430

*Index*

Follicle-stimulating hormone, 114–115, 365, 367
Free-running condition, 297, 298, 301, 307, 314, 317. *See also* Circadian rhythms

Ganglioneuroblastoma, 176
Gastrectomy, partial, and restless legs syndrome, 269
Gastroesophageal reflux (GER), 20, 38, 195, 331–335. *See also* Esophageal monitoring
Gender, effects of
  in children and adolescents, 102, 103, 104, 106–107, 111
  in insomnia, 225
  in sleep apnea, 159
Genioglossus, 166
Gonadotropins, 114–115
Growth hormone, 298, 318–319, 325

Hallucinations, hypnagogic, in narcolepsy, 117
Hamilton Rating Scale for Depression, 246–247, 252, 255, 256, 257, 260
Headache, 155, 161
Head trauma, and sleep disorders, 176–177
Heart rate, 197, 200
  bradycardia, 18, 20, 37, 38, 40, 163, 164, 173
  and childhood snoring, 178
  and circadian rhythm, 41
  monitoring of, 6–7, 9, 17. *See also* Electrocardiogram
  tachycardia, 18, 50, 158, 163
  variability of, 26–28
  *See also* Cardiac arrhythmia; Electrocardiogram
Hemodynamic changes in sleep apnea, 163, 166, 167, 170, 196
Hemoglobin-oxyhemoglobin curve, 172, 189
Hirschsprung's disease, 175, 176
Hodgkin's disease, and sleep apnea, 171
Holter monitor. *See under* Electrocardiogram
Hormones
  in adolescence, 99, 104, 114–115
  cortisol, 298, 318–319, 324
  estradiol, 115
  follicle-stimulating hormone, 114–115, 365, 367

gonadotropins, 114–115
growth hormone, 298, 318–319, 325
hypothyroidism, in infants, 18
luteinizing hormone, 104, 114–115, 365, 367
prolactin, and NPT, 365, 367
testosterone, 115, 365, 367
Hydrocephaly, in an infant, 50
5-Hydroxytryptophan, 269, 276
Hypercapnia, 157, 161, 170, 171, 175, 176, 195. *See also* Carbon dioxide
Hypernychthemeral syndrome, 301–302, 304. *See also* Circadian rhythms
Hypersomnia. *See* Excessive daytime sleepiness
Hypersomnolence, 134, 140. *See also* Excessive daytime sleepiness
Hypertension. *See* Blood pressure
Hypnotic medication, 155, 162, 184, 225–226, 228–229, 231, 232, 235, 276
Hypopnea, 160–166 *passim*, 171
  monitoring of, 196, 199–200, 213, 214, 215, 222
  *See also* Apnea
Hypoventilation, 17, 156, 172, 175–177
Hypoxemia, 18, 20, 36–40, 156, 157, 158, 162, 163, 164, 170–178 *passim*, 195, 332, 375. *See also* Oxygen
Hypoxia, 17, 39, 157. *See also* Oxygen

Impotence, 343–347, 348, 352, 360, 361, 363, 363–368
Infants
  apnea in, 17, 18, 20–31 *passim*, 36–39, 40, 45, 50, 87, 89–93, 159, 162
  and central hypoventilation syndrome, 172, 175
  and circadian rhythms, 41–43, 162
  electrocardiogram in, 17, 18, 19–20, 62, 63, 65–66, 81, 84, 92
  electroencephalogram in, 18, 32–34, 37–38, 62, 63, 71–73, 80, 81, 83–84, 92, 378

electromyogram in, 62, 63, 74–76, 83–84, 86, 87, 92
  eye movements in, 18, 50, 62, 63, 79–84, 88
  heart rate in, 17, 18, 20, 26–28, 37, 38, 40, 50
  monitoring of, 17–50, 61–94
  normative data for, 26–35
  prematurity in, 17–18, 20–42 *passim*, 50, 61–62
  and respiration, 17, 18, 20–45 *passim*, 62, 63, 67–69, 79, 86, 89–93, 155, 172, 199
  scoring of sleep stages and states in, 39–41, 50, 83–84, 92–93
  sleep state organization in, 46–49
Infiltration, and sleep apnea, 168, 170, 171
Infrared method of recording infants' eye movements, 80–82
Inion, 4
Insomnia
  and activity monitoring, 316
  in adolescents, 99
  and delayed sleep phase syndrome, 300, 304. *See also* Delayed sleep phase syndrome
  and depression, 230, 237, 242, 245, 258, 261
  evaluation of, 226–228
  and hypnotic medication, 225–226, 228–229, 231–232
  incidence of, 225–226
  and periodic movements in sleep (nocturnal myoclonus), 269–276 *passim*, 291
  and pupillography, 128, 131–132, 133
  rebound, 228, 232
  and respiration, 155, 156, 158, 160
  and restless legs syndrome, 267–271, 274
  and stress, 225, 226, 227, 230, 235
  *See also* Disorders of initiating and maintaining sleep (DIMS)
Inspiratory effort, in sleep apnea, 168–169

431

*Index*

Intensive care unit, neonatal, 18, 175
Isolation, temporal, 301, 308–309

Jet lag, 299, 302

K complexes, 3, 13, 158, 199, 200, 240, 266, 273, 282
Kyphoscoliosis, 171, 172

Lambda wave, 13
Light reflex, and pupillography, 127–135 *passim*
Light sleep, 13
Luteinizing hormone, 104, 114–115, 365, 367
Lymphoma, and sleep apnea, 171

Manic-depressive illness, 299
Memory, deterioration of, in obstructive sleep apnea syndrome, 161
Menstrual cycle, and adolescence, 99, 104
Methylphenidate, in depression and sleep apnea, 258
Micrognathia (bird-like face syndrome), and sleep apnea, 171
Microphone, in recording respiration, 62, 63, 79, 89–90
Miosis, and sleep, 127
Mixed apnea, 159, 171, 199
MMPI, 230, 275, 364. *See also* Rating scales; Questionnaires
Monitoring
 of activity, 241–242, 304, 316
 of brain waves. *See* Electroencephalogram
 of carbon dioxide (transcutaneous) tcPCO$_2$), 17, 18, 20, 21, 35, 36, 39, 40, 50, 62–92 *passim*
 of eye movements. *See* Electro-oculogram; Eye movements; Rapid eye movement sleep
 of heart rate. *See* Electrocardiogram
 of infants, 17–50, 61–97
 of muscle activity. *See* Electromyogram
 of oxygen (transcutaneous) (tcPO$_2$), 17, 18, 20, 21, 35, 36, 39, 40, 50, 62–92 *passim*
 polygraphic, 1–16
 of respiration, 160–167, 178, 183–209
 of sleep apnea, 161–162. *See also* Apnea; Sleep apnea syndromes
 with strain gauges. *See* Strain gauges
 with thermistors. *See* Thermistors
 video, 82, 84, 286, 291, 379–380. *See also* TV monitoring
 *See also* Ambulatory monitoring
Montage
 definition of, 14
 for epilepsy, 378–379
 in sleep recording, 3, 7
 *See also* Electroencephalogram
Mood scales, 314, 315, 364. *See also* Rating scales; Questionnaires
Mountain sickness syndrome, 157
Mu rhythm (in EEG), 14
Müller maneuver, 163
Multiple sclerosis, and sleep apnea, 171
Multiple sleep latency test, 7, 8, 99, 104, 105, 109–113, 116, 117, 121–122, 145–151
Muscle tone
 in children, 178
 in infants, 18, 38, 39
 of pharynx, 166, 168, 170
 in rapid eye movement sleep, 157
 in sleep apnea, 166, 168, 170
Mydriasis, and wakefulness, 127
Myoclonic jerks, 267
Myoclonus, nocturnal (periodic movements in sleep), 265–291 *passim*
 in depression, 247, 258, 261, 276
 and disorders of initiating and maintaining sleep, 227, 231, 232, 233, 237, 269–276 *passim*, 291
 in elderly patients, 233, 270
 and sleep apnea, 270, 271, 275, 286
 use of EMG in evaluation, 5, 11, 266, 271, 272, 273, 276–291
 use of muscle relaxants in, 276
Myoclonus index (movement index), 273, 275, 282, 284, 290
Myotonic dystrophy, and sleep apnea, 171
Myxedema, and sleep apnea, 171

Naps, daytime
 in children and adolescents, 102, 103, 109, 177
 and circadian rhythms, 301, 302
 and insomnia, 227, 229
 and multiple sleep latency test, 145–150 *passim*
 and nocturnal penile tumescence, 362
 in obese patients, 156
 in sleep apnea, 161–162, 183, 184
 and sleep studies, 246
Narcolepsy
 and adolescence, 99, 109, 116–117
 age of onset, 99, 116–117
 in children, 116–117
 as a familial disorder, 117, 147
 and multiple sleep latency test, 146, 147, 148, 149, 150, 151
 and periodic movements during sleep (nocturnal myoclonus), 270, 271, 277
 and pupillography, 128, 132, 133, 134–135
 sleep onset rapid eye movement sleep periods in, 133, 134, 145, 148, 149
 and stimulant medication, 146
Nasal obstruction, and sleep problems, 156, 188
Nasion, recording from, 4
Near-miss for SIDS, 17, 36–39, 160
Neck trauma, and respiratory problems during sleep, 176–177
Neonatal intensive care units, 18, 175
Neurotransmitters, 365, 368
Night terrors (pavor nocturnus), 111, 374, 375

# Index

Nocturia, 161
Nocturnal myoclonus. *See* Myoclonus, nocturnal
Nocturnal penile tumescence, 343–368
Non–rapid eye movement sleep (NREM)
  in children and adolescents, 103, 107, 108, 109, 115
  definition of, 14
  and electrocardiogram, 194
  and focal activity, 373
  in infants, 175
  and naps, 183
  and oxygen desaturation, 172, 174
  and periodic movements in sleep (nocturnal myoclonus), 270, 282
  and respiration, 155, 214
  and sleep apnea, 160, 162, 165, 170, 175, 196
  *See also* Slow-wave sleep (stages 3 + 4)

Obesity, and sleep, 156, 161, 166, 172
Obstructive sleep apnea, 159–171 *passim*, 188, 195–199, 213, 215, 222, 258, 259.
  *See also* Apnea; Sleep apnea syndromes
Odontoid fracture, 177
Ohmmeter, 66
Ondine's curse, 172, 175–177
Organic brain syndrome, 260
Oropharynx, and sleep apnea, 166, 170
Oximeter, ear, 207–210, 211, 239, 240
  in multiple sleep latency testing, 149
  in sleep apnea monitoring, 185, 187, 189, 191–193
  use with children, 178
Oxygen
  arterial pressure (PaO$_2$), 157, 167
  challenge (hyperoxic), 171, 175
  lack of (desaturation), in sleep apnea, 170, 171, 172, 176, 183, 184, 189, 191, 192, 196, 197, 198, 199, 200
  reduction of (hypoxemia), 18, 20, 36–40, 156, 157, 158, 162, 163, 164, 170, 171, 172, 173, 174, 176, 178, 195, 332, 375
  saturation, 160, 161, 162, 164, 167, 168, 171, 172, 178, 213, 214, 215
  transcutaneous monitoring of, 17, 18, 20, 21, 35, 36, 39, 40, 50, 62–92 *passim*

Pacemaker, cardiac, 214
Paradoxical breathing, in infants, 39, 68, 69, 93
Paradoxical sleep. *See* Rapid eye movement sleep
Parasympathetic system, 127–135, 158, 164
Paresthesia, and restless legs syndrome, 268
Pavor nocturnus (night terrors), 111, 374, 375
Penile prosthesis, 343, 351
Penile tumescence, 343–368
Performance tests, 145, 314–315
Periodic breathing, in infants, 18, 36, 50
Periodic movements in sleep. *See* Myoclonus, nocturnal
Personality changes, in obstructive sleep apnea, 161
Peyronie's plaque, 344, 348, 351
Phase-response curve, 300–301
Phase shift, 298, 299, 300, 301, 302. *See also* Chronobiology; Chronotherapy
pH monitoring, 195, 333–341
Pickwickian syndrome, 166. *See also* Apnea; Obesity
Piezo-electric crystals, 241, 242
Platybasia, and sleep apnea, 171
Plethysmography, 21, 189, 211, 213–222
Pneumonia and pneumonitis, 332
Poliomyelitis, 171, 176, 269
Polycythemia, 176. *See also* Oxygen
Polysomnography. *See* Monitoring
Pontine-geniculo-occipital (PGO) waves, 160
Posture, and respiration during sleep, 156, 157, 178
Pregnancy, and restless legs syndrome, 269

Premature infants, 17–18, 20–21, 24–35 *passim*, 37, 38, 40, 42, 50, 61–62
Pressure transducer, 196
Propranolol, and sleep apnea, 163
Psychiatric disorders, and insomnia, 227, 230, 236
Puberty, 99, 104, 113–115, 117. *See also* Adolescence
Pulmonary artery pressure, 163, 166, 167, 176, 184, 196
Pulmonary aspiration, 332, 334
Pulmonary disorders, 160, 171, 172, 173
Pulmonary edema, in sleep apnea, 163
Pulmonary function tests, and sleep apnea, 184
Pupil (of eye), 127, 128–134, 135–142
Pupillography, 116, 127–142, 145

Questionnaires, 10, 11, 99–100, 102, 111, 113, 227, 290–291, Appendix I
  *See also* Rating scales
Quiet sleep (slow-wave sleep; stages 3 + 4), 14, 25, 80, 83, 84, 87, 90–91. *See also* Slow-wave sleep

Rapid eye movement (REM) sleep, 2–5, 146–151 *passim*, 170–175 *passim*, 245–261 *passim*
  bursts of, and pupillary dilations, 127
  in children and adolescents, 104, 106, 107, 109, 115–116, 117
  and circadian rhythm, 298, 299, 319, 320
  in depression, 245, 249–261 *passim*, 299
  and epilepsy, 373
  in infants. *See* Active sleep
  latency to, 106–117 *passim*, 134, 146–151 *passim*, 245–261 *passim*, 298
  and nocturnal penile tumescence, 345, 346, 347, 351, 355, 357, 306–361, 362, 365, 367
  and periodic movements in sleep (nocturnal

433

*Index*

Rapid eye movement (REM) sleep *(cont.)*
  myoclonus), 268, 275, 281–282
  and respiration, 155–164 *passim*, 170, 175
  in sleep apnea, 160, 162, 170, 183, 184, 196, 198, 200, 201, 237
  at sleep onset, 110–111, 116, 133, 134, 145, 148, 149, 298, 319
Rating scales
  KDS self-rating scales, 246–247, 253, 255, 256
  MMPI, 230, 275, 364
  Stanford Sleepiness Scale, 145
  *See also* Questionnaires
Rebreathing method (Read), 175
Rectal probe, 310, 315–316
Reflexes, polysynaptic, 170
Relaxation training, for insomnia, 229
Renal disease, and nocturnal penile tumescence, 346
Respibands, 214–217
Respiration
  and arousal, 157–159
  changes as a function of sleep state, 83
  and circadian rhythm, 41–43
  in infants, 17, 18, 20–45 *passim*, 62, 63, 67–69, 79, 86, 89–93, 155, 172, 199
  irregularity, 86
  monitoring of, 160–167, 178, 183–209
  during rapid eye movement sleep, 155, 157
  during sleep, 155–179 *passim*
  tracings, 89–91
  use of strain gauges to measure. *See* Strain gauges
Respiratory arrest, 175, 176
Respiratory centers, depressed by hypnotics, 228
Respiratory disorders, 155–167 *passim*, 200–201. *See also* Apnea
Respiratory distress syndrome, 26–28 *passim*, 38
Respiratory inductive plethysmograph (Respitrace), 189, 211, 213–222
Respiratory rate, in infants, 24, 25, 26–28, 36–39, 41,
42–44, 45, 50
Restless legs syndrome, 233, 237, 265, 266, 267–269, 274, 282, 283
Reticular activating system (RAS), 157–158, 160
Retrolental fibroplasia, 17
Reye's syndrome, 176
Rib cage, and breathing, 213–222 *passim*. *See also* Electromyogram, intercostal; Respiration

Saw-tooth waves, 14
Schizoaffective disorders, and sleep, 253, 258, 259
Schizophrenia, and sleep research, 133, 259–260
Scoring of sleep stages, 3, 6, 10, 240
  in adolescents, 105, 106, 115–116
  in infants, 40–41, 83–84, 92–93
  manual for (Rechtschaffen & Kales), 1, 3, 105, 110, 150, 200, 233, 239, 247
  in multiple sleep latency test, 150–151
  and nocturnal penile tumescence, 355, 360
  and periodic movements in sleep (nocturnal myoclonus), 271–273
  in respiratory disorders, 200–201
Secobarbital, 228
Seizures, 37, 38, 39, 45, 175, 232, 373–380 *passim*. *See also* Epilepsy
Sexual function impairments, 170. *See also* Impotence
Short sleepers, 238
Shy-Drager syndrome, 346
Sideropenia, and restless legs syndrome, 269
Sleep apnea syndromes, 155–171 *passim*, 183, 196
  circadian rhythm of, 184
  definition of, 196
  and depression, 170, 247, 258–259, 261
  and electrode placement, 8
  hemodynamic changes in, 163, 166, 167, 170, 196
  normative data for, 159
  and periodic movements in sleep (nocturnal
myoclonus), 270, 271, 275, 286
  screening procedure for, 184–201 *passim*
  *See also* Apnea; Hypopnea; Respiration
Sleep architecture, in depression, 249–257 *passim*
Sleep deprivation, 146, 149, 157, 158, 162, 170, 184, 299, 304, 373–374, 376, 378
Sleep diaries, 227, 302–307
Sleep disorders centers, 226, 229, 230–233. *See also* Association of Sleep Disorders Centers
Sleep efficiency, 245, 249–260 *passim*, 275
Sleep history, 226–227
Sleep hygiene, 229, 304
Sleeping pills. *See* Hypnotic medication
Sleep latency
  in adolescents and children, 103, 106, 109–111, 112, 113, 146
  in depression, 245, 249–256 *passim*
  in hypersomnolence, 134
  in narcoleptics, 146, 147–148, 149, 150, 151
  after sleep deprivation, 146, 149
  testing for, 7, 8, 99, 104, 105, 109–113, 116, 117, 121–122, 145–151
Sleep log, 290–291
Sleep-onset rapid eye movement periods
  in adolescents, 110–111, 116
  and circadian rhythms, 298, 319
  in narcoleptics, 133, 134, 145, 148, 149
Sleep spindles. *See* Spindles
Sleep starts, 265, 266, 281
Sleepwalking, 100, 111, 161, 374
Slow-wave sleep (stages 3 + 4), 3, 8, 9, 13, 14, 15, 25, 80, 83, 84, 87, 90–91, 103, 107, 108, 109, 115, 200, 245, 250–254, 257, 298, 325
Snoring
  in adolescents, 100
  in children, 164, 170, 177, 178, 179

## Index

heart rate changes associated with, 178
and hypnotic medication, 228
and sleep apnea, 161, 168, 170
Spikes (in EEG), 14, 373. *See also* Electroencephalogram; Seizures
Spinal cord injury, and nocturnal penile tumescence, 346, 347, 361
Spinal motoneurons, 172
Spindles (in EEG), 2, 3, 8, 13, 14, 18, 32–34, 37, 200, 240, 266
in infants, 18, 32–34, 37, 84, 87, 90
*See also* Electroencephalogram
Spirobag, 217, 219, 222
Spirogram, 217
Spirometer, 217, 219, 222
Stages of sleep, 2, 14, 15. *See also* Scoring of sleep stages; Slow-wave sleep
Stanford Summer Sleep Camp, 104–105
States of sleep. *See* Non–rapid eye movement sleep; Rapid eye movement sleep
Stiff-man syndrome, 271
Stimulant medication, 146, 155, 231, 258
Strain gauges
for monitoring nocturnal penile tumescence, 348–350
for monitoring respiration in children and infants, 21, 62, 63, 68–69, 89–90, 160, 165, 178
for suspected sleep apnea, 185, 188–191, 196, 199, 202–207, 239
Stress, and insomnia, 225, 226, 227, 230, 235
Stridor, in infants, 175
Strychnine, in treatment of sleep apnea, 170
Sudden Infant Death Syndrome, 17, 36–39, 155, 160
Supine posture, and respiration, 156, 157
Symonds, Sir Charles, 265, 267, 269
Sympathetic activity, 158, 164, 365. *See also* Parasympathetic system
Szymanski actograph, 241

Tachycardia, 18, 50, 158, 163
Tachypnea
in arousal from sleep, 158
in children, 178
in infants, 20, 36, 37, 38, 50
in obese patients, 156
Tanner staging (of adolescents), 104–105, 113–115, 117
and sleep parameters, 107–108, 111, 112, 118–122
Temperature, 24, 41, 89
ambulatory monitoring of, 310, 311, 315–316
monitoring of, in infants, 17, 62, 63, 67, 77, 79, 89
Tension, and insomnia, 229, 235–236, 237, 239, 240–241
Testosterone, 115, 365, 367
Theophylline, in prevention of apnea, 17
Thermistors
for ambulatory monitoring of temperature, 310, 311
for monitoring respiration in infants, 62, 77, 79, 89
in sleep apnea, 160, 165, 185, 188, 189, 196, 199, 202–203, 207, 213, 239
*See also* Airflow; Monitoring; Respiration; Temperature
Theta rhythm (in EEG), 15, 158
Thioridazine, 258
Thoractic effort, in sleep apnea, 188–189, 196, 197, 198, 199, 200
Thorax, disorders of, and sleep apnea, 171, 172. *See also* Apnea; Electromyogram, intercostal; Respiration; Rib cage
Tidal volume, 172, 261–222. *See also* Respiration; Respiratory inductive plethysmograph
Tolazoline, in reducing pulmonary hypertension, 17
Tonsils, enlarged, in children, 164, 171, 177–179
Total sleep time, 100–102, 106, 107, 159
in depressives, 205–257 *passim*
Tracé alternant, in infants, 18, 37, 84–85, *See also* Electroencephalogram
Tracheostomy, 162, 164, 170, 175–176, 177
Tranquilizers, effect on sleep, 231. *See also* Hypnotic medication
Transcutaneous monitoring of blood gases, in infants, 17, 18, 20, 21, 35, 36, 39, 40, 50, 62, 63, 66, 69–71, 89, 91, 92
Transducers, 61, 62, 65–81, 81–82, 160, 195, 196
Tuberculosis, and sleep recording, 174
TV monitoring, 135–140, 309. *See also* Video monitoring

Uremia, 269, 271

Vertex sharp waves (in EEG), 3, 15
Video monitoring, 82, 84, 286, 291, 379–380. *See also* TV monitoring
Visual evoked potential, in infants, 24
Vitamin E, and restless legs syndrome, 269

Whiplash syndrome, and respiratory problems during sleep, 176–177
Withdrawal from drugs, 232, 238, 271, 276. *See also* Hypnotic medication; Stimulant medication
Wrist actograph, 242

Zeitgebers, 297. *See also* Circadian rhythms

435